MANIPULATION, TRACTION AND MASSAGE

THIRD EDITION

This volume is one of the series,
Rehabilitation Medicine Library,
edited by John V. Basmajian.
Originally published as part of the Physical Medicine Library,
edited by Sidney Licht.

New books and new editions published, in press or in preparation for this series:

BANERJEE: Rehabilitation Management of Amputees

BASMAJIAN: Therapeutic Exercise, fourth edition*

BASMAJIAN (ROGOFF): Manipulation, Traction and Massage, third edition*

BISHOP: Behavioral Problems and the Disabled: Assessment and Management

BLOCH AND BASBAUM: Management of Spinal Cord Injuries

BRANDSTATER: Stroke Rehabilitation

BROWNE, KIRLIN AND WATT: Rehabilitation Services and the Social Work Role: Challenge for Change

CHYATTE: Rehabilitation in Chronic Renal Failure

EHRLICH: Rehabilitation Management of Rheumatic Conditions, second edition

FISHER AND HELM: Comprehensive Rehabilitation of Burns

GRANGER AND GRESHAM: Functional Assessment in Rehabilitation Medicine

HAAS ET AL.: Pulmonary Therapy and Rehabilitation: Principles and Practice

INCE: Behavioral Psychology in Rehabilitation Medicine: Clinical Applications

JOHNSON: Practical Electromyography, second edition

LEHMANN: Therapeutic Heat and Cold, third edition*

LONG: Prevention and Rehabilitation in Ischemic Heart Disease

MOLNAR: Pediatric Rehabilitation

REDFORD: Orthotics Etcetera, third edition*

ROY AND TUNKS: Chronic Pain: Psychosocial Factors in Rehabilitation

SHA'KED: Human Sexuality and Rehabilitation Medicine: Sexual Functioning Following Spinal Cord Injury

STILLWELL: Therapeutic Electricity and Ultraviolet Radiation, third edition*

* Originally published as part of the Physical Medicine Library, edited by Sidney Licht.

MANIPULATION, TRACTION AND MASSAGE

Third Edition

Edited by

John V. Basmajian,
M.D., F.A.C.A., F.R.C.P.(C)

Director of the Chedoke Rehabilitation Centre
Chedoke-McMaster Hospitals
Professor of Medicine
McMaster University
Hamilton, Ontario, Canada

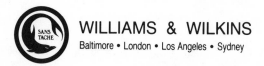
WILLIAMS & WILKINS
Baltimore • London • Los Angeles • Sydney

Editor: John Butler
Associate Editor: Joyce Murphy
Copy Editor: Shelley Potler
Design: James R. Mulligan
Illustration Planning: Lorraine Wrzosek
Production: Anne G. Seitz

First edition, 1960
Reprinted 1963, 1971
Second edition, 1980
Reprinted, 1981

Made in the United States of America

Library of Congress Cataloging in Publication Data

Main entry under title:

Manipulation, traction and massage, 3rd edition

   (Rehabilitation medicine library)
   Includes bibliographies and index.
   1. Massage. 2. Manipulation (Therapeutics) 3. Orthopedic traction. I. Basmajian,
John V., 1921-II. Series. [DNLM: 1. Manipulation, Orthopedic, 2. Massage. 3.
Traction. WB 537 M278] RM721.M29 1985   615.8'2   84-17355 ISBN
0-683-00378-X

(Rehabilitation Medicine Library
First ed. edited by S. H. Licht)

Composed and printed at the
Waverly Press, Inc.

86 87 88 89
10 9 8 7 6 5 4 3 2

Series Editor's Foreword

The rapid and widespread increase of interest in the topics of this book necessitated a new edition in a rather short time. In addition, the volume had become widely used and cited as an authoritative sourcebook. However, Dr. Rogoff, who edited the second edition, felt unable to tackle a third edition because of failing health and handed the mantle of editor back to me. In September 1984, this beloved physician died, leaving an enormous hiatus in the ranks of those who serve handicapped people.

I have selfishly kept the editorship of this volume because this is a book that I particularly like in the *Rehabilitation Medicine Library* series. It is also a book that needed special skills, access to resources, some courage, and even diplomacy in its production. It is a book that will delight some and enfuriate others—which I enjoy; many others would have shied away. Already accepted as one of the "best-sellers" in the *RML* series, this book should take its place alongside of my flagship of the series, *Therapeutic Exercise*. I will be delighted!

JOHN V. BASMAJIAN, M.D.

Preface to the Third Edition

This new edition was made necessary by the rapidly changing attitudes and teaching of the several professions involved, coupled with the warm reception of our second edition. Only five years have passed; in contrast, the interval between the first and second editions was 20 years. This difference reflects fundamental changes in therapeutic approaches on a very broad front.

No longer are the techniques and their theoretic bases the exotic property of select groups. Many general and specialized physicians have come to regard manipulation, traction and massage—particularly manipulation or mobilization—in a new light. Not always favorably impressed and sometimes very antagonistic to these techniques, many members of the traditional medical profession nevertheless want to learn more about the subject of this book. Thus, I shaped it to be a book for those who disagree as much as it is for those who agree to some degree or even wholeheartedly.

"If ignorance is bliss, 'tis folly to be wise." Thoughtful acceptance or rejection of the many ideas in this book may be the beginning of wisdom about this important branch of therapeutics. Anyone who reads it carefully will be better equipped to provide or supervise better care for many patients.

Dr. Joseph Rogoff, who was the editor of the second edition was unable to undertake the considerable new work we contemplated, and, as noted elsewhere, he died during the preparation of the manuscripts. I am most grateful to him for the revival he accomplished in bringing out the second edition, and deeply feel the loss of this wonderful friend. Because of the special nature of this particular volume, I seized the opportunity of editing it myself rather than finding a new editor.

I enjoyed recruiting the new authors needed to effect the changes in emphasis. My considerable shaping of their contributions to fit the existing lightly revised chapters was not all hard labor; some was very exciting. I hope the results will stimulate and educate all readers, and, in fact, the writers, as much as it has done me. To both new and "old" authors, my warmest thanks and to the publishers congratulations for a job well done.

J. V. BASMAJIAN, M.D.

McMaster University, Hamilton
1985

From the Prefaces to the First and Second Editions

The subjects treated in this book share several things in common. Each concerns the application of mechanical forms of treatment, and all rank high on the list of therapeutic procedures that have occasioned extravagant claims, assault, and rejection.

Massage is more than the laying on of hands or bodily contact; it is *personal* contact. Each masseur uses, in addition to his hands, his voice, his assessment of the person massaged (sometimes called "psychology" by masseur and subject), and a knowledge or suppositon of folk medicine. We may group masseurs into three classes: the untrained, the trained, and the educated. The untrained are those who may be found in vacation resorts or attached to athletic teams. They learn massage by watching other "rubbers" give massage. In general, they do no harm medically because they recognize their limitations and will not venture opinions beyond that of folklore medicine (admittedly an occasional danger).

In the second classification are those persons who have taken a few weeks or months of training, during which they have been taught all about massage, anatomy, physiology, disease—in short (very short)—medicine. These people are usually awarded a certificate, sometimes a very impressive-appearing certificate. They usually set up a private practice to fill the prescriptions of referring physicians. Many states now require licensure for private (and even public) massage administration, but such licensure may be based on an inadequate examination given to persons with an inadequate education.

The third class of persons who give massage is limited to qualified physical therapists who have been graduated from schools of physical therapy approved by a national medical association or health ministry. Most qualified therapists work in hospitals, clinics, or the offices of physicians.

Many books and articles have been written about massage; perhaps more than half of these have been by physicians. These writings have seldom been sufficiently objective to be classified as scientific; massage is largely not scientific. In this book, we do not pretend to treat massage from the scientific viewpoint alone because the result would be inadequate for clinical purposes.

Manipulation remains an ugly word in many medical and surgical clinics. When applied improperly it may be dangerous, conceivably fatal when dealing with rotation of cervical vertebrae. If manipulation is performed by an informed physician, the hazard should be no greater than with most valuable therapeutic agents. Manipulations and most other operations requiring the use of the hands are difficult to teach by the printed word or even the printed picture. This book does not presume to make a masseur or a manipulator of anyone without previous knowledge or ability to acquire training from an experienced operator; however, for those who have had or may have the opportunity to watch a skilled worker, this book should serve as a useful reference.

Many physicians prescribe stretching. There are some conditions for which there is no other rewarding approach at the time of this writing; yet, there is little written about the subject. We believe a discussion of stretching belongs in this book because it is performed largely by manually applied forces. We have placed stretching in the section on manipulation because it is probably more closely related to it than to massage or traction. We might say it another way; stretching is manual traction.

Traction is almost as old as massage, yet it is a word which is seldom encountered in ancient writings. The subject was usually discussed in writings on fractures and dislocations. The word traction is lost among descriptions of pulleys, ropes, axles and winches. The traction which is of ancient origin has been used continuously throughout the ages for traumatic bony pathology. As used in this book, traction is concerned largely with minor displacements or pathology not visible on X-ray and in this sense is relatively new—a product of the twentieth century.

New Haven, Connecticut
December 1, 1959

SIDNEY LICHT, M.D.

• • •

My good friends Dr. Sidney Licht and his wife Elizabeth both died recently. They had been my friends for many years, and they greatly influenced my professional and personal life.

Dr. Licht's preface to the first edition is entirely pertinent to the present volume. We have not included the details of certain methods in this edition, such as *Bindegewebsmassage* or Syncardial massage. On the other hand, we have included the original and perhaps sometimes controversial ideas and methods of Dr. Robert Maigne, whose chapters I had the honor of translating. Also, in addition to the authors previously represented, Mr. Jack Hofkosh has contributed a chapter on the technique of "classical" massage as performed by physical therapists; and my former student and present chief, Dr. Catherine Hinterbuchner, has written a complete and carefully researched chapter covering the field of traction.

New York City
1980

JOSEPH B. ROGOFF, M.D.

Contributors

John V. Basmajian, M.D., F.A.C.A., F.R.C.P. (C.)
Professor of Medicine, McMaster University School of Medicine and Director, Chedoke Rehabilitation Centre, Chedoke-McMaster Hospitals, Hamilton, Ontario, Canada

James H. Cyriax, M.D., F.R.C.P.
Honorary Consultant in Orthopaedic Medicine, St. Thomas's Hospital, London, Visiting Professor in Orthopaedic Medicine, University of Rochester Medical Center, New York

James D. Harris, D.O., F.A.O.C.R.M., Board Certified, P.M.&R.
Chairman, Department of Rehabilitative Medicine, Osteopathic Rehabilitation Medicine, Inc., Tulsa, Oklahoma

Catherine Hinterbuchner, M.D.
Professor and Chairman, Department of Rehabilitation Medicine, New York Medical College, Valhalla, New York

Jack M. Hofkosh, R.P.T.
Director, Physical Therapy, Institute of Rehabilitation Medicine, Assistant Professor of Clinical Rehabilitation Medicine, New York University Medical Center, New York, New York

Herman L. Kamenetz, M.D.
Clinical Professor of Medicine, Division of Rehabilitation Medicine, George Washington University School of Medicine and Health Sciences; Professorial Lecturer in Physical Medicine and Rehabilitation, Georgetown University School of Medicine; Formerly Chief and now Consultant, Rehabilitation Medicine, Veterans Administration Hospital, Washington, D.C.

Sidney Licht, M.D. (Deceased)
Formerly Assistant Clinical Professor of Medicine (Physical Medicine), Yale University School of Medicine, New Haven, Connecticut

Robert Maigne, M.D.
Directeur d'Enseignement Clinique, à la Faculté Broussais-Hôtel-Dieu, Paris, France

Richard Nyberg, R.P.T., B.A., B.S., M.Med.Sc.
Physical Therapy Clinician, Instructor, Division of Physical Therapy, Emory University and Institute of Health Sciences, Inc., Atlanta, Georgia

Joseph B. Rogoff, M.D. (Deceased)
Formerly Professor, New York Medical College, Department of Rehabilitation Medicine, Coler Hospital, Roosevelt Island, New York

Khalil G. Wakim, M.D., Ph.D.
Professor of Physiology, Mayo Foundation (Retired), Research Consultant, Mayo Clinic (Retired), Terre Haute, Indiana

C.B. Wynn Parry, M.B.E., M.A., D.M. (Oxon.), D. Phys. Med., M.R.C.P.
Director of Rehabilitation, Royal National Orthopaedic Hospital, Stanmore, Middlesex, England

Contents

Series Editor's Foreword   v
Preface to the Third Edition   vii
From the Prefaces to the First and Second Editions   ix
Contributors   xi

SECTION 1: Manipulation and Mobilization

Chapter **1.** History and Development of Manipulation and
            Mobilization   3
            James D. Harris, D.O.
Chapter **2.** Role of Physical Therapists in Spinal Manipulation . . .   22
            Richard Nyberg, R.P.T., B.A., B.S., M.Med.Sc.
Chapter **3.** Functional Anatomy of the Spine and Associated
            Structures   47
            John V. Basmajian, M.D., F.A.C.A., F.R.C.P.(C.)
Chapter **4.** Manipulation of the Spine   71
            Robert Maigne, M.D.
Chapter **5.** Manipulations and Mobilizations of the Limbs 135
            Robert Maigne, M.D.

SECTION 2: Stretching and Traction

Chapter **6.** Stretching 157
            C.B. Wynn Parry, D.M.(Oxon.), M.R.C.P.
Chapter **7.** Traction 172
            Catherine Hinterbuchner, M.D.
Chapter **8.** Motorized Intermittent Traction 201
            Joseph B. Rogoff, M.D.

SECTION 3: Massage

Chapter **9.** History of Massage 211
            Herman L. Kamenetz, M.D.

Chapter 10. Physiologic Effects of Massage 256
Khalil G. Wakim, M.D., Ph.D.
Chapter 11. Classical Massage 263
Jack M. Hofkosh, R.P.T.
Chapter 12. Clinical Applications of Massage 270
James H. Cyriax, M.D., F.R.C.P.
Chapter 13. Mechanical Methods of Massage 289
Herman L. Kamenetz, M.D.

SECTION 4: What Now?

Chapter 14. Research and Validation 311
John V. Basmajian, M.D., F.A.C.A., F.R.C.P.(C.)

Index 323

Section

I

MANIPULATION AND MOBILIZATION

1

History and Development of Manipulation and Mobilization

JAMES D. HARRIS

Manipulation is defined in *Dorland's Medical Dictionary* as "Skillful or dextrous treatment by the hand. In physical therapy, the forceful passive movement of a joint beyond its active limit of motion." Manipulation is currently an area of great interest for many different groups of medical professionals. The enthusiasm for manual treatment is on the increase in the 1980s, exemplified by such new organizations as the American Association for Orthopedic Medicine. Numerous seminars, books, and videotapes are being used by health care professionals to teach the art of manipulative medicine (8).

Classical Period

Historically, the "hands on" approach to medical care is not new. Although the laying on of hands is well documented in the Old Testament and other historical documents, so-called modern medicine had its birth with the development of the Hippocratic School of Medicine, a logical starting place for this discussion.

Born in Asia Minor in 460 B.C., Hippocrates became a physician and teacher of great skill, and is recognized as the Father of Medicine. The Hippocratic Oath taken by many physicians before entering practice is a tribute to the Father of Medicine, who focused attention on the patient. In his *Aphorisms*, he reminded his students not to meddle with or to hinder nature's attempt toward recovery. The idea of focusing full attention on the patient rather than just on the scientific theory of disease or on elaborate laboratory and radiographic testing has considerable merit.

There were many different schools and philosophies of medicine which affected the course of today's medical care. Even though Hippocrates

3

dominated his time in medicine, there were others who believed that he was too philosophical and who advocated a more practical approach. Their approach was more specifically disease-oriented; they believed that disease was an "outside intruder" that caused the condition which existed within man. However, the Hippocratic School emphasized the study of health in man as an individual and steered attention away from the outside intruders or disease that afflicted man. The theoretical battle in medicine of "inside" vs. "outside" persists today. With the renewed interest in manipulative medicine, the philosophies behind the use of manipulation must be explored.

Hippocrates did not agree with the treatment of lumbar kyphosis of his time. He advocated the use of steam heat, followed by traction from both the head and the foot while the patient lay in a prone position. Pressure was to be sharply applied on the kyphosis while the traction was maintained. The direction of force was dictated by the condition that occurred in the patient. This manner of readjustment proved to be beneficial for selected patients. He also advocated different types of treatment rather than just a single-force thrust: prolonged pressure by sitting on the patient, shaking movements, and a foot being applied to the prominence. A padded board with a long lever arm to apply local pressure across the patient's back (Fig. 1.1) was another device. He related that a thrust without traction could be satisfactory. Hippocrates did not limit manual treatment of patients to the

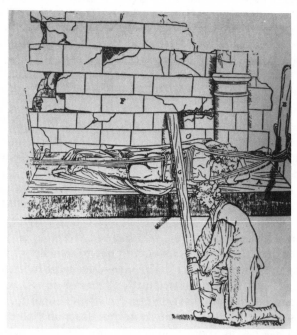

Figure 1.1. Ancient method of treating kyphosis (see text).

low back area. His most famous successor, Galen (A.D. 131–202), preached the use of manual medicine in the treatment of the extremities, as well as for problems in the cervical vertebrae.

In the middle ages, the Arabian physician, Abu'Ali ibn Sina (980–1037), accumulated and wrote a summary of medicine that survived as the authoritative textbook until the 17th century. It included the manual medicine approach to the treatment of backs advocated by Hippocrates. The famous antiquarian Chinese physician, Chang Chung-King, referred to as the Chinese Hippocrates, also advocated treating the patient with manual medicine (12).

Other notables in medicine such as Thomas Sydenham (1624–1689), an Englishman, and Samuel Hahnemann (1755–1843), a German doctor who founded homeopathy, also deviated from the cnidian principle of disease-oriented medicine. Hahnemann developed a medical treatment that often advocated the use of extremely small doses of drugs. This was a counter-movement to the megadoses of medicinal agents that were being used by his contemporaries. Herman Boerhaave (1668–1738), son of a Dutch country pastor, was described as being "poor in money, but pure in spirit." He chose the Hippocratic philosophy of medicine as his guide, and encouraged patient observation rather than disease-oriented medicine (15).

The use of spinal traction, as well as medieval Turkish manipulation during traction, were recorded in the leading textbooks of the Renaissance (Fig. 1.2). Ambroise Paré wrote about "vertebral dislocations" thus:

> "When the vertebrae are dislocated outwards, forming a prominence, the patient should be tied down prone to a board with ropes under the armpits, the waist, and the thighs. He is then pulled and stretched as much as possible from above and from below, but not violently. If traction is not applied, cure is not to be expected. The operator then places his hand on the kyphosis and presses the prominent vertebra in."

John Shultes (1595–1645) advocated Paré's method of treatment. But from the 17th and 18th centuries until the latter part of the 19th century, the treatment by manual means lost favor in the medical profession.

Andrew Taylor Still (1828–1917) (Fig. 1.3) the founder of osteopathic medicine, was a rough-hewn frontier doctor from the midwestern United States. He was an eccentric and nonconformist, but he pursued his beliefs with intensity and devoted himself to the philosophy of medicine and the study of man as a total unit. He did not believe that disease was strictly an outside agent, afflicting evils on the body, but instead considered that disease was a normal body response to an abnormal body situation. During Still's lifetime and to the present, the basic philosophical principle of osteopathic medicine and the term osteopathy has been a focal point of medical controversy and debate (1, 11, 16).

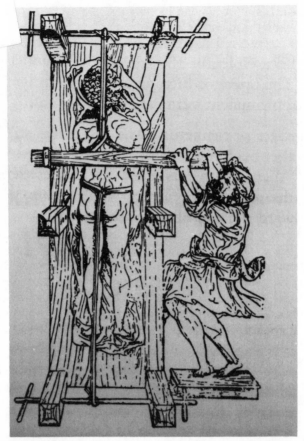

Figure 1.2. Combined suspension and pressure on the lumbar spine by means of a board (The *scamnum Hippocratis*).

Bone-Setters

The contribution of the bone-setters cannot be ignored. In central Europe, the art of bone-setting was handed down from one generation to another. Gypsies of central Europe were known for their bone-setters. The Indians of Mexico employed various manipulative techniques, such as "the shepherd's hug" or the "farmer's push." There also were such techniques as "stamping or trampling," which are practiced in some countries even today. A mystique existed about who had the "great power to heal" or the "right to manipulate." For instance, it was believed that a "stamper" has to be born foot first. Other folklore in many European and Asian countries maintain superstitious beliefs, e.g., that a stamper has to be a virgin or of a certain numerical order of birth (e.g., seventh son).

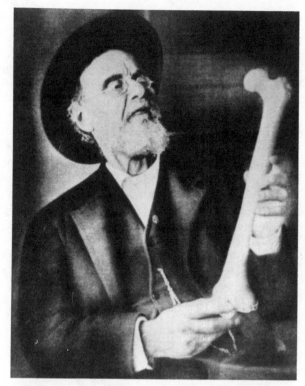

Figure 1.3. Dr. A. T. Still, originator of osteopathy.

Related to the above, "Lomi-Lomi" is an ancient Hawaiian version of massage, over eight centuries old. Its main feature is that the masseur walks on the patient's back, and while he walks, he kneads the flesh and regulates his weight by holding on a bar above the massage table.

In a similar technique in East Africa, women who led camels would lie in a prone position while their cohorts stood on their backs, trampling and kneading with their toes. In European countries such as Norway, Sweden, and Finland, there has been for many years a folklore manual-type of medicine, which appeared to be successful. The technique of "weighing salt" is well documented in Swedish folklore medicine, and time has justified these methods of treatment.

Bone-setters have existed for hundreds of years with their techniques often handed down through families. The first of these bone-setters about whom details exist was a woman called Sarah Mapp, who practiced her skills in Great Britain in the 1700s. She was a very well-known character of her time. She was described by the *London Magazine* (Aug. 2, 1736) as being "enormously fat and ugly," and her nicknames were "Crazy Sally" or "Crosseyed Sally" (13).

Whorton Hood gave the first formal description of the bone-setting craft in the 19th century, as taught to him by Richard Hutton and based on anatomy. In his writings, he insisted that legitimate practitioners failed to meet the desires of the sick. Bone-setting was a major topic at the annual meeting of the British Medical Society in 1882 (13).

Sir Herbert Barker (1869–1950) (Fig. 1.4) of Great Britain enjoyed the support of many individuals, including at least one surgeon who had been president of the British Medical Association. Barker lacked a formal medical education, but practiced in London until 1927. He had learned his skills from his cousin, a bone-setter named John Atkinson, who in turn was taught by Robert Hutton, a nephew of Richard Hutton. The Huttons came from a farming family in England that had practiced bone-setting for over 200 years. Although Herbert Barker was refused an honorary medical degree, King George V honored him with a knighthood. In 1925, Dr. George M. Laughlin arranged for the Andrew Taylor Still College of Osteopathy

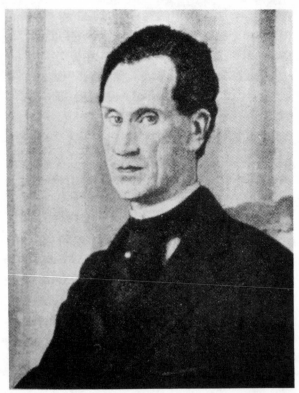

Figure 1.4. The most famous of all bone-setters, Sir Herbert Barker.

and Surgery to give him an honorary D.O. degree, which Sir Herbert referred to as his "American Knighthood." In his autobiography (2), he wrote:

"Strong as the love of service to suffering is among many doctors as a whole, there existed some things much stronger and less worthy in prejudice and jealousy which have from time immemorial darkened the pages of surgical history and smirched its record of noble endeavors ... I am certainly not prepared to be condemned by men who are culpably ignorant of what it is their business to know, and which they are too arrogant, or too prejudiced to learn ... It is still true that the faculty has neglected the study of methods and are today incapable of relieving sufferers who resort to them. Yet they persist still in their refusal to accept the help of those who can instruct them in this beneficial branch of the healing art....

"I cannot afford the time and strength demanded for demonstrations for the benefit of individuals. When I desire to bring the method before the faculty as a whole, secure them a place in the curricula of the medical schools ... obtain for the entire body of students a thorough and practical training in the work ... I contend unreservedly that the method of the manipulative art ... are quite unknown to the general practitioner, and even to the specialist in surgery ... they have no real or effective knowledge even in its rudimentary principles...."

The Lancet in 1925 recognized Barker in an editorial thus: "The medical history of the future will have to record that our profession has greatly neglected this important subject ... The fact that must be faced, that the bone-setters had been curing multitudes of cases by movement ... and that by our faulty methods we are largely responsible for their very existence."

Chiropractic

The history of the chiropractic profession is traced back to Daniel David Palmer (1845–1913) (Fig. 1.5), who practiced his own magnetism business for ten years until 1895. D. D. Palmer wrote his first textbook, "The Chiropractic Adjuster" in 1910, in which he advocated the art of replacing subluxed vertebrae to cure disease. He claimed to be the first to replace displaced vertebrae by using the spinous process and transverse process as levers, which he thought was a revolutionary theory in the healing art. In Palmer's own account, he related that in his readings of the Hippocratic method of treating backs and from his visits to France how he revived this method of treatment. It is reported that his first patient was cured of deafness in September, 1895 by his adjusting a large subluxation of the cervical vertebrae. His son, B. J. Palmer, described this historical event as, "The bump was adjusted, and within ten minutes he had his hearing and has had it ever since."

D. D. Palmer opened the first chiropractic school in Oklahoma City in

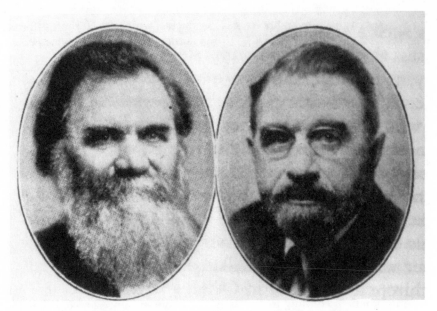

Figure 1.5. David D. Palmer and his son, B. J. Palmer.

1897. He advocated not only manipulating the spinal column, but also the extremities. His followers were known as "mixers" or as adhering to "the Carver method of chiropractic." In later years this included physical therapy, dietetics, megavitamins, and other nonprescription medications.

B. J. Palmer, the son of D. D. Palmer, started his own school in Davenport, Iowa in 1907. It has been reported that he was a student in the Osteopathic College in Kirksville in 1900, but did not finish his course of study; but Dr. Charles Still has reported that Palmer obtained his knowledge from a Mr. Stother, an osteopathic student from Kirksville. B. J. Palmer advocated manipulation of the spine only, and his supporters were called "straights" who followed "the Palmer Method of Chiropractic." In time, the straights lost out to the mixers.

B. J. Palmer was very enterprising; in 1924 he developed the "neurocalometer" which would register variations of skin temperature along the vertebral column. It was used to identify more accurately where the nerves were compressed. This, according to B. J. Palmer, indicated the level of the vertebra in which dislocation had caused the trouble. This instrument was not for sale, but was rented to his graduates and formed an integral part of the teaching of the International Chiropractic Association. The chiropractic doctrine states that chiropractic treatment achieves two ends, "one, to remove the cause which has facilitated the onset of disease and let it gain a foothold in the body; two, to permit a normal flow of life energy from the brain to the tissues, thus preventing the disease from spreading further (13).

In the *British Medical Journal*, chiropractic was described as "a branch of Osteopathy, first, designed to maintain Osteopathic dogma in its most primitive form, and second, maintaining its commercial character." Dr. Morris Fishbein in 1925 staunchly opposed both chiropractic and osteopathic concepts, and his summation was, "Chiropractic is the malignant tumor on the body of osteopathy." In the next half century the training for the chiropractic profession has progressed from a two-week course to a much more extensive syllabus that includes anatomy, physiology, biochemistry, pathology, bacteriology, public health, and hygiene, as well as diagnosis and treatment.

The mixers have defined chiropractic as "the science of healing human ailments by manipulation and adjustment of the spine and other structures of the human body, and the use of such other mechanical, physio-therapeutic, dietetic, and sanitary measures, except drugs and major surgery, as are indicated to care of the human body." Their theory or philosophy underlying spinal adjustment is summed up in five principles: (a) that a vertebra may become subluxed; (b) that this subluxation tends to impinge on the structures (nerves, blood vessels, and lymphatics) passing through the intervertebral foramen; (c) that as a result of such impingement, the function of the corresponding segment of the spinal cord and its connecting spinal and autonomic nerve is interfered with and that the conduction of the nerve impluse is impaired; (d) that, as a result thereof, the nervous tone in certain parts of the organism is abnormally altered, and such parts become functionally or organically diseased, or predisposed to disease; and (e) that the adjustment of the subluxed vertebra removes the impingement from the structures passing through the intervertebral foramen, thereby restoring to diseased parts their normal nervous stimuli and rehabilitating them functionally and organically.

Via newspapers, television, and radio advertisements, the chiropractic profession impresses on the public that subluxation of the spine produces certain diseases, and that the adjustment of these vertebral segments can cure the disease. They claim that chiropractic recognizes the true and primary cause of the disease; but even today some chiropractors discourage vaccination of their family members and choose to treat them by adjustment.

Naprapathy

Naprapathy is an offshoot of chiropractic that started approximately in 1908. Its original school was in Chicago, and it adhered to the principle that ligamentous contracture draws the vertebrae too closely together and causes disease by obstructing nerves and blood vessels. The major premise is that by stretching out these ligaments normal neural and blood flow can be established through a manual thrust type of treatment.

Orthopedic Medicine

James Cyriax, M.D. (Fig. 1.6) has devoted his professional life to orthopedic medicine, the treatment by manipulation, massage, and injection. He has pursued his beliefs with intensity and has written extensively. He defines manipulation as "a method of treatment that consists of different sorts of passive movement performed by the hands in a definite manner for a prescribed purpose." His main purpose for manipulation is the correction of internal derangement. He has lectured extensively on his "parallelogram of force" in reference to the intervertebral disc and advocated extension-type exercises and distractive-type forces to "suck back up" the nucleus pulposus, and certain passive movements to maneuver the displaced fragments of the disc. His choice of maneuver is based on three uncontestable criteria: (a) the most likely one to succeed, (b) the least painful, and (c) the most informative. He works on the premise with a basis of a trial and end-feel, and effect (3).

Cyriax has repeatedly classified osteopathic physicians as lay manipulators, and has requested that osteopaths drop the notion of practicing an alternate system of medicine and to forget anatomical tone in curing visceral disease. "They would have to withdraw from the osteopathic lesion as an

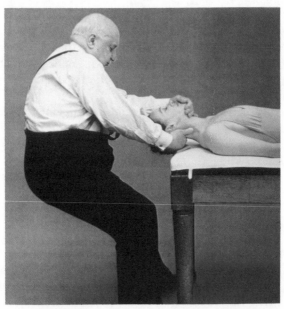

Figure 1.6. Dr. Cyriax treating a patient.

important factor in the development of disease, and agree that fixation of the spinal joint has a local effect only." He also insists that chiropractors who have taken over the panacea effect of manipulation should seek medical guidance and supervision. Cyriax strongly advocates manipulation by physical therapists, as they are taught by doctors and work with doctors, and have a mutual regard established. In his writings he relates that he has taught thousands of people to manipulate through his long stay at St. Thomas' Hospital, and also through his teaching books, videotapes, and guest lectureships. Although the British Chartered Society of Physiotherapists decry the term manipulation and have substituted the word *mobilization*, Cyriax feels that manipulation is a much more preferred term (13).

Cyriax believes that a book written by a Dr. Riadore on *Irritation of the Spinal Nerve* in 1842, probably provided the inspiration for the first osteopath:

"If an organ is deficiently supplied with nervous energy or blood, its function is decreased, and sooner or later its structure becomes endangered. . . .

"When we reflect that every organ and muscle in the body is connected and dependent more or less upon the spinal nerves for the perfect performance of their individual functions, we cannot otherwise prepare to hear of a lengthened catalogue of maladies that are either engendered, continued, or the consequence of spinal irritation."

Riadore also gave the first account for root pain emanating from "contact" at the intervertebral foramen. He recognized disc degeneration.

Manipulation became unethical in 1858 with the passage of the Medical Act in Great Britain. Until then, doctors had sent their patients to bonesetters for manipulation. Dr. James Paget delivered a lecture in 1868 entitled, "Cases That Bone-Setters Cure", in which he pointed out how neglectful doctors were of manipulation, thereby leaving patients with no alternative but to consult laymen. In 1871, the first English book on manipulation appeared, written by a Dr. Hood, about the work of Hutton, the well-known bone-setter (13).

Cyriax on Osteopathy and Orthopedic Medicine

Cyriax in his writings has tried—unsuccessfully—to discredit Dr. Still for his deep religious background, using such terms as "hallucinations" and such statements as "when he was shown that spinal dislocation would cause paraplegia long before it had this effect, he changed his hypothesis to pressure on a nerve."

According to Dr. Cyriax, "*The Lancet* in 1871 collected articles and lectures in book form the same year (surely a gold mine for the first osteopaths); also, Howard March and R. Dacre Fox, both in 1882 and Hugh

Owens Thomas and Sir Robert Jones." However, Cyriax described Edgar F. Cyriax as a prolific author of articles, and claimed that he was the first to describe the displacement of the intervertebral disc as a cause of clinical symptoms (13). He quotes David LeVay: ". . . current medical families such as the Cyriax's arose to occupy themselves in successive generations chiefly with the advancement of mechanotherapeutics. For the first time, these techniques were probably related to a sound knowledge of anatomy and pathology. The bone-setters, their clothes stolen, could only impugn the accuracy with which their very personal tradition had been translated into medical jargon."

In conclusion, Cyriax relates that:

"For hundreds, even thousands of years, manipulative treatment of low back pain has been common practice—by very different methods and with entirely different theoretical aims: Hippocrates straightened a kyphosis; Galen replaced outward dislocated vertebrae; and Ambroise Paré wrote about subluxation of the spine. Patients have been trampled upon by women chosen on sexual grounds (virgins, mothers of seven children, etc.); birth by presentation of the foot has been regarded as a given magical power to the stamper. Sufferers have been given blows on the back with different tools from hammers to brooms and steel yards and have been lifted back to back and shaken. Bone-setters have replaced small bones out of place; osteopaths have treated the 'mysterious osteopathic lesion'; chiropractors have replaced subluxed vertebrae; orthopedic surgeons have manipulated 'subluxation of the sacroiliac joint'; and neurologists have 'stretched the sciatic nerve'. Curiously enough, all concepts and methods have met with some degree of success. Clearly, the mechanism has been a fragment of disc which has become dislocated and was put back into position, or when a protrusion of the disc was 'sucked back' (or perhaps when a jammed or blocked joint was 'unlocked', or perhaps when a nerve root was shifted off the apex of a prolapsed disc)."

In his most recent publication, *Illustrated Manual of Orthopedic Medicine,* (4), Cyriax suggests that orthopedic medicine may have been born in 1929 but only now is it coming of age (Fig. 1.7).

"This was the challenge facing me in 1929. I then found, starting as an orthopedic house surgeon, that patients were divided into two categories—those whose defects showed up on the x-ray, and those whose x-rays were normal. At that time it was the custom to pass the latter on for physical therapy, consisting of various kinds of heat therapy, general diffuse massage, and exercise. It was a question of divided responsibility. No diagnosis was made or attempted in either the orthopedic or physical therapy departments, and the treatments were

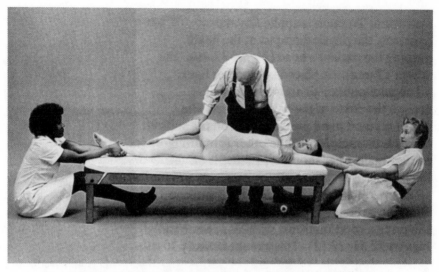

Figure 1.7. Spinal manipulation by Dr. Cyriax and associates.

not given because they were indicated or even specified, but simply because they were available ... Whenever a patient is sent for physical therapy, it must be with the diagnostic certainty, not only that physical therapy is the appropriate recourse, but also that the physiotherapist knows the work, that is, how to treat the right tissue in the right way. In such an informed context, the relationship between physician and physiotherapist becomes complementary; he can inject where she cannot; she can take much time-consuming work off his hands by massage or manipulation. Between the two of them, nearly all patients can be dealt with on the spot; generally the last thing needed is to call in a specialist, least of all a specialist outside the field of soft tissue lesions."

A. T. Still

The roots of manipulative therapy in the United States began with A. T. Still (5), and his philosophy of health care, stressing the wellness and wholeness of an individual. Still's life and political views from early manhood kept him in the center of controversy; he lived in Missouri, a border state, the son of a Methodist minister, and both he and his father were ardent abolitionists. In 1853, the elder Still was appointed a missionary to the Shawnee Indians and with his family moved to Kansas, where Andrew joined his father in the fight against slavery. In 1857 he was chosen by the people of Douglas County, Kansas, to represent them in the Kansas legislature. There, he quickly aroused the anger of the proslavery groups.

Dr. Still, a staunch supporter of Lincoln, enlisted in the Ninth Kansas Cavalry and saw active duty in the war, rising to the rank of Major. The thoughts of slavery and equal opportunity were ingrained in his background and when he founded the American School of Osteopathy, he declared the institution open to Negroes. Always controversial, he fought for women's suffrage as well.

Dr. Still's medical education was typical of the time—much of it by preceptorship, some from formal training. Before the Civil War, he had attended the College of Physicians and Surgeons of Kansas City, but before completing his course he left to enlist. He acquired other related experiences and had literally grown up in the medical field where he helped take care of the Shawnee Indians. In his autobiography (14) he wrote:

> "... one day when about 10 years of age I suffered from a headache. I made a swing of my father's plow lines between two trees, but my head hurt too much to make the swing comfortable; so I let the rope down to about 8 to 10 inches off the ground, threw the end of a blanket on it and lay down on the ground and used the ropes for a swinging pillow. Thus, I lay stretched on my back with my neck across the ropes. Soon, I became easy and went to sleep. I got up in a little while with the headache gone. As I knew nothing of anatomy at the time, I took no thought of how the rope would stop a headache and the sick stomach which accompanied it. After the discovery, I roped my neck whenever I felt those spells coming on. I followed the treatment for 20 years before the wedge of reason had reached my brain and I could see that I had suspended the action of the great occipital nerves and given harmony to the flow of the arterial blood to and through the veins, and ease was the effect."

Still held to the statement of Alexander Pope, "the proper study of mankind is man," to provide himself with material for dissection, he exhumed bodies from the graves of Indians. As he later recorded, "a thousand experiments were made with bones until I became quite familiar with the bone structure." It was a personal tragedy, however, that convinced Dr. Still that the status of medicine was inadequate. In the spring of 1864 there was a severe epidemic of meningitis in which thousands of people died, including three of Still's children. This tragic event served to drive him relentlessly on to the study of man, and led him to develop the philosophy that occupied his mind for the remainder of his life.

In 1874 Dr. Still was ready to present his concepts to the medical world, first to the doctors at Baker University in Baldwin, Kansas. Although he and his brothers and father had donated land to the University, Still was rejected by the University. In spite of his reputation as a good medical doctor and his service in the Civil War, and also his good record as a state legislator, the doors of the University were closed to him.

Dr. Still returned to Missouri determined to continue developing his ideas and incorporating them into his medical practice. He believed that the structure of the body was reciprocal and related to its function. He believed that the body's musculoskeletal system, bones, ligaments, muscle and fascia, form a structure that when disordered may affect a change in the function of other parts of the body. This effect could be created through the irritation and abnormal response of the nerve and blood supply to other organs of the body; the body of man is subject to mechanical disorder (1).

Dr. Still's fame grew and people from all over the United States came to Kirksville, Missouri for treatment by the "lightening bone-setter." The first formal class in the teaching of osteopathic medicine met in Kirksville in November of 1892, under a charter taken out in May of that year. A second charter was issued October 30, 1894, to the American School of Osteopathy. The object of the school was to improve the existing system of surgery, obstetrics, and treatment of disease generally, and place the same on a more rational and scientific basis and to impart information to the medical profession and to grant and confer such honors and degrees to the students that completed courses of instructions (1, 16).

The centennial celebration of osteopathic medicine in 1974 brought out the concept that osteopathic medicine was holistic in nature and was based on five major premises: (a) *unity of the body*—each system both in function and dysfunction depends upon others and influences other systems; (b) *healing power of nature*—there are substances within the body that, when they are in proper balance, preserve health and protect against disease; (c) *somatic component of disease*—the musculoskeletal system is truly the "machinery of life", and its reciprocal communication to other systems of the body is an important anatomical physiological principle of medical care; (d) *structure-function concept*—structure and function cannot be separated in human physiology but there is interdependence; and (e) *manipulative therapy*—its application to restore and maintain normal structural functional relationship of the musculoskeletal system is important (Fig. 1.8), not only to the function of the musculoskeletal system itself, but important also to the neural-hormonal communication with other body systems.

Manipulative therapy was recognized as a potentially useful therapeutic medium for both the maintenance of normal function and the correction of dysfunction. It was pointed out clearly that manipulative therapy and osteopathic medicine must be viewed in totality of their philosophy, not as things set apart. Manipulative therapy, like drugs, surgery, physical therapy, and diet are tools with which the basic fundamentals of osteopathic medicine can be expressed. Manipulation is a therapeutic means, no more and no less, and the American Academy of Osteopathy has set up a program for certification in manipulative skills. Special recognition is given to those who have more or less specialized in structural problems of the musculoskeletal system and special skills in manipulative therapy (1).

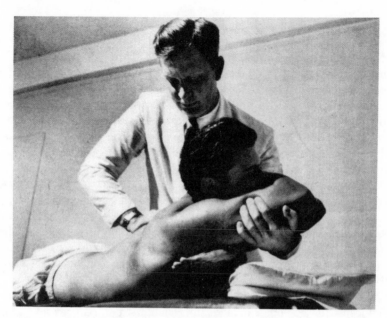

Figure 1.8. An osteopathic physician (Dr. J. Marshall Hoag), treating a patient's back by "mobilizing" the upper thoracic vertebrae (from Hoag [6]).

In 1975 and 1977, the National Institute of Neurological and Communicative Disease and Stroke of the National Institute of Health funded workshops on the research status of spinal manipulative therapy. At the first workshop, 58 scientists and clinicians of national and international status from the United States and eight foreign countries, including doctors of medicine, osteopathy, and chiropractic, and specialists in 11 basic sciences, usually Ph.D.s met. The 1977 workshop was held in 1977 at the Kellogg Center of Continuing Medical Education at Michigan State University sponsored by the College of Osteopathic Medicine, Michigan State University to consider mechanical disorders of the musculoskeletal system (particularly the spinal area) which might cause pain and/or alter physiology both local and at remote points (5).

Since the pioneer paper by Korr (7) many more workers around the world have added their experiments and observations to recent discoveries. The description of what amounts to an intraneural circulation opens the door to much neural biologic investigation, not the least of which is relevant to the neural biologic basis for manipulative therapy.

Manipulation by M.D.s

John McM. Mennell, M.D. has long been a proponent of manipulative therapy in the allopathic medical profession (9, 10). He writes:

"It has always seemed to me that the main reason why the medical profession has been reluctant to accept manipulative treatment of joint pain is because the proponents of manipulative treatment have never clearly emphasized that manipulative maneuvers and treatments are designed solely to restore something which is normal anatomically and physiologically to a joint—something which is unconcerned with voluntary joint movement, but is solely concerned with mechanical joint play, and which is essentially present only in life and absent in death. The prerequisite for successful treatment in any field of medicine is accurate diagnosis. The condition of joint dysfunction is the only pathologic condition that will respond to the treatment of manipulation. So, before manipulative therapy is ever used, the normal range of joint-play movements must be learned as carefully as the range of voluntary movement as now taught and learned in routine anatomy classes. That joint play movements are small, often not more than ⅛ of an inch in extent in any plane, does not mean that they are unimportant."

He further states that

"... manipulating joints is an art and, as with so many arts, not everyone can expect to be able to learn to use it. Perhaps there are two main reasons why joint manipulation has not found the wide acceptance that it merits in the practice of medicine; first, the user has not learned the proper techniques; and second, the user is simply inept at the art. It is so much easier to blame a modality of treatment for failure than it is to blame someone who perhaps never should be using the modality in the first place.... Any pathological joint condition, whether simple joint dysfunction, or some serious joint disease, affects to some extent all the anatomical structures that play a part in the functioning of the joint. All the affected structures need attention in treatment if a return to normalcy is to be expected."

Dr. Mennell further points out, "... so, joint manipulation is one modality of treatment that may or may not have a place in the treatment of a painful joint. If it is not used when it is indicated, treatment will fail to alleviate the patient's symptoms; if it is used when it should not be, treatment will also fail to relieve the patient's symptoms and, indeed, many even make them worse" (9, 10).

Outside the osteopathic profession, manipulative therapy is applied to joint injury, postural imbalance, and neuromuscular rehabilitation. The physiologic basis of manipulation in osteopathic medicine· includes reestablishing normal function of joint relationships, relieving tension and contracture, stimulating improved circulation and tissue drainage, and restoring functional capacity and is well documented. Much interest recently has been directed toward "myofascial trigger zones", and entire texts have been devoted to this topic. It is believed that those who practice manipulative therapy in medicine must have detailed knowledge of functional anatomy including the planes of joint motion, neuroanatomy, neurophysiology, and neurology, along with biochemistry and pharmacology. The purpose of manipulation is not just restoring fragmented disc parts or a herniated nucleus pulposus, but it is to restore or improve structure and function inter-relationships, to normalize function by normalizing structure, to improve circulation including arterial, venous, and lymphatic in localized areas, and to decrease noxious afferent impulses that are being fed into the central nervous system. It also may improve the effectiveness of the body's immune mechanism, develop a helpful psychological attitude and emotional response, and to use the techniques and phenomena of "biofeedback." The time has come for manipulative therapy to achieve its proper place in the total medical care system.

The tool of manipulation is being more liberally used in the allopathic institutions. Different terms have been attributed to manipulative treatment, such as adjustments, mobilization, manipulation, release techniques, and manual medicine. Physicians have the obligation to evaluate the musculoskeletal complaints, diagnose, and set up a treatment program. The question of manipulative treatment has been deliberated over the centuries. If manipulative treatment is indicated, then the physician has the option to treat the patient himself or to delegate this treatment to others. In the United States today, the physical therapist has shown a strong interest in mobilization.

The federal government also has an enormous responsibility in reference to whether manipulative treatment will be paid for. The economics of health care delivery have escalated astronomically. If the physicians are given the responsibility for health care, then they also must have the authority to render the most effective and efficient treatment. Manipulative treatment takes time and energy, as well as learned skill. If there is negative reimbursement for this type of treatment, then it will stagnate and be delegated to lesser trained individuals.

REFERENCES

1. Adler, P., and Northrup, G. *100 Years of Osteopathic Medicine (1874–1974)*. Squibb & Sons Inc., Medical Community, Inc., 1976.
2. Baker, H., *Leaves From My Life*. Hutchinson, N. D. London 1028.
3. Cyriax, J. *The Textbook of Ortopedic Medicine*, Vol. II. Treatment by Manipulation, Massage and Injection, Tenth Ed. Bailliere Tindall, London, 1980.
4. Cyriax, J. *Illustrated Manual of Orthopedic Medicine*. Butterworth's, London, 1983.
5. Gevitz, N. *The D.O.'S*. Osteopathic Medicine in America, John Hopkins University Press, Baltimore, 1982.
6. Hoag, J. M. *Osteopathic Medicine*. McGraw Hill, New York, 1969.
7. Korr, I. M. Axonal delivery of Neuroplasmic components to muscle cells. *Science*, pp. 155, 342, 1967.

8. Laino, C. *Medical Tribune*, p. 16, March 1984.
9. Mennell, J. *Back Pain*. Diagnosis and Treatment Using Manipulative Technique. Little, Brown & Co., Boston, 1960.
10. Mennell, J. *Joint Pain*. Diagnosis and Treatment Using Manipulative Technique. Little, Brown & Co., Boston, 1964.
11. Northrup, G. W. *Osteopathic Medicine & American Reformation*. American Osteopathic Association, Chicago, 1966.
12. Rogoff, J. *Manipulation, Traction and Massage*. 2nd, Ed., Williams & Wilkins, Baltimore, 1980.
13. Schiötz, E., and Cyriax, J. *Manipulation Past and Present*. Heinemann, London, 1975.
14. Still, A. T. Autobiography, Kirksville, 1908.
15. Stoddard, A. *Manual of Osteopathic Practice*. Hutchinson, London, 1969.
16. Young, W. R. (Assoc. Ed.) Osteopaths. *Life*, pp. 108–118, Sept. 29, 1960.

2

Role of Physical Therapists in Spinal Manipulation[1]

RICHARD NYBERG

The practice of physical therapy has undergone tremendous change in the past 20 years, especially in the area of clinical specialization. The most important factor probably relates to the desire of most physical therapists to become proficient in one area of health care. They have recognized the impossible task of trying to excel in all aspects of therapeutic care. The heightened educational awareness of the consumer and the greater demands for excellent service placed upon the physical therapy clinician are also partly responsible for the trend. The result is that today many physical therapists practice in one area such as cardiopulmonary therapy, neurodevelopmental therapy, sports, or orthopedic physical therapy.

The American Physical Therapy Association (APTA) has supported clinical specialization and has created task forces to develop board certification examinations in each specialty area (30). The sanctioning of the board certification exams by the APTA will help identify competent clinicians within specialty areas and will serve to improve the level of health care. The main objective of this chapter is to identify the present and future role of the orthopedic physical therapist (OPT) in spinal manipulation.

As a means of introduction and perspective of involvement by physical therapists in musculoskeletal problems, a few statistics are necessary. In the United States, approximately 38,000 physical therapists are members of the APTA (22). No statistical information is available on the number of

[1] The author expresses appreciation to all who have supported the development of orthopedic physical therapy and specifically to the instructors within the Institute of Graduate Health Sciences, the Clinical Staff at the Atlanta Back Clinic, the Physical Therapy Program at Emory University, Steve Wolf, Ph.D. and Stanley Paris, NZSP, MCSP, P.T., Ph.D.

physical therapists who regularly practice spinal manipulation; however, over 8000 physical therapists in the United States subscribe to the Orthopedic and Sports Physical Therapy Journal of the APTA (23). Members of the Orthopedic and Sports Physical Therapy Section of APTA most likely have had some form of undergraduate, graduate, and/or postgraduate training in manipulation. Almost all undergraduate and basic Master's Programs in Physical Therapy include mobilization training within the curriculum and a number of physical therapy graduate programs offer a clinical specialization track in orthopedic physical therapy. Graduate programs in physical therapy that offer clinical specialization place a strong emphasis upon the manual skills necessary to detect and treat musculoskeletal dysfunction. Most physical therapists at the present time obtain knowledge and skill in manipulation technique by regularly attending postgraduate continuing education programs given by other physical therapists, medical practitioners of manipulation, and osteopaths.

Within the next two to three years the APTA and its Orthopedic Physical Therapy Section probably will have developed board certification examinations. One result of having established the necessary criteria for board certification in orthopedic physical therapy is the identification of the various options in developing knowledge, skill, and proficiency for physical therapists wishing to specialize. Initially, the mechanism by which one prepares for board certification is likely to vary considerably. Clarification as to which method of preparation for board certification works best undoubtedly will be studied extensively by review committees.

Definitions

To understand how and why spinal manipulation is a part of physical therapy practice, a review of terminology is necessary. Since the inception of physical therapy, passive range-of-motion technique has been considered and accepted to be a vital element in maintaining joint function. The definition of passive movement is motion that is not under voluntary control but occurs in response to an external or outside force (7). Passive motion therefore can be considered a classical movement performed by a physical therapist for the purpose of maintaining or promoting range of motion. Passive movement has been a part of physical therapy practice and will continue to be so.

Manipulation is generally defined as any manual operation or maneuver (27). More specifically, manipulation is a skilled therapeutic passive movement designed to restore joint motion or tissue extensibility. Manipulation justifiably falls into the category of passive motion and as a natural consequence of this physical therapists became involved in manipulative technique. Manipulation performed by physical therapists is not a new development within the profession, but in relation to the formal practice of manipulation among manual medical practitioners and osteopaths, physical therapists doing manipulative technique are newcomers. In the United States, the physical therapy profession is itself only 60 years old (33).

The nature of any health practice tends to have different areas of focus at any one particular time and such is the case with physical therapy. The past 20 years have seen a tremendous shift in emphasis toward manual therapeutic practice in orthopedic physical therapy. Some of the change is accounted for by patient experiences because clinical success and failure helps shape the way a physical therapist practices. Part of the change also relates to the growing scientific basis of manipulation and the increasing acceptance of manipulation as a useful tool among the medical field. The fact that an immediate result sometimes follows a manipulative procedure is perhaps also an attractive option for a physical therapist who needs instant feedback on performance.

Role of the Orthopedic Physical Therapist

Before introducing a classification system on the types of manipulation, the role of the OPT must be identified. The OPT is trained to detect motion impairment in the musculoskeletal system. Abnormal movement, within either a joint or soft tissue, can take two forms. Hypomobility means motion restriction whereas hypermobility means motion instability. The ability of an OPT hinges upon an evaluation which focuses on identifying resistance to motion and/or range of motion. Therefore, a qualitative and quantitative assessment of movement is performed. The basic underlying foundation for an OPT's evaluation lies in biomechanics and neurophysiology. Physical therapy education places considerable emphasis on biomechanics and neurophysiological science; as a result, motion evaluation is a skill possessed by most physical therapists.

An effective working relationship between the OPT and the primary medical physician requires proper role identification. The OPT is trained to evaluate for motion abnormality. The OPT has sufficient anatomical knowledge to understand the pathologic basis for the condition, but is not accountable for identifying by diagnosis the tissue source of pain. The physical medicine specialist, rheumatologist, orthopedist, neurologist, neurosurgeon, and osteopath first diagnose, and then determine the nature of the musculoskeletal pathology and rule out disease processes. Diagnostic procedures such as routine x-rays, myelograms, discograms, EMGs, nerve conduction velocity tests, and CAT scans require physician interpretation and analysis. The OPT must be aware of the importance of diagnostic tests and utilize the information from each test to formulate or adjust physical therapy treatment. The physician, on the other hand, must understand physical therapy strategy and technique, use the appropriate diagnostic tests and develop a medical approach in handling the orthopedic problem.

The physician/surgeon and OPT communicate to determine if the patient is responding to conservative treatment or whether surgery is necessary.

A clear understanding of the roles of the OPT and physician in managing musculoskeletal dysfunction enables both effective and quality patient care. Mutual agreement on their functions also leads to an effective working relationship in which both health practitioners contribute in the area of their strengths. Physician realization that a competent OPT has expertise in manipulation, exercise, posture, and preventive-care concepts may provide relief of a major burden in health management.

Types of Manipulation

The word manipulation takes on many different meanings among health practitioners and lay people. The ambiguity and lack of clear definition of manipulation results in communication problems which ultimately lead to misconceptions. To some, manipulation is the use of a vigorous high speed manual maneuver which repositions displaced bones into place and results in a pop or crack. To others, manipulation is a gentle, refined motion which increases movement in a joint. The language of manipulation is in need of further specification and definition. The following section deals with the various forms of manipulation used by the OPT. The purpose is to define each manipulation type clearly so that the language of manipulation can be understood, and communication among manipulative therapists and other practitioners enhanced.

An overview of manipulation types is given in Table 2.1. The first differentiation to make is that manipulation can be *general* (regional) or *specific* (localized).

A **general spinal manipulation** is a stretch performed to more than one joint and usually more than one spinal segment. The manipulative force is transmitted to a number of segments, some of which may have normal

Table 2.1
Types of Manipulation

General (Regional)	Specific (Localized)
Indirect	Direct
Noncontact	Contact
Cyclic Loading	Sustained loading
Nonthrust	Thrust
Graded oscillation—1–4	Surgical
Progressive stretch	General
Continuous stretch	Specific
Muscle energy technique	High velocity
Functional technique	Overpressure
Counterstrain	Locking

motion or perhaps even exhibit hypermobility. Therefore, the disadvantage of general spinal manipulation is the possibility of increasing motion in an already unstable joint. The obvious indication of general manipulation is in improving motion in an area of the spine which is generally stiff.

Specific spinal manipulation intends to stretch only one segment or one spinal joint. One of the aims of specific spinal manipulation is to minimize force transmission through uninvolved spinal segments. Proponents of specific spinal manipulation claim that the technique is safer and more effective than the general technique because only the involved segment or joint is manipulated. On the other hand, an OPT applying specific spinal manipulation to an incorrectly identified normal spinal joint may not be helping the condition.

The evaluation of motion impairment entails determining which direction(s) a spinal joint is restricted. For example, the inability of L3–4 to rotate and side-bend to the left may be due to a restriction in the cephalad and anterior motion of the right inferior process of L3. Figure 2.1 demonstrates the arthrokinematic behavior of L3 and L4 during left rotation.

Direct manipulation involves a stretch in the direction of the motion restriction or barrier (13). In the case of L3–4 where the right inferior process of L3 does not slide cephalad and anterior, a direct manipulation would move into the restricted range and stretch. Osteopathic manipulators state that direct technique engages the motion barrier. Direct techniques are logical and effective, but sometimes painful.

Indirect manipulation technique involves stretching in the opposite direction of the motion restriction (24). An OPT using indirect technique on an L3–4 left rotation restriction would move the right inferior process of L3 caudal and posterior to create right rotation. Indirect manipulation involves moving away from the motion barrier. At first, the concept of indirect manipulation may appear strange. To understand the concept of indirect manipulation, consider how a stuck, skewed drawer in a chest is pulled out of the chest. Often the movement which frees the drawer and

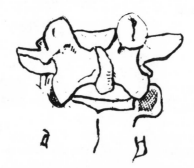

Figure 2.1. Left rotation of L3 on L4 viewed from behind.

allows the drawer to be pulled out is, in fact, an inward push. In other words, the drawer is pushed in first, before pulling it out—an indirect technique. A restricted spinal joint may work in the same manner. Indirect manipulation is usually safer than direct manipulation and has less tendency for an adverse reaction. A general rule of thumb when in doubt is always to choose an indirect approach. On the other hand, unlocking a fixed joint but not creating increased motion in the needed direction is possible when using an indirect technique.

Manipulative techniques can also be classified as being *contact* or *noncontact*.

Contact manipulation technique requires hand or finger placement on the involved segment. Contacts are frequently made on the spinous processes, lamina, facet joint, and sometimes the transverse processes in the cervical spine. In the thoracic and lumbar spines the only accessible contact points are the spinous and transverse processes. Contact is recommended for enhancing specificity, assisting in force transmission and control, and for monitoring tissue response. Occassionally, additional leverage is required in effecting a joint release and so contact needs to be away from the involved segment.

Noncontact techniques do not require hand or finger placement on the lesioned segment. The major indication for noncontact manipulation is when greater force is necessary to achieve a joint release. Frequently greater manipulative force requires leverage which is obtained by using distal contacts on the extremities. Opponents of noncontact manipulation insist that noncontact techniques are unsafe and not specific.

The OPT decides whether a restricted segment will respond to *cyclic loading* or *sustained pressure*. **Cyclic loading** is the alternate loading and unloading of a joint for the purpose of gaining increased range of motion. Cyclic loading is a rhythmical activity usually performed at a certain set speed depending on what is comfortable for the patient. As a result of cyclic loading, a progressive increase in joint movement occurs. As the tissues become extensible the joint undergoes the full available range of motion during each cycle until normal motion is restored. Cyclic loading can be likened to the "try, try again" philosophy. Sometimes an irritable joint structure prefers not to be carried passively through an entire range of motion in the attempt to increase movement. Acute conditions, therefore, may not respond to cyclic loading.

Sustained pressure manipulation involves a slow, gradual, continuous, progressive force which ultimately creates additional segmental movement. The advantages of a sustained pressure technique include an increased sensitivity to tissue response, an immediate feedback mechanism which allows the OPT to adjust the manipulation force or direction, and the beneficial physiological-hydraulic effects of sustained pressure on viscoelastic tissues. One disadvantage of using sustained pressures occurs in the situation of a long-standing joint adhesion. Adhesion formation in or around joints sometimes requires a high velocity manipulation in order to break loose.

The next distinction within manipulation procedure concerns *thrust* and *nonthrust* technique.

Thrust manipulative technique requires a high velocity, low amplitude motion which is delivered at the end of the pathologic limit of an accessory range of motion (12). The thrust technique requires skill in force application especially in regard to amplitude. The inherent safety valve in thrust manipulation is the fact that the motion excursion involves an extremely low amplitude. Appropriate patient selection is a critical factor in successful treatment, perhaps more so than the actual application of the technique. The OPT should keep in mind that not all patients are psychologically, structurally, or biomechanically suitable candidates for thrust manipulation. In addition, the length of time of the motion impairment as well as the stage of the condition needs careful scrutiny. A 20-year joint restriction of significant magnitude will most likely react adversely to a sudden thrust manipulation. Preparation of the surrounding joint tissues is often an important preliminary step. Thrust manipulations are necessary to snap an adhesion, alter vertebral position, normalize segmental motion, and reduce pain.

The three types of thrust manipulation used are described below.

Surgical thrust manipulation is performed under general anesthesia. The patient under general anesthesia with loss of sensation and depression of nerve function has no mechanism to protect a joint structure and therein lies the danger in surgical thrust manipulation. The obvious advantage is that involuntary muscle guarding around an affected joint is eliminated; as a result, resistance to passive movement is due solely to the limitations of the joint itself.

General thrust manipulation involves a high-velocity, low-amplitude stretch to more than one joint and possibly more than one spinal segment. Multisegmental manipulation is sometimes recommended in the thoracic spine when three or four segments in a row become fixed. Precaution is to be taken in other spinal areas when using general manipulation because of the possibility of having a joint hypermobility.

Specific thrust manipulative technique involves *three criteria*:

1. The first is the use of spinal locking procedures designed to minimize force on uninvolved spinal segments and to maximize force on the involved segment. To accomplish spinal locking, the mechanical behavior of the spinal motion segment must be understood. Often, to achieve locking, the facet joints on one side of the spine are apposed. Approximation of the two articular processes theoretically opposes further motion at the segment. Facet apposition is one method used by the "specificity therapists" to protect

neighboring joint instabilities. Another mechanism by which spinal locking is attained is through ligamentous-myofascial tension (29). The OPT creates this tension: by locking the spine above and below the lesioned segment the manipulative force is concentrated mostly at the site of segmental dysfunction.

2. The second criterion involves the use of a high velocity movement. The faster a performer is able to pull a tablecloth, the less likely is the table setting affected. Similarly, the quicker the manipulative thrust the less chance of affecting adjacent spinal levels. A skilled manipulative therapist has quick-acting hands capable of high speed activity.

3. The third criterion for specific thrust manipulation deals with overpressure. All thrust techniques require overpressure in the sense that the movement is performed at the end of the available joint range. In specific manipulation the overpressure is of very low amplitude. The larger the manipulative excursion, the greater the possibility of engaging an adjacent segment. Specific thrust manipulation through the use of spinal locking procedures, high-velocity movement, and low-amplitude overpressure is a subject of controversy among manipulators. The theoretical intention is admirable, but whether spinal specificity in manipulation actually occurs is unknown.

Nonthrust manipulation or **mobilization**, is a gentle, persuasive pressure performed within the available accessory range or at the end of the accessory range (11). Inherent within a nonthrust manipulation is a patient feedback mechanism. Because the motion is relatively slow, controlled, and gentle, the patient can report about the effect of the technique during the time of application. Various types of nonthrust manipulation are used to restore segmental motion in the spine and perhaps reduce pain.

Graded oscillation technique is a form of nonthrust manipulation whereby alternate pressure, on and off, are delivered at different parts of the available range (17). The amplitude of the oscillation may also vary according to the purpose of the technique. Oscillatory technique is graded on a 1 to 4 scale based on the amplitude of the motion and part of the range being reached (Fig. 2.2). The vibratory nature of the graded oscillation technique is an excellent way to activate sensory mechanoreceptors. Activation of mechanoreceptors may help reduce pain and improve proprioceptive function.

Progressive stretch mobilization involves a successive series of short-amplitude, spring-type pressures or a series of short-amplitude stretch movements (26). The pressure or stretch is imparted at progressive increments of the range (Fig. 2.3). Progressive stretch is also graded on a 1 to 4 scale as is graded oscillation. The major indication for the use of progressive stretch nonthrust manipulation is mechanical and/or soft-tissue restriction.

Continuous stretch is a sustained, gradual-increase stretch or pressure

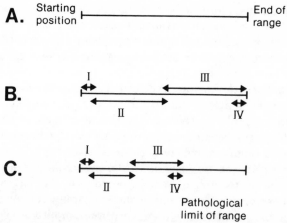

Figure 2.2. Graded oscillation ranges. *A*. total range. *B*. For each of 4 grades, the *arrows* depict amplitude of each of the movements and the position they occupy in the range. *C*. When pathology limits the range of movement, the grades are also reduced in range.

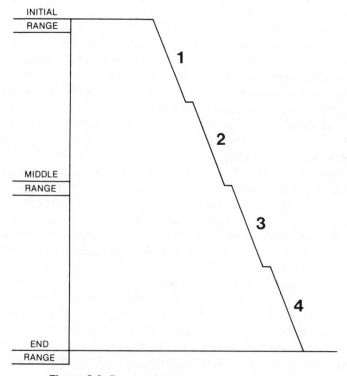

Figure 2.3. Progressive stretch mobilization.

without interruption. Maintaining a stretch or pressure throughout the manipulation procedure is the recommended technique when immediate tissue feedback is desired. Adaptively shortened periarticular soft-tissue structures are most likely to be affected through the use of continuous stretch technique. Improving extensibility of the periarticular soft tissues about a spinal joint by collagen fiber realignment and viscosity change allows for improved joint mobility.

Muscle energy is a nonthrust manipulation technique that requires muscle contraction on the part of the patient in order to normalize muscle function and/or increase joint range (10). In osteopathy, muscle energy is the use of the muscle force from a precisely determined position in a specific direction against a distinct counterforce. Muscle energy usually involves three phases—contraction, relaxation, and stretch; it can be performed either as a direct or indirect technique. Most authorities agree that localization of the force to the affected spinal level is more important than the amount of force and counterforce. In fact, very light force is often desirable in obtaining the desired result. Physical manipulations using proprioceptive neuromuscular technique often employ hold-relax-stretch procedures to obtain an increase in range of motion and normalize muscle function about a joint. The hold-relax-stretch technique is comparable to the muscle energy technique in both application and affect.

Functional technique proponents claim that active-assistive positioning of a joint away from the motion barrier of restriction and into a position of ease allows normalization of neurophysiologic activity about the joint (4). By normalizing myofascial activity, the persistent reflex muscle guarding is inhibited and relaxation is promoted about the joint. Functional technique involves working with the patient's respiratory mechanism and sensing tissue relaxation during the exhalation phase. As tissue relaxation occurs the operator maneuvers the spine into a different position of joint ease. Functional technique is a subtle nonthrust manipulation which requires skill and sensitivity. Individuals with reflexogenic protective muscle-guarding or spasm and resultant joint dysfunction respond to functional technique quite well. On the other hand, chronic and rigid joint fixations are usually less receptive to the functional approach.

Counterstrain is another type of nonthrust manipulation. The procedure involves localization of a sensitive myofascial trigger point and a positioning of the muscle and related joint into a position of comfort (5). Pressure is applied into the trigger point while the muscle and related joint are maintained in the position of maximal relaxation. The abnormal reflex and resultant muscle spasm are inhibited by the trigger point pressure and opposite counterstrain created by the positioning. The pressure is applied for 90 seconds and is followed by a slow passive return to neutral so that the abnormal reflex is not reinstated. The counterstrain technique is also best suited for joint lesions which come about from a self-perpetuating tonic-reflex muscle spasm.

In summary, manipulation by an OPT takes on many forms. The type of technique selected is dependent on many patient factors: age, body build, sex, type of problem, stage of condition, length of time of the condition, type of personality, and general health state. The OPT must become skilled in the selection and performance of all manipulative types. Certain patients may only respond to particular types of manipulative procedure and, therefore, one must be experienced with all types. The language of manipulation has been unclear in the past. If health practitioners using manipulation are to communicate effectively, a classification scheme for different manipulations and clear definitions for each type are necessary.

Spinal Evaluation and the OPT

Before deciding on a treatment plan and whether a manipulative approach is required, the OPT conducts an evaluation. The evaluation involves a biomechanical and neurophysiologic assessment of the patient's physical condition. Details of the evaluation process are not necessary, however, an overview of the major components of the evaluation is presented.

An assessment of pain location, intensity, frequency, and duration is done through initial observations and history. Some OPTs rely heavily on pain description in determining treatment strategy while others depend on functional ability (movement). The OPT who trusts pain as a sole indicator of improvement needs to be extremely knowledgeable in pair physiology and psychology in order to judge patient status accurately. For example, the multisegmental nature of spinal innervation often interferes with correctly identifying the segmental source of pain by analysis of pain location (37). In other words, referred pain from the S1 myotome may actually be the result of an L2–3 spinal irritation. The psychological aspects of chronic pain behavior are also an important aspect in determining the patient's condition. The way one reacts to pain is dependent on a multitude of factors which range from culture, religion, family, social environment, personality type, and coping mechanisms (28). The functional approach, on the other hand, focuses more on movement and functional level and less on pain.

A structural evaluation attempts to identify gross alignment problems that may create areas of abnormal tissue tension tone. Spinal posture is analyzed during the structural evaluation. The effects of faulty spinal posture or any deviation of major spinal alignment on spinal motion as well as the relationship of spinal posture or deviation to the region of pain are noted. Spinal structure governs function. The extent to which this relationship is true during the evaluation often determines the seriousness of the condition. Basically, the structural evaluation helps focus in on the possible areas of motion dysfunction.

Active spinal movement tests are analyzed after the structural evaluation. The purpose of testing active movements is threefold:

1. Active movement-testing requires voluntary motion on the part of the patient. Therefore, the patient's ability as well as willingness to move is assessed, i.e., indirectly the pain tolerance of the patient is determined. A patient with a high pain tolerance may exhibit greater range despite pain than a patient with a low pain tolerance.

2. Another purpose for active movement testing is pain reproduction. Identification of active movements which duplicate the patient's symptoms may be extremely valuable in deciding on a treatment plan. For example, if forward-bending at the lumbar spine is painful though backward-bending is not, then instruction to avoid forward-bending and promote backward-bending might be warranted.

3. Analysis of active movements also helps assess gross spinal motion behavior.

Three aspects of spinal motion require attention. The first is range of motion. How much movement occurs during side-bending, forward-bending, backward-bending, and rotation? The second aspect concerns motion direction. Do forward- and backward-bending take place in the midsagittal plane or does a deviation to one side occur? Does side-bending occur in the frontal plane and rotation in the horizontal plane? Movement deviations away from the correct body plane are due to biomechanical abnormalities such as a segmental motion restriction on one side. The third aspect is motion control; this is exhibited when spinal movement occurs at a smooth, uninterrupted, constant rate. Any evidence of a change in motion speed that comes about because of a spinal hitch or judder may indicate a motion-related problem. Motion control or the quality of movement is a component of the degree of resistance offered as one recruits each spinal level.

Impairment of all aspects of spinal motion, range, direction, and control is likely to have more pathomechanical significance than impairment of just one aspect, such as range of motion. Analysis of active movements, therefore, requires an evaluation of all three parameters. Active movement testing further assists the OPT in centering in on the problem area(s).

Palpation testing comes after active movement testing. Again, three aspects of palpation require mentioning. Palpation helps determine the condition of tissues. By evaluating temperature, moisture, tissue texture, tone, and tension the OPT can define the stage of the condition. For example, a warm, moist area on the spine that exhibits hypertonus and reflex contraction to palpation may indicate an acute condition in an active inflammatory process and the initial stage of repair.

Local tenderness to palpation with associated changes in tissue thickness or tone, evidence of hypertonus or reflex muscle contraction, changes in skin temperature and moisture along with motion abnormality are all clinical manifestations of a facilitated segment. Facilitation occurs when a disturbance in sensory input results in a lowering of firing thresholds for the nerve cells located in a particular segment(s). Thus, the neurons in facilitated segments are hyper-responsive to impulses from any part of the body (15). Palpation testing enables the OPT to identify facilitated segments.

Vertebral palpation is a means by which the OPT can find positional faults. Positional changes such as anterior or posterior vertebral displacements, forward- or backward-bending faults or rotational faults that affect spinal motion are considered to be significant pathomechanical problems. The OPT is to be aware of possible vertebral anomalies in shape and size which may be falsely interpreted to be a positional fault. X-ray confirmation of vertebral position is sometimes valuable for confirmation purposes.

Specific mobility assessment is the third part of palpation testing. The procedure utilized is called **passive intervertebral motion testing (PIVM).** Digital palpation on a facet joint or at an interspinous space is used to feel the motion which is passively induced by maneuvering the spine or extremities. PIVM testing is a skill that is developed by continuous practice and concentration. Patient relaxation is a prerequisite for reliable testing. The OPT uses light palpation to feel the motion at one spinal segment or joint. Envisioning the perceived motion is sometimes helpful. Remembering that the palpating finger acts as a sensory electrode is another important key in successful PIVM testing.

PIVM GRADING SCALE (TABLE 2.2)

The most common grading scale used by the OPT is the 0 to 6 scale (9). *Three* indicates normal motion behavior in terms of range and resistance.

Table 2.2
Passive intervertebral motion (PIVM) grading scale

Grade	Description	Criteria
0	Ankylosed	No detectable movement within the segment; requires stress film radiology for confirmation
1	Considerable restriction (hypomobility)	Significant decrease in expected range; significant resistance to movement
2	Slight restriction (hypomobility)	Limitation expected in range, some resistance to movement
3	Normal	Expected range for body type; uniform movement throughout range
4	Slight increase (hypermobility)	Some increase expected in range; less than normal resistance to movement
5	Considerable increase (hypermobility)	Excessive range (but eventually restricted by capsular and ligamental structure)
6	Unstable	Excessive range (as in Grade 5) but without the restraint of capsular and ligamental structure

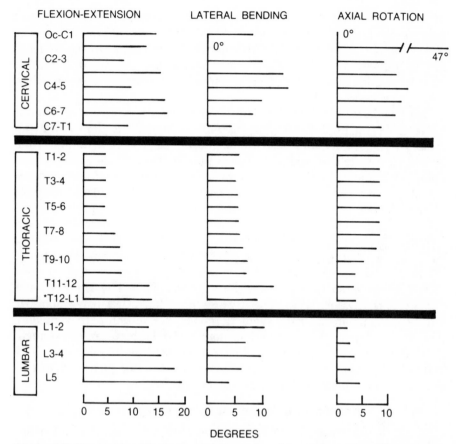

Figure 2.4. Composite of the representative values for rotation at the different levels of the spine in the traditional planes of motion. It is designed to allow a ready comparison of the motion in the various regions of the spine, as well as the different types of movement in each region. *The figures for the T12–L1 interspace are derived from interpolations (from White and Panjabi [34]).

Grades of *2 or less* signify motion restriction. The range of motion is less than normal and the resistance through the available range is increased. Grades of *4 or above* denote an increase in range of motion and less resistance to motion. Judgments are based on knowledge of normal segmental range as well as the relative changes from one motion segment to the adjacent segments. Figure 2.4 shows degree values of spinal segmental motion as calculated by White and Panjabi.

The OPT, therefore, may choose to use a manipulation technique on segments which are graded to be 1 or 2. The type of manipulation technique chosen is somewhat determined by the segmental grade given. A grade 1 limitation, for example, may respond slower to nonthrust manipulation than a thrust manipulation, but is less likely to result in an adverse reaction such as swelling or pain. The results of PIVM testing often confirm the observations made during the active motion exam. Some OPTs rely more heavily on visual assessment of active spinal movements to determine whether manipulation is necessary, whereas others depend more on palpatory tests such as PIVM.

The remainder of the OPT's evaluation includes provocation testing for nerve involvement, i.e., straight leg raising, as well as a review of all radiologic, laboratory, and electrical diagnostic tests. Positive findings from all tests are correlated and a treatment plan outlined. Goals are set and a prognosis given. A manipulative approach to a biomechanical, pain-related, spinal problem should show some results in terms of increased range of motion, decreased resistance to motion, improved proprioceptive function or decreased pain within five treatment sessions. This does not imply that a chronic low back degenerative disc condition of 15 years will be completely cured in five treatments. The suggestion made is that some type of change should happen within five treatments.

A summary of an OPT's evaluation has been given. The essential components of the evaluation were briefly presented. Each OPT may emphasize a different component of the evaluation or have a certain pathologic bias. The one similarity across evaluations done by OPTs, however, is thoroughness. Without a complete evaluation to determine dysfunction, the OPT stands little chance in helping the recovery process and greater chance in causing harm or delaying the recovery process.

Rationale for the Use of Spinal Manipulation

Spinal manipulation, in whatever form, entails the laying on of hands which historically always has been part of the healing arts (31). Perhaps not universally accepted among medical practitioners, manipulation seems to have advanced from what many believed to be unorthodox medicine to a more commonly accepted practice. At the present time, scientific justification of the use of spinal manipulation is equivocal. The OPT uses theoretical rationale and clinical study to justify manipulation. A part of the rationale for the use of spinal manipulation as a healing art is that it requires touch, but the powerful psychologic effect of tactile sensation can be ignored or denied. The following section discusses three possible mechanisms by which spinal manipulation may work.

MECHANICAL EFFECTS

The effects of immobilization of joints have been extensively studied by many investigators. Joint restriction is the result of a loss of extensibility in the periarticular soft-tissue structures about the joint, i.e., capsules, ligaments, connective tissue, and myofascia. The periarticular biochemical changes of soft tissue resulting from enforced immobilization, immobilization after injury, or perhaps lack of use, involve the loss of glycoaminoglycan (GAG) molecules. A parallel loss of water content occurs in response to the decrease in GAGs. Authorities contend that the water between collagen fibrils serves as a diffusion medium for cellular transport and as a lubricating mechanism to allow for greater extensibility. A loss of fluid volume between collagen fibers along with the stationary attitude of the fibers allows the fibers to approximate, thereby increasing the potential for abnormal cross-link formation (35). One histologic study demonstrates an increased number of adhesions between collagen fibers after 10 weeks of immobilization. Motion may also be inhibited by an abnormal waveform deposition and arrangement of new collagen fibrils which resists tensile force (1). In summary, joint stiffness is the result of: (a) a loss of the normal lubricating mechanism between collagen fibers due to decreased numbers of GAGs; (b) the approximation and stationary attitude of collagen fibers which leads to an increased number of adhesions; (c) the smaller crimp angles found in the collagen fibrils (3).

Restoration of extensibility to the joint capsule and ligaments as well as the myofascial tissues about the joint is a significant part of spinal manipulation theory by OPTs who favor passive motion through the use of manipulation. Movement may, in fact, inhibit a contracture process by stimulating GAG synthesis thereby maintaining lubricating efficiency and normal three-dimensional spatial patterns in the matrix (2). Most OPTs would agree that some form of general or specific exercise is necessary after spinal manipulation to restore fully and maintain the critical fluid barrier between collagen fibers.

Rupture of the abnormal cross-links which form between fibers (8) is the second possible way in which spinal manipulation may work. Intra- and extra-articular joint adhesions may be broken as a result of a specific manipulative force. Most OPTs speculate that thrust manipulation is effective in rupturing joint adhesions because of the high velocity used in the technique. The possibility of normal capsular tissue being overstretched or torn by thrust manipulative technique must be considered. Therefore, repetitive use of thrust technique on a patient at the same segmental level is not advisable. The potential end result of repetitive thrust manipulation is joint instability which ultimately may lead to early degenerative joint changes such as articular cartilage wear, capsular thickening, and bony hypertrophy. On the other hand, the benefit of thrust technique in creating joint release and freedom of motion cannot be ignored.

Restoration of normal positional relationships of vertebrae is a third possible mechanism by which spinal manipulation works. To accept that spinal manipulation may reposition a vertebra one must first believe in an underlying assumption that vertebrae abnormally displace. Not all clinical practitioners in orthopedic physical therapy are willing to accept the vertebral displacement supposition. Nonetheless, the possible mechanisms behind vertebral displacement include segmental instability, joint incongruence from degenerative bony changes, or significant muscle spasm. The objective, therefore, is to use spinal manipulation to correct vertebral position.

Reduction of a disc protrusion is the fourth possible mechanical effect of spinal manipulation. Considerable controversy surrounds the possible benefits of spinal manipulation for patients with known disc protrusions. Clinical evidence exists to support spinal rotary manipulation for patients with small disc protrusions (18). Reduction in the size of small disc protrusions was demonstrated on two patients with positive epidurograms after having rotational spinal manipulation. In both cases, a complete relief of symptoms occurred. OPTs who argue in favor of spinal manipulation for disc protrusions claim that the torsion stress created by the rotary manipulation exerts a tensional force on the posterior longitudinal ligament and annulus fibrosis which, in turn, applies pressure to the posterior disc contents; the torsional force developed within the spine, therefore, produces a centripetal force within the disc which reduces the bulging disc material.

Disc Protrusion

Rotary manipulation did not prove to be effective in reducing disc protrusions in a clinical study on 39 patients with known disc protrusions determined by myelogram (6). Although over half of the patients reported relief of sciatic pain within 24 hours after manipulation, none had any demonstrable change in myelographic re-examination. Significant improvement in straight leg raising was also demonstrated after manipulation. In addition, eight of ten patients with lateral spinal shifts in posture showed improvement in spinal position. Interestingly, the authors did not question the relevance of the assumed underlying pathology (disc protrusion) as determined by the myelogram. The question clearly in need of explanation is the mechanism of pain relief after rotary manipulation of the spine if the disc is not affected. Perhaps the other pain-sensitive structures within the spine need additional consideration when analyzing the etiology of back pain. Most OPTs would agree that rotary thrust manipulation is a relative contraindication for patients with large disc protrusions or herniations.

The popularity and acceptance of the extension concept among OPTs is widespread. Proponents of the extension principle theorize that the hydrodynamic balance within the intervertebral disc is disturbed after a disc derangement. The posterior annular fibers have been stretched or torn and fluid has migrated posteriorly into the weakened area. The fluid volume, therefore, has increased in the posterior compartment of the disc. Spinal manipulation which promotes backward-bending at the involved level supposedly drives the fluid anteriorly within the disc and reduces the posterior intradiscal pressure. The posterior annular fibers are relieved of the increased fluid pressure and thus, allowed to approximate and heal (20). The beneficial clinical results achieved by the use of the extension program on certain select patients cannot be argued; however, the theoretical scientific basis for the technique needs further validation.

Whether spinal manipulation is able to reduce a disc protrusion or herniation remains a question mark for most orthopedic physical therapists. If, in fact, spinal manipulation is effective in correcting a discogenic problem, one must still determine how long will the reduction last. If a disc is reduced by spinal manipulation, does the disc stay reduced permanently or is the effect only temporary? Furthermore, does the patient have a role in maintaining the correction and preventing reinjury? OPTs, as well as all physical therapists, no matter what philosophical differences exist regarding pathologic bias, share one common bond—patient responsibility. With respect to prevention of reinjury the OPT believes that spinal manipulation is a part of the entire management plan and that the ultimate responsibility in spinal health lies with the patient. As a result, patient education in the form of posture, exercise, and functional activity receives high priority.

Total management. One point that requires clear elucidation concerns the use of modalities and other manual techniques by the OPT. If a passive procedure such as spinal manipulation is to be helpful, the patient's myofascial tone should not offer resistance. Various massage and soft-tissue mobilization techniques are utilized to optimize the effects of spinal manipulation. The less resistance offered by the surrounding myofascial tissues the less force is required in manipulation. Soft-tissue mobilization and massage, therefore, are often used as preparatory or preliminary steps to spinal manipulation. One must keep in mind that the soft-tissue component is sometimes the primary condition and when so, the soft-tissue techniques are no longer preliminary, but actually corrective. The use of electrical nerve and muscle stimulation is also a common procedure among OPTs. Usually electrical stimulation is given in conjuction with moist heat or cold. Consequently, the outcome of any one physical therapy treatment cannot be evaluated by one factor alone. The possibility of multiple treatment effects causes problems in clinical research.

NEUROPHYSIOLOGIC EFFECTS

Pain. Aside from the described mechanical effects, spinal manipulation is believed to produce changes in neurophysiologic activity in tissues. With respect to pain, OPTs refer to the work of Wyke and Freeman to substantiate a scientific basis for pain relief after spinal manipulation. Through experimental study, Wyke and Freeman, have determined the existence of four types of synovial joint receptors (38). Types I, II, and III are classified as mechanoreceptors which function to convert mechanical stimuli into electrical energy. Mechanoreceptors offer positional and kinesthetic information from the respective joint structure to the central nervous system. Type IV receptors are nociceptors and are responsible for signaling pain.

According to the Gate Control Theory proposed by Melzak and Wall in 1965, mediation of incoming stimuli through afferent nerve fibers from the various body tissues, somatic and visceral, occurs in the cells of the substantia gelatinosa in laminas two and three of the spinal cord (21). Mechanoreceptor discharge has an inhibitory effect on the presynaptic cells of the substantia gelatinosa which, in turn, depresses nociceptive activity. Wyke states that the perception of pain from an irritated spinal structure is inversely related to the amount of mechanoreceptor activity from the embryologically associated spinal tissues (37). Mechanical force generated from spinal manipulation is transmitted to the affected spinal segment and may activate mechanoreceptor endings. In essence, mechanoreceptor discharge would assist in closing the gate to pain. OPTs recognize pain determination as a central summation phenomenon and a function of postsynaptic neuronal regulation as well as presynaptic influence (21).

Proprioception. An additional consideration to the OPT is the possibility of spinal manipulation affecting proprioceptive function. Capsular or ligamentous injury from overstretch, repeated trauma, disuse, and accelerated aging changes results in a loss and deactivation of mechanoreceptors. The proprioceptive role of the affected segment is adversely affected as a result (36). Spinal manipulation may help activate inactive receptors and thus, improve postural and kinesthetic awareness. Reviving inactive mechanoreceptors and restoring proprioceptive control reduces the chance of reinjury and hence is an important consideration in preventive care.

Tone. In accordance with the facilitated segment concept, a joint lesion may cause the segmentally related musculature to become hyper-responsive. According to one hypothesis, the fusimotor neuron (Gamma) discharge to the affected intrafusal muscle fibers is being sustained at high frequencies. Consequently, the intrafusal fibers are kept in a chronic shortened state and the muscle spindle becomes hypersensitive to incoming stimuli. The spindles reflexly control the tensional state of the extrafusal muscle fibers. Local muscle spasm is sometimes palpated in the area of dysfunction and reflex muscle contractions are occasionally elicited after pressure. The joint surfaces become tightly apposed and an increased resistance to motion, usually in one direction, results (14).

During spinal manipulation, the affected joint is moved and muscles about the joint are stretched. A barrage of afferent impulses is generated from the mechanical force of the manipulation which may order the central nervous system to reduce the fusimotor neuron discharge. Stretching of the muscle by spinal manipulation may also transmit tension to the tendon. The golgi tendon organs may then inhibit fusimotor neuron discharge and serve to relax both intrafusal and extrafussal fibers (14). Another possible mechanism by which spinal manipulation may normalize myofascial tone is reflex inhibition from Type III mechanoreceptors in the joint capsule (25). Apparently, the Type III mechanoreceptors have a reflex inhibitory affect on the associated musculature about the joint. Although the spinal reflex inhibitory theory is not supported by the work of Wyke, many OPTs sense palpable change in local paraspinal muscle tone after spinal manipulation.

Craniosacral Therapy Technique proponents propose another neurophysiologic effect by which spinal manipulation works. They claim that specifically directed, gentle pressures to various bones of the cranium and sacrum influence the volume of cerebrospinal fluid within the spinal canal and skull. "Redistribution" of cerebrospinal fluid is believed to have a mechanical affect in stretching tight membranes, normalizing joint mobility, and lubricating inflamed, irritable nerves or spinal tissues. Enhancing fluid flow through an involved segment may soothe and bathe hypersensitive tissue and thus decrease pain (32). Support for the craniosacral theory is demonstrated in the work by Mays (19); injection of autogenous cerebrospinal fluid into the lumbar subarachnoid space in selected postlamectomy chronic pain patients resulted in pain relief within 10 to 15 minutes and lasting about 15 minutes. Manual pressure to redirect cerebrospinal fluid is an interesting concept which is gaining popularity among OPTs.

Psychologic Effects

Treatment strategy by the OPT is determined by the objective physical findings and by the subjective report of pain described by the patient. The patient's pain behavior and description sometimes suggest a strong emotional factor in the problem. The OPT recognizes that emotional and stress-related factors contribute to pain perception and that pain is a poorly measured clinical phenomenon. Effectiveness of a manipulation approach therefore must be based on two components—objective clinical changes such as range of motion and the patient's report of pain.

The tactile nature of spinal manipulative therapy is acknowledged to have a powerful psychologic effect. OPTs attempt to provide a rational explanation for the effectiveness of spinal manipulation by mechanical and neurophysiologic mechanisms, but often they do not appreciate fully the degree to which the laying on of hands as a placebo factor contributes to pain relief. While OPTs prefer to believe that spinal manipulation is effective at least partially on a physical basis, they accept the placebo role of tactile healing.

Further reinforcement of the placebo effect of spinal manipulation is exhibited through the interest and concern of the evaluator during the examination. After having been thoroughly assessed, patients are often impressed by the expertise of the OPT. Psychologically, they experience a sense of satisfaction and relief because the condition has been closely examined, and in some cases, the pain is reduced after the evaluation alone.

In thrust manipulation, an audible sound frequently occurs. The pop or snap usually offers assurance to the patient that a correction has been made. In physical therapy, psychologic dependence on such joint sounds is not encouraged. Association of joint noise with the correction of the problem may place the OPT in a situation where the patient desires repetitive thrust manipulation, a treatment strategy not advocated.

Application of Spinal Manipulative Technique by the OPT

The criteria for successful application of spinal manipulation are presented in Table 2.3. The following section will briefly discuss each factor in relation to the actual application of spinal manipulation.

Appropriate Choice of a Technique

The choice is largely governed by the stage of the condition, the type of dysfunction, and the personality of the patient. Generally speaking, acute conditions do not respond to forceful, large-amplitude movements. Because pain relief is often the objective in acute conditions, many OPTs select a graded oscillation technique of small amplitude to stimulate mechanoreceptors. Chronic conditions may need a stretch or progressive stretch manipulation to improve joint motion.

A joint dysfunction with a considerable myofascial component may respond to a muscle energy technique because of the active muscle contraction required in the technique. An adhesive joint condition which has a rather abrupt end feel to passive motion may be receptive to a thrust manipulation which breaks the adhesion. Technique selection is also determined by the psychologic set of the patient. A frightened, anxious, somewhat timid

Table 2.3
Criteria for Manipulation Technique

Appropriate choice of technique

Rationale for chosen technique

Appropriate sequencing of techniques

Appropriate adjustments of technique

Appropriate time length

Evaluation of effects of technique

Technique criteria
    Patient position
    Therapist position
    Specificity of locking
    Hand placement
    Recruitment of tissue (force velocity or development)
    Sensitivity to tissue response
    Force direction
    Force control
    Amount of force
    Force amplitude

---

individual is likely to respond to gentle manipulative therapy and not to an aggressive approach. In fact, a corrective release of a joint fixation by thrust manipulation sometimes may lead to an increase in pain because of the resultant anxiety and muscle tension produced by a panicky patient.

RATIONALE

Establishing rationale for the use of a particular manipulative technique is important in clarifying its objective. For example, is the technique principally being used for the mechanical, neurophysiologic, or psychologic effects? The answer to this question undoubtedly assists in the appropriate selection of the technique.

Sequencing

A treatment plan may entail a series of manipulative procedures. How one sequences the treatment may affect the outcome. A facilitated segment may respond favorably to 20 minutes of soft-tissue mobilization followed by a specific nonthrust continuous-stretch manipulation. The hyperexcitable tissues are relaxed by the soft-tissue work and the joint irritability is lessened. The use of a nonthrust continuous-stretch manipulation allows instantaneous sensory feedback regarding tissue response and is less likely to result in additional facilitation. Conversely, a progressive stretch manipulation performed without reducing the tone of the hypersensitive tissues is likely to create further irritation because of the spring-like nature of the technique.

ADJUSTMENT OF TECHNIQUES

The ability of an OPT to adjust manipulative techniques during a treatment or during a series of sessions is dependent upon experience and expertise. Knowledge of various techniques is important in allowing flexibility in approach. Skill and proficiency in many techniques is necessary in order to substitute one manipulation for another when the condition warrants. No substitution exists for the long, hard hours required to become a skilled and adaptable manipulator. Some OPTs are extremely talented in the application of certain techniques but have obvious shortcomings in other techniques. A truly talented OPT is skilled in all manipulative approaches.

TIME AND EVALUATION

Probably the most difficult aspect of manipulation to analyze is length of time necessary to achieve the desired result. Clearly, if the sole intention of manipulation is to relieve pain, the OPT relies on the testimony of the patient during and after application of the technique. The problem evolves from the assumed mechanical effects. How long does one apply a nonthrust continuous stretch manipulation? How many repetitions of a nonthrust progressive stretch manipulation are essential in increasing range of motion? No scientific answer exists. The OPT must rely on palpation and observational skills. If one feels the resistance to stretch decrease as one applies a particular manipulation technique and a sense of ease in the motion one is satisfied that the technique is successful. Some OPTs verify palpable findings by repeating active and passive motion tests. Increased range of motion, as determined by passive intervertebral motion testing or active movement analysis after spinal manipulation is a sign of the effectiveness of the technique.

If the primary intention of a manipulation is to affect the visco-elastic properties of the periarticular soft-tissue structures, sustained pressures are advisable. The viscous nature of the ground substance within connective tissue requires time for permanent change to occur. The valid amount of time is not substantially established; however, one study of the effectiveness of low-load, prolonged stretches on knee joint contractures successfully used one-minute stretches with 15-second rests for 15 minutes (16). Any less time is likely to affect only the elastic property of the tissue, which then returns to the original shape or configuration.

TECHNIQUE CRITERIA

The specific criteria for the manipulation technique is also provided in Table 2.3. Correct body position of both patient and therapist is essential in promoting relaxation and technique safety. Whenever possible, the specificity concept should be adhered to. Fixating areas of the spine which do not require manipulation helps to protect against creating a segmental instability.

Hand placement is essential in obtaining the desired objective and in promoting comfort during the application of the technique. The hand and wrist making direct contact on the involved area needs to be relaxed. Force is generated from the entire body and arm and not from tension in the hand. The way in which one places the hand often determines how the force is transmitted to the spinal segment.

The OPT tries to recruit tissues sequentially from the superficial to the deep by appropriate force development and speed. The rate at which force is developed is a function of the response of the tissues. The OPT must be sensitive to the reaction of the surrounding soft-tissue layers. Palpable detection of a reflex muscle contraction prohibits further stretch or pressure.

The direction of force is decided upon when the manipulative technique is chosen. Direct manipulation moves into the motion barrier while indirect technique moves away from the motion barrier. Aside from the spring-type manipulative techniques, the OPT uses smooth, controlled forces which are applied at low, even rates. The patient feels comfortable and has a sense of control over the procedure. Force development and control are essential elements in force dissipation.

The amount of force varies according to sex, age, stage of the condition, general health of the patient, type of dysfunction, degree of the dysfunction, and the manipulative style of the OPT. The greater the force used, the greater the chance of an adverse reaction. The philosophy concerning force amount may be best summarized by: the skill of a manipulator is inversely proportional to the amount of force used in the technique. Advocates of this philosophy use as much force as is required, but as little as necessary. Physical therapists agree that a natural, safe, physiologic tissue change occurs when the body is subjected to a slowly applied, gentle force as opposed to a strongly applied, quick force.

The amplitude of the force is often a function of the stage of the condition as well as the degree of the dysfunction. A chronic, stiff joint needs frequent and repetitive motion throughout the entire available range once movement is restored. Active exercise and passive movement both play a part in maintaining joint range in chronic conditions because of the degree of the restriction.

Conclusion

Physical therapy practice has made substantial changes in recent years and its nature has become well delineated. The scope has widened and as a result, clinical specialization became unavoidable. The role of the orthopedic physical therapist (OPT) has been defined and the relationship of the OPT to other medical disciplines presented in this chapter. The rationale for the use of spinal manipulation was provided and theoretical explanations were offered. Finally, the criteria for successful application of spinal manipulation technique were identified and discussed. We recognize the danger of trying to generalize for a large population of individual therapists, but we believe that the chapter provides some clarification of the role of the OPT and spinal manipulation.

REFERENCES

1. Akeson, W. H., Amiel, D., Mechanic, G. L., et al. Collagen cross linking alterations in joint contractures: Changes in the reducible cross links in periarticular connective tissue collagen after nine weeks of immobilization. *Connect. Tissue Res.*, 5:15. 1088.
2. Akeson, W. H., Amiel, D., Woo, S. L-Y. Immobility effects of synovial joints: The pathomechanics of joint contracture. *Biorheology*, 17:95, 1980.
3. Betsch, D. F., and Baer, E. Third International Congress of Biorheology Symposium on Soft Tissues Around a Diarthrodial Joint. *Biorheology*, 17:83, 1980.
4. Bowles, C. H. Functional technique: A modern perspective. *J. Amer. Osteop. Assoc,.* 80:326, 1981.
5. Brandt, B., and Jones, L. H. Some methods of applying counterstrain. *J. Amer. Osteop. Assoc.*, 75:786, 1976.
6. Chrisman, O. D., Mittnacht, A., and Snook, G. A. A study of the results following rotary manipulation in the lumbar intervertebral-disc syndrome. *J. Bone Joint Surg.*, 46-A:517, 1964.
7. *Dorland's Illustrated Medical Dictionary*, 25th Edition. W. B. Saunders, Philadelphia, 1974.
8. Enneking, W., and Horowitz, M. The intra-articular effects of immobilization on the

human knee. *J. Bone Joint Surg.*, *42-A:*973, 1980.

9. Gonnella, C., Paris, S. V., and Kutner, M. Reliability in evaluating passive intervertebral motion. *Phys. Ther.*, *62:*436, 1982.

10. Goodridge, J. P. Muscle energy technique: Definition, explanation, methods of procedure. *J. Amer. Osteop. Assoc.*, *81:*249, 1981.

11. Grieve, G. P. *Mobilization of the Spine*, Third Edition. Churchill Livingstone, Edinburgh London and New York, 1979.

12. Heilig, D. The thrust technique. *J. Amer. Osteop. Assoc.*, *81:*244, 1981.

13. Klapper, R. E. Direct action techniques. *J. Amer. Osteop. Assoc.*, *81:*239, 1981.

14. Korr, I. M. Proprioceptors and the behavior of lesioned segments. In: *Osteopathic Medicine—Clinical Review Series*. Edited by Stark. E. I., pp. 183–200.

15. Korr, I. M. Symposium on the functional implications of segmental facilitation—research report, I. The concept of facilitation and its origins. *J. Amer. Osteop. Assoc.*, *54:*265, 1955.

16. Light, K. E., Nuzik, S., Personius, W., et al. Low load prolonged stretch vs high-load brief stretch in treating knee contractures. *Phys. Ther.*, *64:*330, 1984.

17. Maitland, G. D. *Vertebral Manipulation*, Third Edition. London, Butterworths, 1973.

18. Matthews, J. A., and Yates, D. A. H. Reduction of lumbar disc prolapse by manipulation. *Br. Med. J.*, *20:*696, 1969.

19. Mays, K. S., et al. Relief of postlaminectomy syndrome in selected patients by injection of autogenous cerebrospinal fluid. *Spine*, *6:*274, 1981.

20. McKenzie, R. A. *The Lumbar Spine—Mechanical Diagnosis and Therapy*, Spinal Publication, Aukland, New Zealand, 1981.

21. Melzack, R., and Wall, P. D. Pain mechanisms: A new theory, *Science*, *150:*971, 1965.

22. Membership statistics. *Phys. Ther.*, *63:*1816, 1983.

23. Minutes, Business Meeting of the Orthopaedic Section. *J. Orthop. Sports Phys. Ther.*, *3:*89, 1981.

24. Mitchell, F. L., Moran, P. S., and Pruzzo, N. A. *An Evaluation and Treatment Manual of Osteopathic Muscle Energy Technique.* Mitchell, Moran and Pruzzo Associates, 1979.

25. Paris, S. V. Mobilization of the spine. *Phys. Ther.*, *59:*988, 1979.

26. Paris, S. V. Spinal Course Notes. Unpublished Information.

27. *Stedman's Medical Dictionary*, 21st Edition. Williams & Wilkins, Baltimore, 1970.

28. Sternbach, R. A. Psychophysiology of pain. *Intern. J. Psychiat. Med.*, *6:*63, 1975.

29. Stoddard, A. *Manual of Osteopathic Technique*, Eighth Edition. London, 1974.

30. Task Force Report. Certification of Advanced Clinical Competence will come before 1978 House, Bulletin of the Orthopedic Section, APTA, Vol. 3, No. 2, Summer 1978, pps 6–7.

31. Taylor, T. F. K. Editorial. The laying on of hands. *Aust. N.Z.J. Med.*, *8:*587, 1978.

32. Upledger, J. E., and Vredevoogd, J. D. *Craniosacral Therapy*, Eastland Press, Chicago, 1983.

33. Vogel, E. E. The beginning of "modern physiotherapy." *Phys. Ther.*, *56:*15, 1976.

34. White, A. A. III, and Panjabi, M. M. The basic kinematics of the human spine. A review of past and current knowledge. *Spine*, *3:*12, 1978.

35. Woo, S. L-Y, Matthews, J. V., Akeson, W. H., et al. Connective tissue response to immobility. *Arthritis Rheumatism*, *18:*257, 1975.

36. Wyke, B. Conference on the aging brain, cervical articular contributions to posture and gait: Their relation to senile disequilibrium. *Age Ageing*, *8:*251, 1979.

37. Wyke, B. Neurological aspects of low back pain. In: *The Lumbar Spine and Back Pain.* Edited by Jayson, M., Grune & Stratton, Inc., New York, 1976.

38. Wyke, B. The neurology of joints. *Ann. Roy. Coll. Surg. Engl.*, *41:*25, 1967.

3

Functional Anatomy of the Spine and Associated Structures[1]

JOHN V. BASMAJIAN

Vertebral Column

VERTEBRAL BODIES AND INTERVERTEBRAL DISCS

Each vertebral *body* is a short, cylindrical block of bone flattened at the back and possessing a slight "waist." Many vertical lamellae of spongy bone in its interior enable it to resist compression; its outer covering of compact bone is very thin. Adjacent bodies are firmly united to one another by an *intervertebral disc* roughly one-fifth to one-third as thick as the neighboring bodies. This disc is composed of concentric rings of fibrocartilage and a central mass of pulpy tissue, the *nucleus pulposus*, which represents the remains of the notochord. The disc, being under pressure, bulges, i.e., it is convex at its periphery. Discs are "shock absorbers" giving resilience to the column, and they are relieved of pressure only when the body is recumbent. Being the nonrigid portion of the column, they also give it its flexibility. When the body is erect and in the "normal" position, the various parts of each disc are under uniform pressure, but when the vertebral column is flexed, extended, or bent sideways, one part of a disc is under increased compression whereas another part of the same disc is under tension.

An *anterior* and a *posterior longitudinal ligament* extend the length of the column, one down the fronts, the other down the backs of the vertebral bodies; they are firmly attached to the discs (which they reinforce) and they guard against excessive movement of the flexible column.

---

[1] The illustrations for this chapter are reproduced with permission of the publishers (Williams & Wilkins, also publishers of this book) from *Primary Anatomy*, 8th edition, by J. V. Basmajian, 1982.

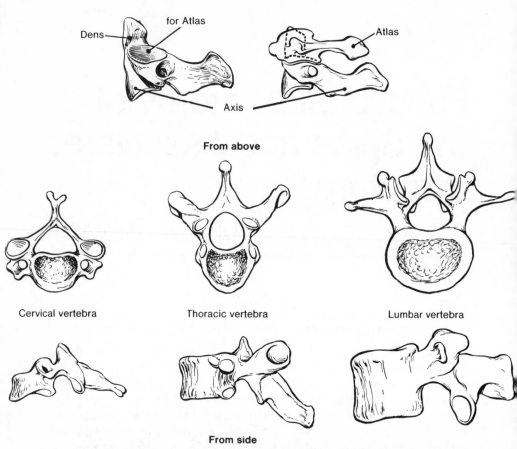

Figure 3.1. Cervical, thoracic, and lumbar vertebrae (from Basmajian [2]).

VERTEBRAL ARCHES

A vertebral arch springs from the upper part of the back of its vertebral body (Fig. 3.1) and each half is made up of two parts: (a) a very short rounded bar projecting backward from the body and known as the *pedicle*; and (b) an oblong plate with sloping surfaces known as the *lamina*. The lamina is continuous with the pedicle and meets its fellow of the opposite side in the midline. The hole thus framed in behind each vertebral body is the *vertebral foramen*; the succession of foramina makes up the *vertebral canal* in which the spinal cord and its coverings reside.

A typical vertebra begins to ossify before birth from three centers of ossification; these ultimately unite to form the adult bone (Fig. 3.2).

PROCESSES

At the angular junction of pedicle and lamina on each side there are three processes, one upward (superior), one downward (inferior), and one lateral-

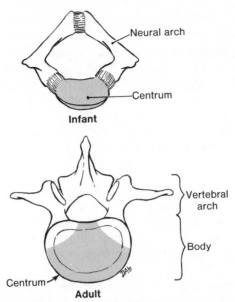

Figure 3.2. Three centers of ossification joined by cartilage form the vertebra in infant. These unite to form an adult vertebra, but the "body" is not the same as the centrum, nor the "vertebral" arch the same as the neural arch (from Basmajian [2]).

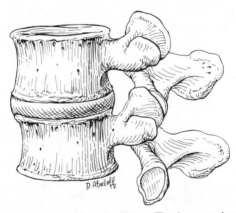

Figure 3.3. Two lumbar vertebrae in articulation. The lower pair of processes grasps the upper and prevents rotation. Note the boundaries of the intervertebral foramen, the exit for a spinal nerve (from Basmajian [2]).

ward (transverse). The *superior* and *inferior processes* meet and form joints with similar processes from adjacent vertebral arches; their chief function is to prevent undesirable movements between adjoining vertebrae (Fig. 3.3). The *transverse process* is chiefly for attachments of muscles although in the thoracic region a rib abuts against the transverse process and is steadied by it.

Where the two laminae meet in the midline posteriorly, there projects backward a *spinous process* which is for attachment of muscles.

Because a vertebral arch springs from the upper part of its vertebral body, a deep notch is visible below the pedicle when the vertebra is viewed from the side. When two adjacent vertebrae are in position, the notch becomes a hole—the *intervertebral foramen*—which gives exit and entrance to spinal nerves and vessels (Fig. 3.3). The intervertebral foramen is bounded above and below by pedicles; it is bounded in front and behind by joints (intervertebral disc and bodies in front, articular processes behind).

SACRUM

Five vertebral bodies, united by four ossified intervertebral discs, are easily distinguishable on the concave anterior surface of the curved triangular bone that comprises the sacrum. The body of the first of these vertebrae has a prominent, oval, upper surface with a distinctly forward slope. To it is attached a thick disc that unites it to the body of the fifth lumbar vertebra.

Two parallel rows of four pelvic (anterior) *sacral foramina*, in line with intervertebral foramina above, serve to separate the sacral vertebral bodies from the parts of the bone lateral to these openings and known as the *lateral masses* (Fig. 3.4). The thick upper part of each lateral mass, smooth above and in front where it is continuous with the side of the first sacral vertebral body, is called the *ala* of the sacrum. On the side of each ala are two areas. In front is a large ear-shaped area by means of which the sacrum articulates with the hip bone on each side. This area is called the *auricular surface* and

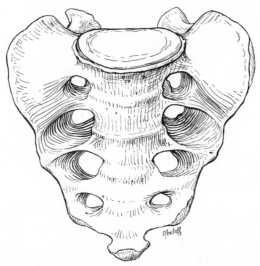

Figure 3.4. Sacrum from front (from Basmajian [2]).

the articulation is the *synovial sacroiliac joint*. Above it (when the bone is correctly oriented) is an equally large rough area known as the *tuberosity*; it is for a mass of strong, short ligaments that further unite the pelvic girdle to the sacrum and that constitute the *fibrous sacroiliac joint*. Below the level of the auricular surface the whole sacrum tapers rapidly since the lower part of the bone bears no weight.

Behind, the bone is convex and much rougher; here the two rows of *dorsal sacral foramina* (in the same vertical plane as the anterior ones) serve to separate the laminae, which are all fused together, from the lateral mass on each side (Fig. 3.5).

At the upper end of the bone, there projects a pair of large superior articular processes that face one another and embrace the inferior ones of the fifth lumbar vertebra. The triangular upper opening of the sacral canal lies between them and is bounded behind by the paired laminae.

An irregular vertical ridge down the back of the lateral mass of each side represents transverse processes, while a similar ridge medial to the dorsal foramina represents articular processes. Four bony tubercles in the midline represent spinous processes.

At the lower end of the bone, there is a pair of small processes, the *sacral*

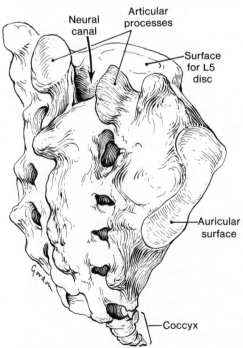

Figure 3.5. Sacrum and coccyx viewed obliquely from behind and right side (from Basmajian [2]).

cornua (horns). Between them is the lower end of the vertebral canal which is closed in life by a tough fibrous membrane.

The extent to which the vertebral (sacral) canal is closed by bone in the lower half of the sacrum is very variable; in other words, the lowest vertebral arches are frequently incomplete or absent.

COCCYX

The irregular coccyx (Fig. 3.5) consists usually of four fused vestigial vertebrae, the first of which is by far the largest. The body of this first coccygeal vertebra is united to the lower end of the sacrum by a fibrocartilaginous intervertebral disc; the vertebral arch is represented by two upwardly projecting horns or *cornua* which meet those of the sacrum. Below this vertebra the bone is nodular and represents the vestigial human tail. It can be felt quite easily in the living person.

Functions and Differences in the Vertebral Column

WEIGHT-BEARING AND SIZE OF BODIES

Weight borne by individual vertebrae increases progressively as the series is descended; vertebral bodies, in consequence, become more massive as they proceed from the cervical to the lumbar region; discs must increase in size in conformity with the bones (Fig. 3.6). (These statements are true only in animals that walk erect; the general tendency among quadrupeds is for vertebrae actually to decrease in size as the column is "descended.")

MOVEMENTS

Movements between individual vertebrae take place (a) at the discs, and (b) at the joints between the (paired) articular processes of the vertebral arches. Movements at the discs are greatest where the discs are thickest; movements at articular processes are greatest where the joint surfaces are largest.

In the lumbar region, both of the above conditions exist and here movements are freest. In these lumbar movements, lumbar discs accept considerable strain. If to the normal lumbar movements of flexion, extension, and side-bending, rotary movements were added, the resulting torsion of the discs might be more than they could stand. For this and other reasons, the dispositions of the joints between lumbar articular processes restrict rotation (Fig. 3.3). These joints are "interlocking," i.e., the superior articular processes of the vertebra below grip the outsides of the inferior articular proceses of the vertebra above. In this region, bending forward and backward can be freely performed; sideways bending is much less free and rotation is severely limited. Even with this safeguard, lumbar discs rupture more readily than any others.

In the thoracic region, the discs are relatively thin, the opposing surfaces

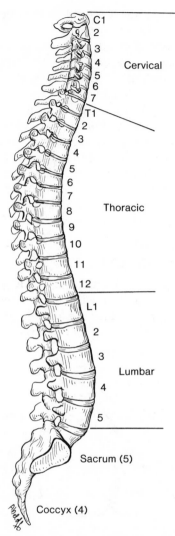

Figure 3.6. Vertebral column from right side. Note intervertebral discs between bodies (from Basmajian [2]).

of the articular processes on the vertebral arches are small and flat and face backward and forward; no type of movement is entirely prohibited, yet movements in all planes are slight. Nevertheless, because there are 12 vertebrae in this region, the total mobility between the first and the last is considerably greater than might be thought. The transition from the more mobile lumbar vertebrae to the less mobile thoracic vertebrae is unfortunately rather abrupt, and it is the 11th or the 12th thoracic vertebra that is most commonly fractured.

In the cervical region, the discs are relatively thicker than those in the thoracic region, and the articular surfaces of the processes—facing at first upward and downward but gradually changing to a forward and backward direction—are small but relatively larger also. Thus, the seven cervical vertebrae permit movement in all planes as do the thoracic ones, but the range is considerably greater. In addition to their rather free movements of flexion, extension, and side-bending, the cervical vertebrae engage in movements of rotation (twisting or torsion). But it has been observed that such a combination of movements throws excessive strain on the discs. Perhaps this accounts for why the periphery of the upper surface of a typical cervical vertebral body is built up markedly at the sides and slightly at the back; it slopes away in front (Fig. 3.7).

The first and second cervical vertebrae are very specially modified, for they carry the skull and aid in its movements. They will be discussed separately, below.

VERTEBRAL FORAMINA

The caliber of the spinal cord varies very little from end to end, but it has two local enlargements associated with the sites of origin of the great nerves destined for the upper and for the lower limbs; these are the cervical

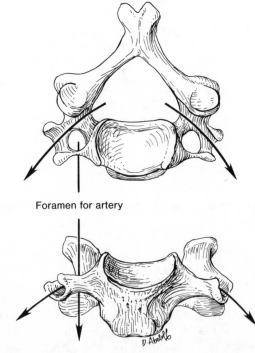

Foramen for artery

Figure 3.7. A cervical vertebra from above and from in front (see text). *Curved arrows* lie in gutters for spinal nerves (from Basmajian [2]).

and the lumbar enlargements. With these facts in mind it is easy to understand why it is that: (a) the vertebral foramina are relatively and actually large in the cervical region, where they are also triangular; (b) they are small and circular in the thoracic region; (c) they are actually, but not relatively, large in the lumbar region where, again, they are triangular.

TRANSVERSE PROCESSES AND JOINTS FOR RIBS

A very special feature distinguishes the thoracic vertebrae: they carry the ribs. The head of a rib meets the vertebral column at the side of a disc and at the adjacent edges of two vertebral bodies. In its excursion around the trunk, the rib at first sweeps backward to abut against the front of the tip of a transverse process. The presence, therefore, of little joint surfaces, the one on the body and the other on the transverse process, proclaims a vertebrae to be rib-bearing and thoracic.

A special feature distinguishes cervical vertebrae also. Each transverse process has a hole or foramen in it, the bar of bone in front of the foramen being, in effect, an undeveloped rib (Fig. 3.7). This "rib" is in line with the true ribs in the thoracic region, so that the foramen obviously is the space between the rib and the transverse process in the thorax. Through the series of foramina, vessels (vertebral artery and vein) thread their way upward to aid ultimately in the blood supply of the brain. Lateral to the foramen, the issuing spinal nerve rests in a bony gutter formed by the two elements of the compound transverse process.

Sometimes one of the normally undeveloped ribs (usually the seventh) becomes greatly enlarged and like a true rib—a "cervical rib," which may cause symptoms.

SPINOUS PROCESSES

The "spines" are anchors and levers. They are distinctive for each region: cervical ones have double tips, i.e., they are bifid; thoracic ones are long, slender, pointed, and tend to project more downward than backward; lumbar ones are massive, square-cut, and project straight backward.

CURVES OF THE VERTEBRAL COLUMN

During intrauterine life, the body of the fetus is noticeably flexed, and this applies to the vertebral column as well as to the other structures. Soon, two primary curves, both with their concavities forward, are recognizable, one involving the presacral vertebrae, the other the sacrum itself.

In a structure such as the vertebral column, which is built up of superimposed bodies and discs, these curves must be expressions of differences in thickness between the fronts and the backs of the individual bodies and discs. Furthermore, when it is the bones (bodies) that are chiefly concerned, the curve is likely to be permanent; when the discs also or alone are concerned, the resulting curve can be temporarily abolished.

The two permanent or primary curves persist as thoracic and sacral (pelvic). The *secondary curves* develop in the cervical and lumbar regions, and there the relatively thick discs that these regions possess take a considerable part. These secondary curves are convex forward and are subject to temporary elimination. The cervical curve would seem to develop in response to the need for holding the head up. The lumbar curve develops so that the center of gravity of the body will not lie in a plane in front of the hip joints during the sitting or standing positions.

Where the last lumbar vertebra (fifth) meets the sacrum there is an abrupt change; this is provided for by the last lumbar vertebral body and especially the last lumbar disc being much thicker in front than behind, i.e., they are wedge-shaped. Occasionally, an accident occurs here and the lumbar body (fourth and fifth) slips forward—spondylolisthesis; the accident is said to be due to a developmental failure of the neural arch to be fixed to its body, but because the separation is rarely (if ever) at the site of union of arch and body, it seems more probable that it is due to a bilateral fracture of the arch. The fifth lumbar vertebra is often "sacralized" (bodies united by bone) in older persons.

The normal curvatures of the column are rather more pronounced in the female than in the male, and in both sexes there is usually a slight lateral curvature to one side said to be associated with right- or left-handedness. An excessive lateral curvature is known as scoliosis.

Atlas and Axis

The first cervical vertebra, the atlas, has lost its body and consists simply of a ring of bone made up of two *lateral masses* joined in front and behind by the *anterior* and *posterior arches of the atlas* (Fig. 3.8). The upper surface of each lateral mass is elliptical, concave, and articular. The long axis of the ellipse runs mainly anteroposteriorly, but the two ellipses are so placed that they are nearer one another in front than behind, i.e., the anterior arch is shorter than the posterior. On the concave surfaces of the lateral masses, the occipital condyles rock and slide in the nodding movement of "Yes." The lower surface of each lateral mass is circular, flat, and articular and rests on a similar surface of the axis.

Lateral to each lateral mass is the very large and widely set transverse process, containing the foramen previously noted as transmitting the vertebral vessels. This process projects so far laterally that it may be felt on deep pressure behind the mandible just below the ear.

Medial to each lateral mass and encroaching somewhat on the anterior part of the very large vertebral foramen, there is a pronounced tubercle to which is attached the very strong *transverse ligament of the atlas* stretching to the tubercle on the other side. The vertebral foramen is divided by this ligament into a smaller anterior compartment and a larger posterior one.

The second cervical vertebra, appropriately named the axis, is distinguished by a blunt, tooth-like process, the *dens* or odontoid process, pro-

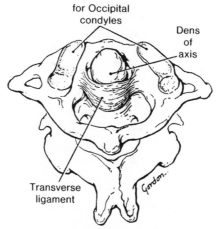

Figure 3.8. Atlas and axis in articulation viewed from behind and above (from Basmajian [2]).

jecting upward from the body (Figs. 3.1 and 3.8). It is in reality the body of the atlas which has become divorced from the atlas and has joined the body of the axis. This dens projects upward into the anterior compartment of the vertebral foramen of the atlas and provides a mechanism, consisting of a pivot and a collar, whereby the head and atlas can rotate around the dens in the "No" movement. On each side of the dense is a large, flat, and circular joint surface for the support and rotation of the atlas.

The *foramen magnum* in the midline of the base of the skull lies halfway between the posterior edge of the palate and the inion. Its outline is made rather pear-shaped by the encroachment of the paired *occipital condyles* on the sides of its anterior half. These oval lumps of bone have a smooth inferior surface which is convex from front to back and give the impression of a pair of rockers from a rocking chair. They rest in concavities on the upper surface of the first cervical vertebra and by sliding back and forth produce much of the nodding motion of the head signifying "Yes."

Joints of the Vertebral Column

Two series of joints unite the individual vertebrae of the spinal column: (a) the fibrocartilaginous joints (synchondroses) uniting adjacent bodies; and (b) the synovial joints uniting adjacent vertebral arches. Because synchondroses are functionally more limited in their movements than synovial joints, it follows that the extent of movement enjoyed by the joints of the vertebral arches is primarily determined by the extent of movement permitted at the discs (Fig. 3.9).

SPECIAL LIGAMENTS

The *anterior* and *posterior longitudinal ligaments*, binding the fronts and the backs of the vertebral bodies to one another throughout the length of

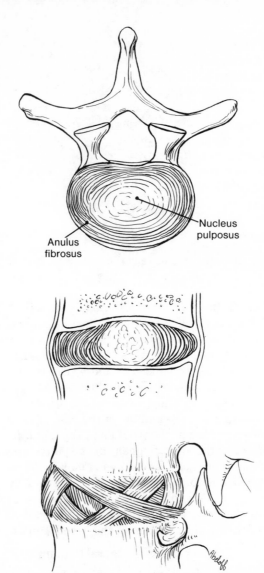

Figure 3.9. Cross-section and vertical cut surface of a lumbar intervertebral disc and a dissection of outer obliquely crossing fibers of annulus fibrosus (from Basmajian [2]).

the column have been noted earlier. The vertebral arches possess restraining ligaments also. One group consists of the *ligamenta flava*—so called because they are rich in yellow elastic fibers—and they stretch between the adjacent laminae of the vertebral arches; being elastic these ligaments tend to restore the spinal column to a neutral position after it has been flexed. They also serve, with the laminae, to cover in the spinal cord posteriorly and so protect the contained spinal cord. A second group unites adjacent spinous processes as *interspinous ligaments*. Contiguous with these posteriorly are longer fibers which stretch the length of several spines and are, in consequence, *supraspinous ligaments*. These have the same effect as the ligamenta flava. Undoubtedly, they relieve the back muscles of considerable work.

In the neck, the supraspinous ligaments are so enlarged as to produce a midline ligamentous partition separating the thick muscles of one side of the back of the neck from those of the other. It is known as the *ligamentum nuchae* (L. = of neck).

Joints of the Ribs

Synovial joints occur at the heads and the tubercles of the ribs (Fig. 3.10). The capsule of each is thickened in front and is known as a *radiate ligament* because it fans from the rib head (or costal cartilage) to the adjacent

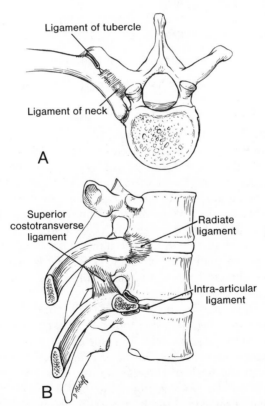

Figure 3.10. Joints and ligaments between ribs and vertebrae A, from above; B, from side (from Basmajian [2]).

vertebral bodies and disc (or sternum). In the interior of each joint is an *intra-articular* ligament that binds the head (or costal cartilage) to the disc (or sternum) and divides the cavity into upper and lower compartments.

The synovial joint at the rib tubercle occurs where the rib, in its backward sweep, abuts against the transverse process of the vertebra with which it numerically corresponds. Each small joint is reinforced, and the rib more firmly bound to the transverse process, by two ligaments, one on each side of the joint. The strong medial one is simply called the *costotransverse ligament* (or *ligament of the neck*); it lies horizontally disposed and it fills the space between the back of the neck of rib and front of the adjacent transverse process of the vertebra. The lateral one is the *lateral costotransverse ligament* (or *ligament of the tubercle*); it is a short but strong cord that passes horizontally lateralward from the tip of the transverse process to the back of the rib just beyond the tubercle. A third and rectangular ligament stretches vertically from the neck of the rib to the transverse process next above. It often produces a flange on the neck of the rib and is known as the *superior costotransverse ligament*.

The heads of ribs, 1, 11, and 12 reach the spinal column not at the side of a disc but at the side of vertebral bodies 1, 11, and 12.

Muscles of Axial Skeleton

MUSCLES OF THE VERTEBRAL COLUMN

Dorsal or Posterior

When the muscles of the upper limb girdle (Fig. 3.11) are removed from the back, the underlying intrinsic muscles are seen to occupy a pair of broad gutters situated one on each side of the vertebral spines and extending laterally as far as the angles of the ribs, the transverse processes of the cervical vertebrae, and the mastoid process. The territory is limited above by the under, horizontal surface of the occipital bone at the back of the head; below it is limited by the back of the sacrum and by the posterior spines of the iliac crests which project somewhat behind the sacrum. The muscles are covered behind by a tough sheet of fascia coextensive with them, and when this is removed the paired muscular columns are exposed (see Figs. 3.12–3.15).

Here, there are scores of muscles or muscle bundles, but they can be organized into more or less definite groups. First of all, the mass of intrinsic muscles is divided into a superficial and a deep group.

Erector spinae is the name for the *superficial group*. It arises by a strong aponeurosis from the back of the sacrum and adjacent parts of the iliac crest as a single muscle. As the fibers mount the vertebral column, they extend over several segments and in general divide into three columns: (a) a lateral one inserted into (and helping to form) the posterior angles of the

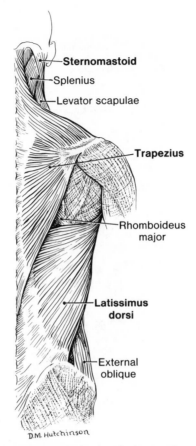

D.M. Hutchinson

Figure 3.11. These large upper limb muscles (extrinsic muscles of back) cover intrinsic muscles of back (from Basmajian [2]).

ribs and, after many overlapping relays of muscle bundles, reaching the cervical transverse processes—*iliocostalis*; (b) a middle column inserting into thoracic transverse processes and, after similar relays on cervical transverse processes, reaching the mastoid process—*longissimus* (L. = longest, see Figs. 3.13, 3.14, 3.16). (c) Confined to the thoracic region is a small column lying medial to the above-named ones and alongside the tips of the spinous processes to which it attaches—*spinalis*.

The *deep group*, collectively named the *transversospinalis*, lies deep to longissimus along most of the length of the vertebral column. In reality, it consists of a multitude of small muscles in (two or) three layers, whose fibers all run obliquely from the region of transverse processes to the region of spinous processes. Naturally, the muscles of the deepest layer—*rotatores*—have the shortest span, running from one lamina to the next. The

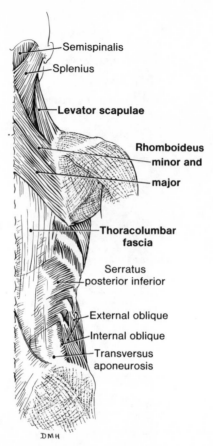

Figure 3.12. Next layer of extrinsic muscles of back. Intrinsic muscles partly revealed (from Basmajian [2]).

most superficial layer, *semispinalis*, is not found below the thoracic region; its bundles have the longest spans (three to six vertebrae), and the upper ones reach the occipital bone. Between these two is a fleshy muscle, *multifidus*, which begins below from the sacrum (deep to the aponeurosis of erector spinae) and, by short relays (two to three vertebrae), it finally reaches the first cervical spinous process (see Fig. 3.15).

Until now we have ignored three superficial muscles, each of which partly covers the large mass of muscle described above: (a) *splenius*, (b) *serratus posterior superior*, and (c) *serratus posterior inferior* (Fig. 3.13). (a) is described below; (b) and (c) are muscles of the thorax.

Muscles at Back of Neck. Just below the skull, several massive muscles fill in the back of the neck where they are separated from their fellows of

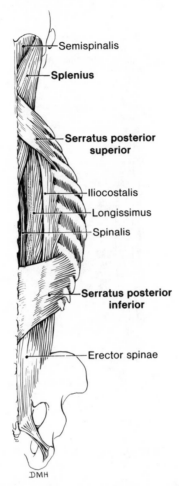

Figure 3.13. Erector spinae and its immediate relations (from Basmajian [2]).

the opposite side by the *ligamentum nuchae*, already described. The two most important are the *splenius* (L. = a bandage) (Figs. 3.13, 3.15) and the *semispinalis capitis* (Fig. 3.14). They arise from lower cervical and upper thoracic vertebral arches and are inserted on the skull, the splenius running obliquely to the mastoid process and adjacent occipital bone, the semispinalis running vertically to the occipital bone and, with its fellow, covering deeper and smaller muscles now to be noted.

Muscles of Suboccipital Region (Fig. 3.16). On each side, they are:

1. Obliquus capitis inferior (inferior oblique)—running almost horizontally lateralward from the spine of the axis to the transverse process of the atlas.

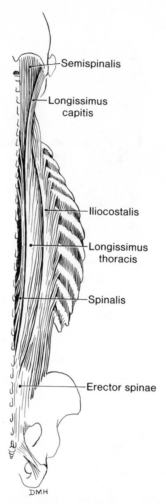

Figure 3.14. Superficial layer of erector spinae splitting into its three columns of muscles as it ascends (from Basmajian [2]).

2. Obliquus capitis superior (superior oblique)—running almost horizontally backward (in the sagittal plane) form the transverse process of the atlas to the occipital bone.
3. Rectus capitis posterior major—running upward and backward from the spine of the axis to the occipital bone.
4. Rectus capitis posterior minor—insignificant, lying deep and medial to 3, and running from the "spine" (posterior tubercle) of the atlas to the occipital bone.

The first three form a triangle (suboccipital triangle).

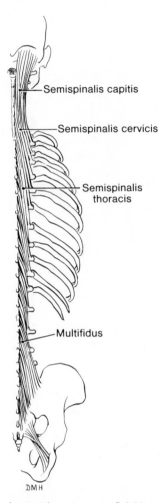

DMH

Figure 3.15. Oblique muscle layers deep to superficial layer. (Rotatores, the deepest layer, not seen.) (From Basmajian [2]).

Nerve Supply. All of the intrinsic muscles of the back are supplied by posterior branches of the spinal nerves which issue in series from the intervertebral foramina.

Ventral or Anterior Vertebral Muscles

The muscles on the fronts of the vertebral bodies are found only in the neck and in the lumbar region.

On each side of the midline a flat muscle known as the *longus cervicis* clings to the fronts of the bodies of the cervical and upper three thoracic

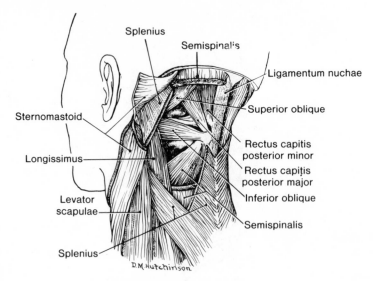

Figure 3.16. Dissection of suboccipital region of the left side (from Basmajian [2]).

vertebrae; it runs in relays to the atlas (Fig. 3.17). Lateral to the upper part of the longus cervicis another muscle, the *longus capitis*, runs from the cervical transverse processes to the occipital bone in front of the foramen magnum. Uniting the anterior arch of the atlas to the occipital bone directly above is a pair of short quadrangular muscles on each side, the medial one being the *rectus capitis anterior*, the lateral one, the *rectus capitis lateralis*.

In the lumbar region a powerful muscle, the *psoas major* arises from the sides of the lumbar vertebrae and is inserted on the femur. It is a composite muscle much more concerned with femoral movements than with vertebral, as proved by electromyographic studies (1).

Nerve Supply. The ventral muscles all are supplied by the anterior branches (rami) of the spinal nerves in their vicinity.

Actions and Functions of Muscles of Back

It is obvious that the dorsal muscles extend or straighten the column and that their unilateral actions assist in bending the column to the same side (1).

The *multifidus* and other oblique muscles associated with it are concerned with local movements of the vertebral column, e.g., rotary movements (twisting) of groups of vertebrae. The *splenius and semispinalis capitis* extend the head and, if contracting without their fellows of the opposite side, turn the head, tilting the chin up and to the same side. The ventral muscles of the neck flex both the neck and the head. Their unilateral actions help turn the chin down and to the other side (1).

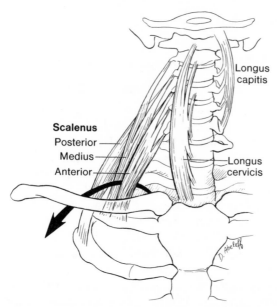

Figure 3.17. Left longus capitis; right longus cervicis; and the right scalene muscles—anterior, medius, and posterior. *Arrow* indicates course of subclavian artery between scalenus anterior and scalenus medius (from Basmajian [2]).

All of the small suboccipital group extend the head, but the inferior oblique also turns the face to the same side.

A great many other muscles situated far afield also have important actions on the vertebral column. For example, the whole "rectus" group flexes the column; unilateral action of the oblique muscles of the abdominal wall bends the trunk to the same side and twists it to the opposite side. In short, almost any muscle, one of whose attachments is to the axial skeleton, can directly or indirectly influence the vertebral column (1).

In walking, the vertical muscle masses on the two sides of the vertebral column contract alternatively. Those on the same side as the foot that is leaving the ground are contracting while those on the opposite side may or may not also contract; sometimes the imbalance of activity is the reverse, for no apparent reason.

The *posture of the vertebral column*, including the neck, is regulated by the intrinsic muscles of the back but, contrary to a widely held belief, these muscles are not the prime movers; nor are they necessarily all in constant activity. During relaxed standing most of the muscles are only slightly active most of the time. Individual groups become more active when balance is threatened. When one holds a moderate forward-bending position, the muscles become very active. They relax completely when one bends the back as far forward as possible because the ligaments of the vertebral column assume the load. Muscles are never used where ligaments suffice (1).

Related Muscles of the Neck

SCALENE AND STERNOMASTOID MUSCLES

There are three scalenes (Gr. = uneven) on each side, *scalenus anterior, scalenus medius*, and *scalenus posterior* (Figs. 3.17 and 3.18). The scalenus anterior arises by tendinous slips from the fronts of the transverse processes of the cervical vertebrae (except the highly modified atlas and axis). The slips fuse into a flat muscle which descends obliquely lateralward to be inserted into the upper surface of the first rib.

The *scalenus medius*, rather larger than the scalenus anterior, arises from the backs of the same transverse processes plus that of the axis. It then runs parallel to, but behind, the anterior; it also is inserted into the upper surface of the first rib. The scalenus posterior is but the posterior part of the medius and its fibers reach the second rib.

Regarding movements of the neck, the scalenes pale into insignificance beside the sternomastoids. Their greatest and most important use is to suspend the thoracic inlet and to maintain its level; they raise the first rib and indirectly the lower ribs during the inspiratory phase of breathing, being particularly active in forced inspiration (1).

The sterno(cleido)mastoid (Fig. 3.18) runs obliquely down the neck and stands out like a heavy cord when the face is turned to the opposite side.

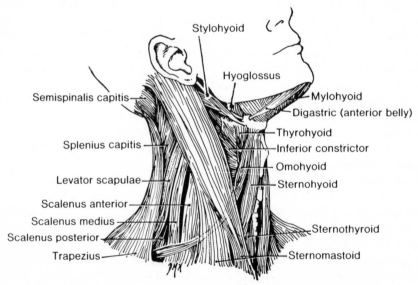

Figure 3.18. Muscles of front and side of neck (from Basmajian [2]).

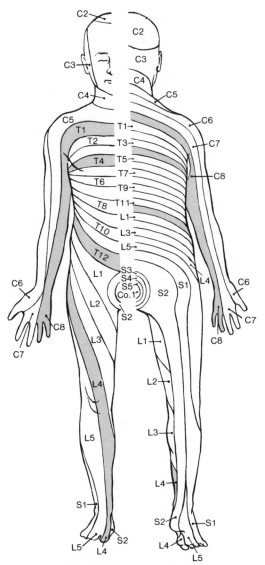

Figure 3.19. Dermatomes: the strips of skin supplied by the various levels or segments of the spinal cord (from Basmajian [2]).

When right and left sternomastoids contract simultaneously, the head and neck are flexed. Unilateral contraction tilts the chin up and to the other side—the position assumed in torticollis (wryneck), due to shortness or spasm of one sternomastoid. The sternomastoid usually does not initiate the simple turning of the head to one side; as a rule it comes into action only during the later part of that movement.

Dermatomes and Myotomes

The human torso shows evidence of its segmental development in that its nerve supply is by an orderly series of spnal nerves. The strip-like area of skin supplied by one pair of spinal nerves is known as a dermatome (Gr. = skin-slice) and these dermatomes have been mapped by different investigators by varying techniques and with somewhat varying results. In Figure 3.19, it will be noted that there is a regular sequence of dermatomes on the limbs, too, becauase the limbs are outgrowths from the torso in the cervical and lumbosacral regions. Physicians and other persons dealing with patients having nerve injuries must be familiar with the general pattern of the dermatomes.

Although the segmental origin of skeletal muscles and their nerves is less apparent, the myotomes (Gr. = muscle slices), which parallel the dermatomes in general distribution, can be traced and are important, too.

REFERENCES

1. Basmajian, J. V. *Muscles Alive: Their Functions Revealed by Electromyography*, 4th Edition. Baltimore, Williams & Wilkins Co., 1979.
2. Basmajian, J. V. *Primary Anatomy*, 8th Edition. Baltimore, Williams & Wilkins Co., 1982.

4

Manipulation of the Spine

ROBERT MAIGNE

Vertebral manipulations, when applied in carefully chosen cases and when correctly performed, are an excellent treatment for many common spinal disorders. They rightly deserve the interest of physicians, rheumatologists, physiatrists, and orthopedic surgeons.

Their reputation is often bad. This is due partly to their misuse by laymen who have tried to use manual techniques as a miracle cure for various disorders, and partly to doubtful pathogenic interpretations. Manipulations have been used to treat vertebral subluxations, vertebral "blockings" in a bad position, articular adhesions, sacroiliac subluxations or sprains, etc. In short, each maneuver was justified by the existence of a particular pathology, belied later on by the advances in radiology and by a better knowledge of spinal pathophysiology.

Some diagnostic techniques, used by manipulators and based on a particular palpation, defied common sense by reason of their subtlety, while the use of coarse and stereotyped manipulations by others, done in all directions and for all cases, were totally illogical.

Nevertheless, with a good knowledge of indications and contraindications, a selection of effective and harmless maneuvers, and with a codification of their use, manipulations must have their place in our therapeutic arsenal.

If their mode of action, apparently so simple, is still not well understood, it is because we are not sufficiently aware of the nature of some conditions which are relieved by them—often better and faster than by other measures.

So, to explain the cases of vertebral pain which are helped by manipulation, the "minor reversible intervertebral derangement" hypothesis has been proposed by the author.

This working thesis appears to correspond to clinical facts. These minor reversible derangements can be determined by careful clinical examination of the spine (20, 22, 29, 32). They are often accompanied by some changes in the tissues supplied by the corresponding posterior and anterior primary rami of the spinal nerve (20, 22, 29, 32): Systematic palpation of the skin and the subcutaneous tissue by the "pinch and roll" method will reveal this involvement of the dermatome of the nerve. Palpation of the muscles of the

71

myotome of the nerve may reveal the presence of cordlike structures which are tender to palpation.

These conditions may be responsible for "misleading" pain. There is great consistency both in topography and in the relief obtained by vertebral treatment in these cases. Confirmation can be obtained by anesthetizing the involved nerve roots, which will result in temporary relief, even though remote from the area of manipulation. There are, however, no specific x-ray abnormalities present.

It appears that many of these tissue pains, especially those of muscle, have been noted in the past (5, 54). However, various explanations given of the origin of the pain differ from that described here. The local treatments proposed, in fact, have been useful. But the recognition of the spinal origin of the pain, when it does exist, leads to more rapid and effective treatment and contributes to an understanding of the origin of musculoskeletal pain. The effectiveness of manipulative treatment evidently leads to questioning some theories concerning the pathology of pain of the spine or the extremities.

It has been said that the only effect of manipulation is psychotherapeutic. But we must notice that bad manipulations or manipulations done in the wrong direction can exaggerate or provoke exactly the same symptoms that they can help when they are properly done.

Basic Principles of Manipulation

DEFINITIONS AND DIFFERENT TYPES OF MANIPULATION

Manipulation involves forced passive movement, carrying the elements of an articulation beyond the usual range of motion to the limit of the anatomical range. Thus for the spinal area it involves movements of rotation, lateral flexion, flexion, and extension, either isolated or combined, done on the desired vertebral segments.

Manipulation must be a very precise orthopedic act whose coordinates are determined by the examination. It is also a treatment with very clear indications. There are three steps, which comprise proper positioning of the patient and operator, correct "taking up of the slack," and the manipulative thrust itself.

For example, in manipulating the neck the physician will hold the supine patient's head between his hands; this is the "positioning." The neck is then rotated to the left until there is the impression of having reached the end of the possible range of motion. A slight additional tension is the taking up the slack. If from this point the neck is brought back to the starting position and the movement repeated several times, a series of "mobilizations in left rotation" have taken place. If in extreme left rotation, a sudden slight and very short thrust of the physician's right wrist is used to obtain supplementary rotation, there is then the impression that some resistance has given way and that the segment of the vertebral column has gone a few degrees of range further. This thrust is accompanied by a characteristic "cracking noise." It must be always carried out from the point of "tension." It must be a very small movement. A large movement is violent, not measurable, painful, and dangerous (Figs. 4.1 and 4.2).

Manipulation must be perfectly controlled by the operator. In order to do it well, experience is necessary. Manipulation should be entirely painless. It can be carried out at any level of the spine by a well-trained operator on

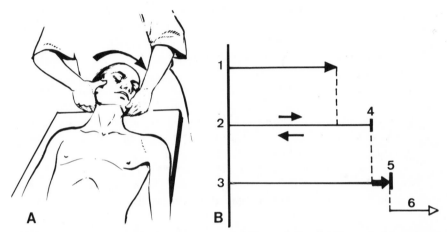

Figure 4.1. (A) Manipulation: the physician causes the patient's neck to undergo rotation to the left (see text). (B) *line 1*, extent of voluntary range; *line 2*, extent of passive range—the extreme limit (4) equals the tension-set, which when repeated is mobilization; *line 3*, starting with tension-set, a sudden and brief thrust produces manipulation (5). Additional displacement leading to dislocation (6).

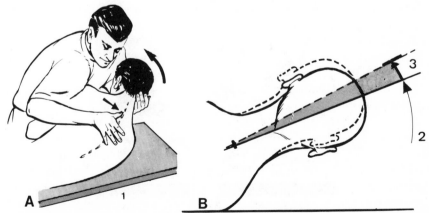

Figure 4.2. Manipulation in lateral flexion; *A1*, position-set; *B2*, tension-set; *B3*, manipulation.

a normal patient, without any of these *forced* movements being either painful or disagreeable.

Manipulation can be either direct or indirect.

For direct manipulation, the patient should be prone, and manipulation is carried out by direct pressure over the vertebral column using the "heel" of the hand or the pisiform. The movement may be in the lateral or medial direction (Fig. 4.3) and must be followed by a very quick release. This technique cannot be measured, and is frequently disagreeable for the patient. Direct manipulation has only limited usefulness.

For indirect manipulation, the operator uses the body as a lever to move the vertebral column. For example: with the patient in lateral decubitus, opposite pressures upon the pelvis and the shoulder will result in twisting of the dorsolumbar spine. In a similar manner it is possible to manipulate any vertebral segment (Fig. 4.4)

It is well to understand that gently progressive movements of this type can be used for mobilization. They have the advantage of being tried before being carried through completely. It is important to be able to judge whether the movement is painless or not. This is extremely important in the system of manipulation described in this chapter.

The precision of these maneuvers can be increased by using semi-indirect techniques. Here, as in indirect manipulations, the manipulation occurs at a distance. More precise localizing of the manipulation can be determined

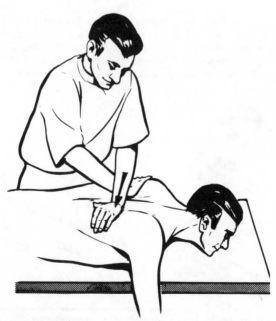

Figure 4.3. Direct manipulation, by direct pressure over the transverse or spinous processes—limited usefulness.

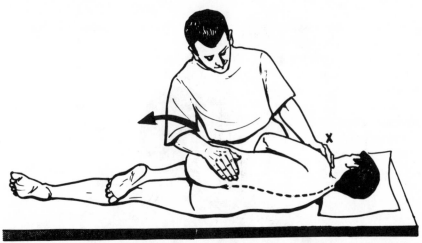

Figure 4.4. Indirect manipulation—in this case, using the pelvis and shoulders as levers to cause rotation of the lumbar spine while stretching into flexion.

by the operator, using pressure and counterpressure, which sometimes act at a different level from that being moved. It is thus possible to move the desired segment in the same or the opposite direction (Figs. 4.5 and 4.6).

There are many different techniques which permit a trained operator to manipulate any vertebral segment in any direction or combination of directions.

Manipulation causes a characteristic *cracking sound* similar to finger cracking. This sound appears to be caused by cavitation, because of negative pressure in the synovial fluid during joint separation. The dissolved gas in the synovial fluid is then released and causes the cracking noise. When the released gas is completely redissolved in the synovial fluid (15 to 30 minutes) the cracking sound can be reproduced. This noise therefore does not prove that a maneuver was successful, and even less that anything has been replaced. Its only interest is that it occurs in the desired articulation.

A trained manipulator can cause this cracking sound in a normal subject (without causing any pain) in any vertebral segment in any direction—all without hurting.

RULE OF NO PAIN AND OPPOSITE MOVEMENT

The manipulative system described here differs from many others. The movement which causes pain is determined and the opposite movement is then used, if it has remained free and painless. This is the "rule of no pain and opposite movement" (26, 33, 38). It means that the manipulative thrust should be in the opposite direction to that which provokes pain in the involved vertebral segment.

This refers to the movement brought about by the manipulation on the involved vertebral segment and not by spontaneous active movements. For

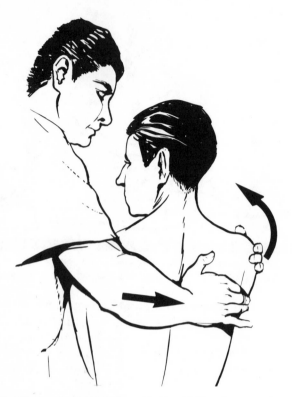

Figure 4.5. Semi-indirect manipulation: The example given is that of an assisted manipulation in left rotation by placing the operator's right hand over the transverse process of the vertebral segment to be manipulated. This maneuver allows precision and controlled progression.

example, traumatic torticollis, which prevents the patient from turning his head to the right but permits turning the neck to the left without pain and limitation, will not be helped by forced rotation of the neck to the right; on the contrary, forced rotation to the left will be helpful. This point is extremely important because this permits one always to act without causing pain.

When two or three directions are blocked, manipulation should be carried out in all the "free" directions, either successively or with a multidirectional technique. It then becomes very easy to plan the manipulation. For this purpose a six-branched star-shaped diagram corresponding to the six elementary movements of the spine can be used. These are left rotation, left lateral flexion, right rotation, right lateral flexion, forward flexion, and extension. Any of the above-described branches are eliminated if a movement is painful or blocked. Manipulation is done only in free directions. If all the branches of the star are blocked no manipulation is possible (Figs. 4.7 and 4.8).

This system permits us to determine technical contraindications to ma-

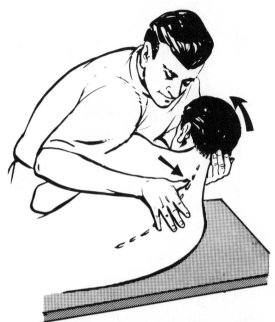

Figure 4.6. Opposed semi-indirect manipulation, the contrary of Figure 4.5, is accomplished by using the thumb as counterpressure over the spinous process of the adjacent distal vertebral segment in order to cause lateral flexion.

nipulation. Thus, there are cases in which manipulation might be considered as valid treatment because the involvement is mechanical in nature and the state of the spine permits it, but it cannot be used because the rule of no pain and opposite movement over-rides it.

Usually at least three directions should be free for the manipulation to have any chance of success. Most often there is no problem in applying this rule; it is usually easy to determine which movements are free and which are painful. There are, however, conditions helped by manipulation which do not permit a clear determination of painful movements. This is particularly true in certain cases with longstanding involvement. Here, other means must be used in order to apply the rule of "opposite movement and no pain."

For the neck, repeated mobilizations in the various directions may be used with the usual manipulative techniques (without thrusting); done in one direction they will decrease the tenderness of the posterior facet, and the local spasm of the muscle, and done in the opposite direction they will increase both.

The manipulative thrust will be done in the painless direction.

For thoracic and lumbar areas it is convenient to use lateral pressure upon the spinous process, which results in rotation of the vertebra. This

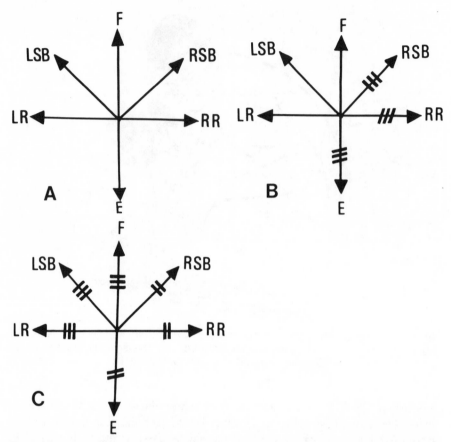

Figure 4.7. The "star" diagram and the rule of no-pain and opposite movement (see text). Thus, at *A*, left and right rotation, left and right lateral flexion, and flexion and extension are the six possibilities. At *B*, manipulate in left rotation, left lateral flexion and flexion. At *C*, there is no free painless direction, and no manipulation is possible. F, flexion; E, extension; LR, left rotation; RR, right rotation; LSB, left side-bending; and RSB, right side-bending.

may be painful in one direction and not in the other. For example, pressure over the left lateral aspect of a spinous process causing left rotation may be painful while the opposite direction is painless. Right rotation will be the direction of manipulation.

Manipulation is not just a movement which, if successful, will miraculously cure the patient. Although this sometimes happens, it is not usual. Treatment is usually carried out with less spectacular results, but success is nevertheless real and useful.

TREATMENT SESSION

A treatment session has several steps. Treatment must be titrated to prepare the tissues progressively and the patient for the final maneuver.

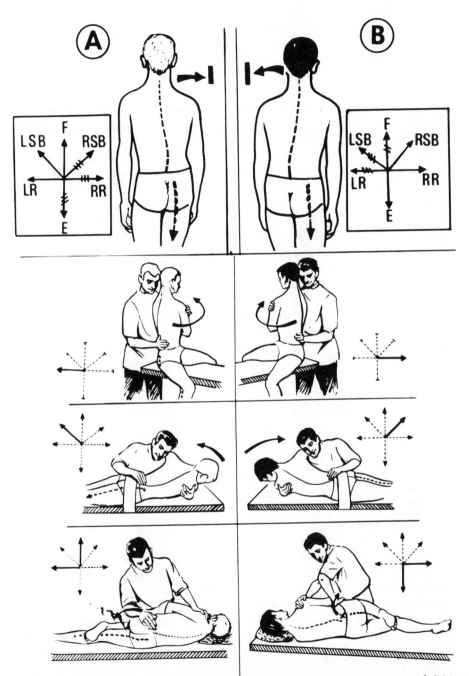

Figure 4.8. Using the rule of no-pain and opposite movement in two cases of right sciatica: (*A*) Here right rotation, right lateral flexion and extension are painful. (*B*) In this case, it is the opposite movements which are blocked and painful. In these two cases the manipulation will be in opposite directions in order to follow the "rule."

All this should permit the operator to appreciate the local tissue reaction to the maneuvers. A treatment session comprises three stages: local and general maneuvers of tension release, oriented mobilization maneuvers, and the final thrust.

Good positioning of operator and patient is essential, otherwise it is impossible to manipulate properly. The trained clinician will then go through the three manipulative stages successively. These are placing in position, taking up the slack, and finally the manipulative thrust itself.

The result of this first maneuver can immediately be noted by the patient, who may subjectively consider himself entirely or partially healed. There are objective signs which are easy to appreciate (for example, amelioration of the Lasègue sign in case of sciatica, of forward flexion for lumbago, of movements of the neck for torticollis, and so on). Re-examination of the patient will now reveal changes in free movements.

Afterward, a second manipulation can be performed which can use a different free direction as a principal coordinate. Repeating the examination may now indicate a third manipulation which might be in another direction which the preceding maneuvers may have freed. It is generally not advisable to do more than three or four consecutive maneuvers upon a vertebral segment. But the treatment may sometimes consist of a single maneuver, while at other times a series of six or seven might be required, according to the response obtained and to the case being treated. This practical aspect, which is difficult to describe, requires experience.

The desired result may be obtained with the first session; more frequently two or three are required, while in some chronic cases even four to six might be needed. The time between each session depends upon the case and the operator's technique and the manner in which he applies the technique, whether he goes more or less far in the thrust. In some cases, the spacing might be for two sessions per week or one session every two weeks. A trained manipulator can quickly determine in two or three sessions whether he has a reasonable chance of success. Much depends upon the discipline of the patient. When the patient has been helped very quickly there is a tendency not to observe the recommended precautions.

There are some reactions to the treatment, but these are minor in character. Stiffness after a manipulation is not unusual after the first session, even if the manipulation was quite gentle. These reactions are usually quite moderate and easily treated with aspirin. The reactions may last from 6 to as much as 48 hours, and can be noted in perhaps a third of the cases. In some rare cases they can be quite painful. They do not occur in later sessions; if they do occur they are very much less than the first time in both intensity and duration.

REACTIONS TO TREATMENT

It is not rare to have a temporary exacerbation of the original symptoms after the first manipulation. The pain may disappear completely and immediately, definitively or temporarily. Pain may reappear in the following days and may be helped by a second manipulation. In other cases, several hours after the treatment, the pain, having entirely disappeared, can return to a more severe degree and now be accompanied by stiffness. Here the acute pain may remain for 6 to 24 hours, and then disappear again without returning.

Sometimes the patient may have the impression, immediately after the manipulation, that the relief was slight or absent. A day or two later there may be definite diminution of the pain, sometimes preceded by a reaction. In some very chronic cases the improvement may not be noted for several days after the manipulation.

These reactions are much fewer after the second session and rare after the third. If they appear at each session, with no improvement of the treated condition, then the treatment should be stopped and the diagnosis reviewed. These temporary exaggerations of the treated pain, which are almost unavoidable reactions, should not be confused with exacerbations of the pain caused by incorrect manipulation or manipulation done on the wrong cases.

If the manipulation is not correctly done, the patient will have pain during the sessions. There should be a free interval between the session and the reaction. This interval is usually about 6 to 18 hours, during which time the patient may feel better. On the other hand, if the increased pain was due to an incorrect indication or technique, the pain will occur immediately after the manipulation, without any free interval, and will continue to increase rapidly. Although the reaction may last 24 to 48 hours in the first case, in the second case the pain may persist for days and even weeks and will be quite resistant to any treatment. It is clear that although reactions are possible, especially after the first manipulation, aggravation can follow any session.

It is frequent for a patient who has had sciatica for two or three months to be spectacularly relieved by the first session of manipulation, and then, if he becomes active instead of being on bed rest for a day or two, to have a more intense reaction than usual. This might prevent the good result which could have been obtained, and might even result in increasing the initial symptoms. In any case, a bad result instead of a good one will be obtained.

The patient must be warned of the precautions to be taken after manipulative treatment.

Besides the painful reactions there are sometimes sympathetic reactions. These can be immediate, perhaps instantaneous. It is quite frequent that after manipulation (even quite mild) the patient may show increased sweating of the axillary area or the body. This may occur at each session no matter how close together or far apart the sessions are. It results from the action of the maneuver upon the sympathetic system and should not influence the course of the treatment. Sometimes, the menstrual periods may be changed, resulting in an earlier occurrence of the menses. In other cases abdominal bloating may occur and last several hours.

POSSIBLE ADJUNCTIVE TREATMENTS

While manipulation in most cases can be used alone, it may be useful to add anti-inflammatory and analgesic medications. These help the result and diminish the reactions which sometimes occur, especially after the first session.

Corticosteroid injections into the apophyseal joint may be a useful complement to the manipulation, especially in those cases in which manipulation has not completely eliminated the joint tenderness. It is the most useful treatment when manipulation is contraindicated.

Immobilization using a collar or plaster jacket is sometimes quite useful, especially in those acute cases in which manipulation results in clear but quite fleeting improvement.

Therapeutic exercises are frequently a useful complement for maintaining a favorable result of the manipulation. Manipulation must be viewed as *one treatment among others* to be used with the others for the best relief of the patient. It is a useful method which should not be neglected.

Minor Intervertebral Derangement (20, 32, 33)

It is generally accepted that manipulation is concerned with the correction of a dysfunction of one or more vertebral segments. Most schools of thought consider that this dysfunction is associated with segmental hypo- or hypermobility. The diagnosis of hypo- or hypermobility is usually made by palpation; however, sometimes "mobility" x-rays may be used as an additional aid. Manipulation is directed only to the treatment of hypomobility.

For the author, the important finding is not the loss of mobility but the presence of pain elicited by direct pressure over the involved segment. The maneuvers are pain free when applied to asymptomatic vertebral segments; this remains true even in the presence of x-ray changes which may show degenerative, arthritic, or discal lesions either with or without loss of mobility. The involved segment is considered to represent a *"minor intervertebral derangement"* which can usually, though not always, be reversed by manipulation.

DEFINITION

The definition of the minor intervertebral derangement (MID) is: isolated pain in one vertebral segment, of a mild character, and due to a minor mechanical cause. This situation is independent of the radiologic and anatomical condition of the segment. A vertebral segment which has more or less severe arthrosis or disc involvement can function in a perfectly normal manner, can be painless, and can cause no symptoms. Here, because there is radiologic evidence of involvement, it cannot be called MID.

On the contrary, a vertebral level can be painful while having a normal static and dynamic radiologic appearance. This is the most frequent case.

When the painful segmental area is the consequence of a mechanical, postural, traumatic, or static disturbance, and when manipulation makes it disappear, it can be considered an MID which is reversible.

Although there are many possible hypotheses concerning the nature and mechanism of this involvement, whether due to reflex or mechanical causes, it is possible by clinical evaluation to determine exactly which vertebral level is involved and which is responsible for the local pain, from irritation of the corresponding spinal root. There are many painful conditions whose spinal origin is clear, for example, a patient may have vertebral pain after an awkward movement, after an effort, or secondary to a poor position. The standard clinical and radiologic evaluation frequently remains "normal" inasmuch as this examination does not reveal the precise signs of vertebral movement, and even less the determination of the responsible vertebral level.

The segmental examination will permit the determination of the segment which presents this painful dysfunction and also the determination of the correct maneuver for manipulation.

This examination consists of: (a) direct pressure over the spinous process, (b) lateral pressure over the spinous process, (c) pressure over the apophyseal joint, and (d) pressure over the interspinous ligament.

SIGNS

All these maneuvers for diagnosis are painless on a normal segment. All (or some) are painful over an affected segment. If x-ray and clinical evaluation determine that there is no generalized or localized pathology, and if the involvement is mild and of a mechanical origin, then an MID is present. Direct pressure over the spinous process (Fig. 4.9) is one of the

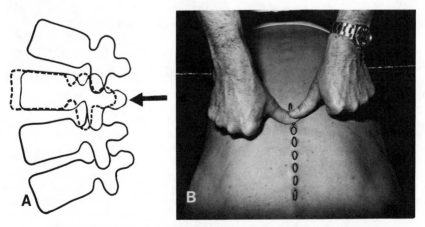

Figure 4.9. (*A and B*) Direct pressure over the spinous process.

usual methods. Slow pressure over the spinous process reveals a deep pain, and, at times, may reproduce or increase the spontaneous pain previously present. Lateral pressure over the spinous process is carried out in an appropriate position, from right to left and vice versa. In the usual case, the maneuver is painful in only one direction, and only over the involved vertebra. This maneuver causes rotation of the vertebra. It is possible to increase the sensitivity of the examination by providing simultaneous counterpressure over the spinous process immediately above and below, in the opposite direction (called contrary lateral pressure) (32, 33) (Fig. 4.10). This permits the precise localization of the segment involved in the MID.

Pressure over the interspinous ligament (Fig. 4.11) of the involved vertebral area is usually more painful than over others. This sensitivity may be evaluated by using a keyring.

MID always involves one of the two zygoapophyseal joints. The exami-

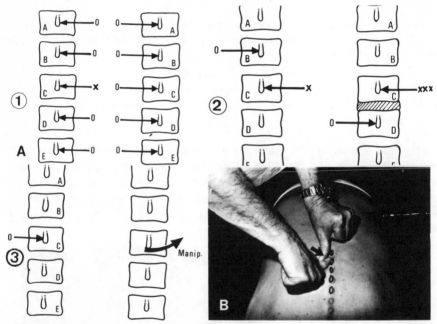

Figure 4.10. (A)*1*, Lateral pressure over the spinous process (especially useful in lower thoracic and lumbar areas). Lateral pressure over the spinous process at *C* is painful from right to left (*X*) but is painless in the opposite direction, which is the direction for manipulation. *2*, Lateral and opposed pressure; pressure is painful only at *C* from right to left. In order to know if the MID is between *B* and *C* or *C* and *D* it is necessary to give counterpressure over *B*, then over *D*. Here the pain originally triggered over *C* is unchanged by counterpressure on *B*, but is changed (*XXX*) by counterpressure over *D*, thus, segment *CD* is involved. *3*, Manipulation in the painless direction is therefore in left rotation. (*B*) Lateral pressure over the spinous process at the thoracic and lumbar levels.

nation of these articulations is more or less easy according to the level involved and is especially useful at the cervical level (Fig. 4.12).

The cervical spine is evaluated with the patient sitting, head bent forward for examination by axial pressure over the spinous process. The patient is supine for examination of posterior facet pain, which is the most characteristic sign of minor mechanical cervical derangement. This is usually associated with signs of corresponding root irritation (Fig. 4.13).

For the thoracic spine, the patient should be seated or, even better, lying across the table. At this level it is very important to avoid the error in evaluation caused by the frequent sensitivity of the mid-dorsal cutaneous

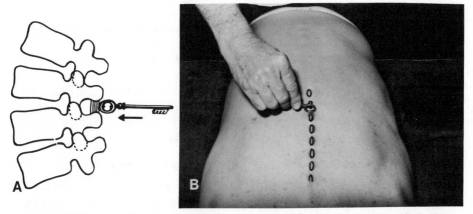

Figure 4.11. (*A and B*) Pressure over the interspinous ligament, usually applied with a round keyring.

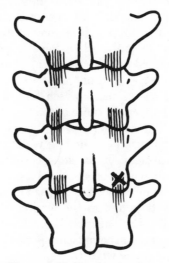

Figure 4.12. The facet point.

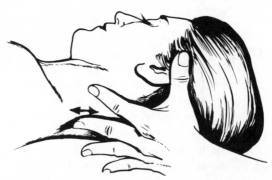

Figure 4.13. Seeking the cervical facet tenderness (see text).

area. Direct and lateral pressure over the spinous process might then appear to be painful when really it is the skin which is painful to pressure. This skin sensitivity is usually caused by involvement of the lower cervical spine (interscapular pain of cervical origin) (32, 38).

For the lower thoracic and lumbar spine, the patient should also lie across the table. Particular attention should be paid to the maneuver of lateral pressure to the side of the spinal processes, which should be carried out slowly and gently segment by segment (Fig. 4.14).

"Metameric Celluloperiosteomyalgic Syndrome"

The usual signs of involvement of the spinal nerve include sensory signs in the corresponding cutaneous region with hyperesthesia or hypoesthesia or even anesthesia, and later motor involvement in the corresponding myotome, including weakness and paralysis. Besides these, there may be decreased or absent deep tendon reflexes, and even at times involvement of sympathetic innervation. Actually, when considering the minor mechanical spinal pathology, true painful root involvement is not very frequent.

On the other hand, careful and systematic palpation may frequently reveal localized or grouped sensory changes. These are found in the cutaneous planes of the muscles and of the tendons, innervated by the nerve root corresponding to the segment which had demonstrated the signs of MID. These sensory changes are those of the metameric celluloperiomyalgic syndrome (Maigne). The recognition of this syndrome is an important element in the comprehension of common vertebral pain, and is important for diagnosis and treatment. It explains certain apparently paradoxical therapeutic results which can be obtained by vertebral manipulation in some painful conditions of tendons or in pseudovisceral pain.

This syndrome may be noted in the territory of both the anterior and posterior rami. Its manifestations include localized painful cutaneous areas, painful cordlike structures in the muscles, periosteal tenderness.

Figures 4.15 and 4.16 show what this syndrome might be at the level of

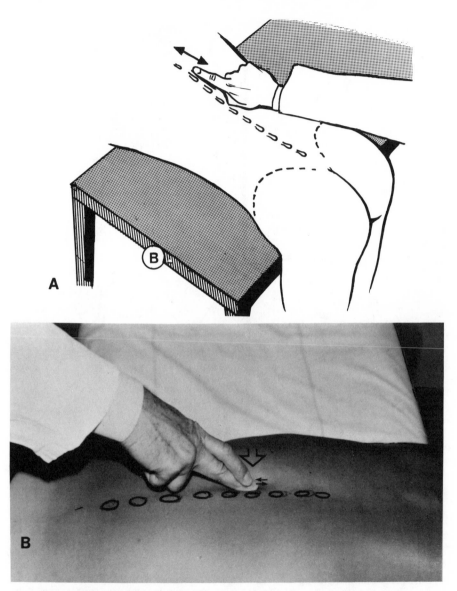

Figure 4.14. (*A and B*) Seeking the facet point in the thoracolumbar area.

the L5 and S1 roots, Figure 4.17 for roots C6, Figures 4.18 and 4.19 for roots T9 and T12. The signs of the radiculocelluloperiomyalgic syndrome can occur in groups or isolated. They may accompany cases with clinically evident root pain with sensory reflex or motor disturbances, and then disappear at the same time as these conditions. It may sometimes persist

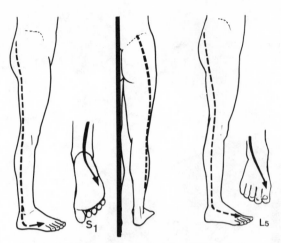

Figure 4.15. Area of pain in L5 and S1 sciaticas.

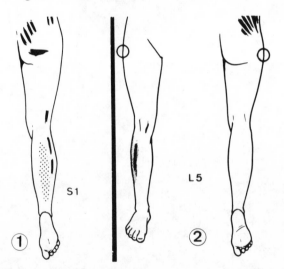

Figure 4.16. Metameric celluloperiosteomyalgic syndrome in sciatica. (*1*) S1, subcutaneous tenderness (indicated by *light lines*). The indurated and tender muscle bundles are those of the gluteus maximus, the gluteus medius, the pyriformis, the distal portion of the biceps femoris, and portions of the lateral gastrocnemius. (*2*) L5, tensor fasciae latae, gluteus medius, toe extensors: subcutaneous tenderness; tenderness at the trochanteric tendinous insertion of the gluteus medius. Note that all of these findings may be present at the same time.

as a painful state which can only be helped by appropriate treatment of the localized condition. However, this syndrome could be the *only manifestation of minimal root or facet irritation*. In this case there will be no pain in a root distribution. The involved area will have the same cutaneous, muscular, and tendinous involvement described above. Relief can be obtained, at least for the time being, by anesthetic injection of the root.

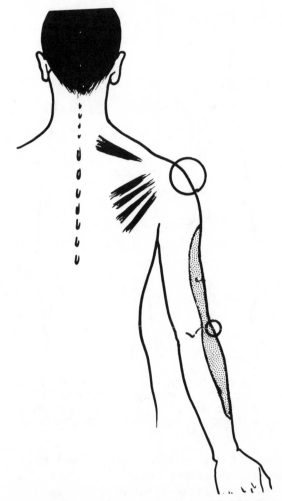

Figure 4.17. Metameric celluloperiosteomyalgic syndrome at C5–6 level; *shaded area*, zone of subcutaneous tenderness; *darker lines*, infraspinatus muscle bundles which are indurated and tender; *circles*, periosteal and tendinous pain—infraspinatus, supraspinatus, biceps, lateral epicondyle, radial styloid.

An MID (with or without radiculalgia) is usually accompanied by specific findings in the territory of the corresponding spinal nerve. These sensory changes are those of the author's "radicular cellulotenoperiosteomyalgic syndrome." These include:

1. Pain and often thickening of the skin and subcutaneous tissues over part or all of the corresponding dermatome. This is detected by the "pinch-roll" maneuver.

2. The presence of hard tender muscle cords which are detected by palpating the muscles in the corresponding myotome.

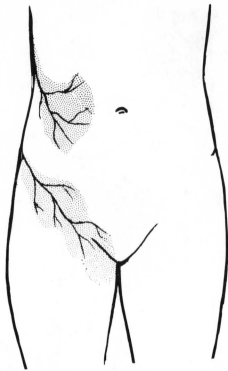

Figure 4.18. A zone of subcutaneous tenderness in the abdominal wall may be the only sign of chronic root irritation, with the only subjective evidence being a deep spontaneous pseudovisceral pain. This is a common cause of diagnostic error. The illustration is that of a T9 and T12 involvement. The pinch-roll is very painful.

3. Tenderness of the periosteum (especially at tendon insertions) detected by palpation at the corresponding sclerotome.

These signs can be found in the territory of the dorsal ramus of the spinal nerve (of which the pinch-roll is the only clinical sign); and not quite so commonly, in the territory of the ventral ramus of the spinal nerve.

The manifestations of the cellulotenomyalgic syndrome may be:

1. *Silent*, and cause no painful symptoms; or
2. *Misleading Pain*:

    (a) *Vertebral*—but at some distance from the involved vertebral segment.

    Examples: —low back pain originating from the thoracolumbar junction,
             —dorsal pain originating from the cervical region.

    (b) *Pseudovisceral*—through skin tenderness over the dermatome on the anterior part of the trunk.

    (c) *Pseudoarticular*—through tenderness of the tendon and periosteum.

    Example: —epicondylitis of cervical origin (C6–C7)—65% of cases,
             —tenderness of the greater trochanter of vertebral origin (L5),

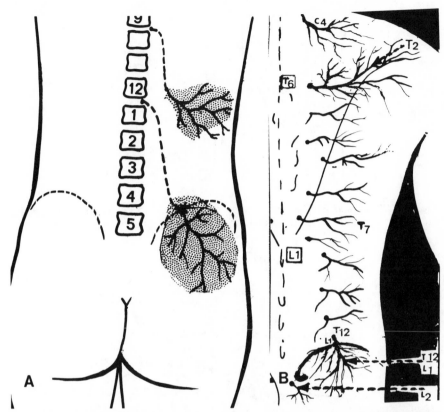

Figure 4.19. (A) Painful subcutaneous syndrome of the cutaneous rami of the posterior root branches. (B) Superficial exit area for the cutaneous rami of the posterior root branches (from Hovelacque, modified by Maigne). The importance of the posterior branches of C4, T2, T12 with L1, and the frequent absence of the cutaneous branches C5-6-7-T1 and L3-4-5 have been described.

—false pain in the knee (L3, L4),

—tenderness over the periosteum of the pubis T12, L1.

These cases are diagnosed by detecting the existence of pain and tenderness at the relevant vertebral level, most often caused by a minor intervertebral derangement.

SKIN AND SUBCUTANEOUS TISSUES

Painful conditions caused by irritation of the roots corresponding to the cutaneous areas of the thorax or abdomen may be responsible for misleading pseudovisceral pain. Localized painful dermatologic conditions caused by involvement of a particular dermatome may be revealed by the maneuver of the pinch-roll (Fig. 4.20). The cutaneous fold is pinched and rolled between the thumb and index finger (20, 22, 29). Compared to adjacent and

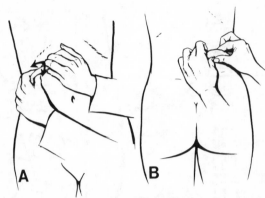

Figure 4.20. (*A and B*) The pinch-roll evaluation, used to demonstrate the area of subcutaneous tenderness. The skin fold is thickened, granular, and very tender.

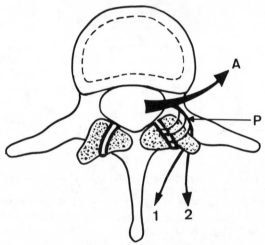

Figure 4.21. The anterior (*A*) and posterior (*P*) spinal roots (according to Lazorthes [19]). The medial (*1*) and lateral (*2*) rami of the posterior root.

opposite areas it appears thickened, grainy, and very sensitive. The involved zone has a variable surface of between 2 and 10 cm or even larger. The areas involved can be in the dermatome of the anterior or posterior ramus (Fig. 4.21). All of this cutaneous territory should be carefully explored, while comparing the findings with the neighboring and opposite zones. Localized cutaneous involvement may be noted in some sciaticas, and may sometimes be a part of other chronic painful conditions. The most frequent area where this condition may be present is at the level of thorax and abdomen. The patient may complain of pain considered to be of gynecologic, digestive, or renal origin. This may then be the only evidence of nerve irritation provoked by the MID which can be revealed by the examination. It is a very frequent cause of diagnostic error (Fig. 4.18) and could lead to unnecessary treatment and even surgery.

The role of the posterior ramus has been considerably underestimated in the mechanism of common vertebral pain. Back pain due to involvement of the posterior rami T12 or L1 has been described by the author (35). Posterior ramus irritation is essentially revealed by a band of unilateral localized tenderness isolated in the midst of normal territory. The pinch-roll maneuver in this zone reproduces, more often than not, the patient's spontaneous pain. This band of tenderness is usually a few centimeters in width, and spreads obliquely to the lateral portion of the back. It should be recalled that the cutaneous territory of the posterior rami at the dorsal and lumbar levels is usually located at four levels or more below the level of exit (19, 32). For example, the skin in the area of the iliac crest and of the lateral fossa is innervated by posterior rami T11, T12, L1, L2 (Fig. 4.19).

It is thus possible to describe an unrecognized and frequent anatomical origin of low back pain: the "thoracolumbar junction" (35, 37, 39).

The superficial tenderness found in all or part of the dermatome is most probably of neurotrophic origin and is due to chronic root irritation. It may sometimes be relieved almost immediately by anesthetic injection of the responsible nerve. This is especially obvious in involvements of posterior rami T11, T12, or L1.

MUSCLES

Palpation of the muscles may reveal the existence of hard cordlike structures, with a diameter varying from a few millimeters to 1 or 2 cm, and about 5 cm long, and very sensitive to pressure. These are found in some muscles innervated by the involved root. Just as in superficial pain, the root involvement can be responsible for pain which is resistant to treatment and diagnosis, and results in the persistence of the original radicular pain (e.g., sciatica). These bundles are always located in the same muscle of the same root, and always in the same part of the muscle. They may be noted, for example, in the lateral portion of the gastrocnemius in S1 involvement, in the rectus femoris for L3–4, or in the distal portion of the biceps femoris for S1. They are particularly frequent in the gluteal muscles in irritative lesions of L5, S1 (Fig. 4.16). The treatment should be first vertebral and then local: anesthetic injection into the indurated area, stretching, and sometimes deep massage are all useful.

The mechanism is rather difficult to understand if the pain is considered to be due to peripheral nerve involvement. Electromyographic examination shows no clear changes. Nevertheless, the relationship with "cramp" is quite reasonable, because the muscles which are involved frequently show fasciculations. It might be considered that the cords are in a kind of "subcramp" state as shown by palpation indicating motor root involvement.

TENDONS

Tenoperiosteal pain forms the third section of the metameric celluloperiosteomyalgic syndrome. Some tendons and tenoperiosteal areas innervated by irritated roots can be very sensitive and mimic a tenosynovitis. This may be the only clinical manifestation of root irritation and it sometimes can be relieved by a single vertebral treatment.

For example, in L5 sciatica there is, rather frequently, marked sensitivity at the insertion of the gluteus medius on the greater trochanter, which will be relieved by manipulation. In the same manner, shoulder tendonitis or lateral epicondylitis may really be of cervical origin. It is therefore useful to determine systemically whether there is irritation of cervical roots at levels corresponding to the innervation of the muscle or tendon being considered: supraspinatus, biceps, infraspinatus (C5, C6), etc. (Fig. 4.13). Involvement in the cervical area occurs in 60% of lateral epicondylitis or tendonitis of the shoulder region. A single cervical treatment can then bring immediate proof of this etiology (Figs. 4.16 and 4.17).

Pathophysiologic Hypotheses of Manipulation

The physiopathologic basis for manipulation relies upon the hypothesis of the reversible minor intervertebral derangement (reversible MID) already mentioned.

The manifestations of this reversible MID, as described above, can be treated by appropriate manipulation. The exact nature of the MID is unclear, and appears to be entirely a clinical manifestation. However, the MID can be noted only in the mobile portion of the spine. The notion of the "mobile segment" given by Schmorl and Junghanns (48) is an important one.

The mobile segment consists of all the anatomical structures between two adjacent vertebrae and thus includes the disc anteriorly, the posterior articulations posteriorly, and the supporting elements in between, consisting of the common anterior ligament, the common posterior ligament, the ligamentum flavum, the interspinal ligament, and the supraspinal ligaments. In addition there are also the appropriate muscles and nerves (Figs. 4.22 and 4.23). The functioning of the mobile segment and its resistance to injury greatly depend upon the condition of the intervertebral disc. When the disc is injured, other structures inevitably will be involved. The proper functioning of the mobile segment requires perfect synergy of the involved muscles. An awkward or unexpected movement may lead to improper division of forces, and some elements of the mobile segment may thus undergo traction or compression greater than their resistive capacity.

The different elements of the mobile segments are innervated by the posterior ramus of the spinal nerves, and by the sinuvertebral nerves.

The posterior ramus innervates all of the spinal articulations, with the exception of the atlanto-occipital and atlanto-axial articulations, which are

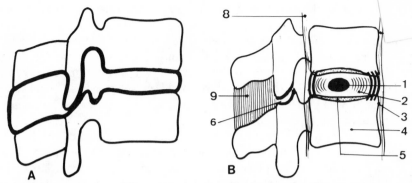

Figure 4.22. (A) The mobile segment (Junghanns). (B) The elements of the mobile segment; *1*, nucleus pulposus; *2*, innermost (transitional) layers of the annulus fibrosus; *3*, zone of attachment of Sharpey fibers; *4*, vertebral body; *5*, cartilaginous area; *6*, zygoapophyseal articulation; *7*, common anterior ligament; *8*, common posterior ligament; *9*, interspinous and supraspinous ligaments.

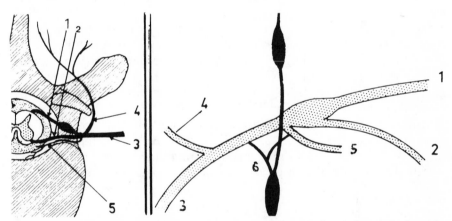

Figure 4.23. The sinuvertebral nerve: *1*, dorsal root; *2*, ventral root; *3*, anterior branch; *4*, posterior branch; *5*, sinuvertebral nerve; *6*, sympathetic rami communicantes.

innervated by the anterior rami of the corresponding nerves. The posterior rami have a very close relationship to the posterior articular area. For this reason, these rami are vulnerable to arthritic or traumatic lesions of these articulations. The posterior rami also innervate all the paravertebral muscles, all the interspinous ligaments and the cutaneous areas of the back (Figs. 4.18 and 4.21).

The sinuvertebral nerve is formed by the junction of a spinal and a sympathetic root. It is distributed segmentally by an ascending root to the vertebral body, to the lamina, and to the subjacent disc by a few inconstant branches (the only branches to have a descending pathway) to the common posterior ligament, to the epidural tissues, and to the dura mater, to the common anterior ligament and to the superficial fibers of the annulus fibrosus (19).

The elements of the mobile segment are interdependent functionally. When these constituents are in good condition, pressures and forces are harmoniously distributed. This is not so when there is a lesion of one of the elements, especially of the disc. The spinal muscles, whose function is automatic, have a particular and very important role in the mechanisms of vertebral pain and of manipulation.

In a certain number of cases the MID seems to be caused by mechanical lesions, even minimal ones, of the disc. A disc lesion, which may by itself be asymptomatic, may be responsible for bad pressure distribution (especially if it is lateral or posterolateral and may lead to posterior articular dysfunction. Thus the superior and inferior articulations may then function in a condition of excessive constraint, and may become painful, especially after a bad position or a false movement or effort (Figs. 4.24 and 4.25). In other cases it could be a mild strain of a facet joint. But in all these cases the reflex muscle spasm is preeminent, and the local signs of MID are the same.

For example, in a mild sprain, the ankle is automatically "locked" by muscular action in order to avoid painful movements, resulting in a limp. But if the pain provoked by this movement is overcome, it is then possible to force the painful foot to have a normal movement, and to avoid the limp. None of this is possible in the spine. The victim of a lumbago may, overcoming his pain, walk while smiling, but his spine will nevertheless remain stiff and twisted. Vertebral muscles cannot be commanded in the same manner as the muscles of the limbs. This makes the importance of the reflex element of the intervetebral derangement quite obvious. Any vertebral pain—whether posterior articular, discogenic, or other—may pro-

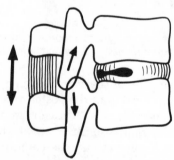

Figure 4.24. Disc lesions, even when asymptomatic, can lead to dysfunction of the segment, thus resulting in or causing an intervertebral derangement. Posterior blocking by the disc can itself be symptomatic from the pressure over the common posterior ligament, but it can also be asymptomatic. In any case it upsets the proper function of the mobile segment and results in interference with the posterior articulations and the interspinous ligament.

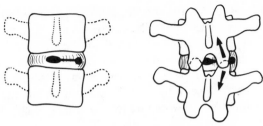

Figure 4.25. The lateral intradisc blocking is always asymptomatic in itself, but can trigger a painful posterior articular dysfunction and thus open the way for chronic facet involvement.

voke a protective reflex and disturb the harmonious functioning of the ensemble of the spinal elements. This inevitably leads to an avoidance of painful pressure and movements of the involved segment, which will be fixed and thus tend to perpetuate the dysfunction. On the other hand, any movement which causes a false movement of the segment will reinitiate the process. There is thus little tendency for the condition to improve spontaneously. Weight bearing and increased postural tonus should be avoided by rest in order to obtain, as rapidly as possible, a return to a normal situation.

However, by means of manipulation, it is possible to re-establish normal function. In all MIDs, regardless of cause, there is element of muscle spasm. Manipulation constitutes a powerful, well-directed stretching of these muscles which provokes a reflex inhibition of the spasm, and this undoubtedly is the essential action of the manipulation.

Systematic spinal examination demonstrates the presence of silent MIDs. The signs are present but pain is either absent or only occasionally present and very mild, especially after efforts or with fatigue. These MIDs are therefore not beyond the threshold of tolerance. Such a derangement can become symptomatic if increased by a mechanical cause such as effort, bad position, etc. It can also be revealed when local tolerance is decreased by an external cause, such as cold, or when general tolerance is decreased by intercurrent illness, fatigue, or depression.

The notion of threshold is important for the understanding of chronic painful vertebral pain. Depending on it, the same MID will be silent or the cause of pain.

Indications and Contraindications for Manipulations

Manipulations are useful when vertebral pain or pain of vertebral origin of a mechanical nature is present. Manipulation is a therapeutic method which requires a correct diagnosis. It should not be used unless the mechanical origin can be demonstrated. It is necessary to eliminate the presence of infection, inflammation, tumor, fracture, etc., which obviously are absolute contraindications. In addition, manipulation is not applicable to all cases of pain of mechanical origin. It is of course necessary to evaluate the vertebral column both clinically and radiographically. Postural tests should be used, especially before cervical manipulation. As noted above, insistence upon the rule of no-pain and opposite movement is always necessary. Also as mentioned above, preliminary evaluation should note positive indications for manipulation. The study of manipulation can be the key which unlocks a new approach to minor mechanical vertebral pathology.

As detailed below, certain aspects of spinal pathology have led the author to postulate some theories which may not be acceptable to all. Fortunately, as mentioned below, other authors have noted similar facts, although their interpretation may not be identical. Thus, the descriptions which follow will demonstrate that the "ordinary" dorsal pain usually has a cervical origin, and that ordinary low back pain, always considered of lumbosacral origin, has often its origin at the T11–12–L1 level (35). Common ordinary headaches are frequently due to involvement in the upper cervical region. Shoulder and tendon pain in shoulder and elbow can have a spinal origin, and so can muscle pain elsewhere, while pain which is apparently of visceral origin may in reality originate in painful subcutaneous or muscular tissues whose nerve is irritated at the spinal level.

CERVICAL REGION

Manipulations are a frequently effective treatment for various painful cervical conditions. These can be acute, subacute, or chronic, with or without radicular pain. Manipulation is also useful in some conditions not usually considered of cervical spinal origin, such as some headaches, shoulder pain, lateral epicondylitis, etc.

Acute and Chronic Cervical Pain

Torticollis can sometimes be helped by manipulation; the muscular component is most important here. Therefore the maneuver must be mild, slow, and progressive, more like stretching. Manipulation should only be done with absolute respect for the no-pain principle. However, some cases of acute torticollis do not have a mechanical origin, even when they seem to have been triggered by an awkward movement. Sometimes the involvement might be that of viral myalgia, and thus not treatable by manipulation.

Other acute painful cervical conditions may be due to inflammatory involvement of the capsular structures of the cervical joints and should not be manipulated. The rule of no-pain would prevent the use of manipulation here. Acute cervical pain of intervertebral disc origin may sometimes be a possible but rather rare indication. Great care should be taken in cases of this sort. The use of a cervical collar is essential in all cases with acute cervical pain.

Chronic cervical pain, whether a sequel to trauma or accompanying an arthrosis (which plays the role of "rust" and makes MID more possible), is an excellent indication for manipulation. From the very first session—essentially consisting of mobilization—one can frequently note partial or transitory improvement. An average of three to four sessions will be necessary, and follow-up sessions one to three times yearly are advisable. The maneuvers should be precise and at the right level,. always respecting the rule of no-pain and opposite movement.

Rotation and lateral flexion are the essential directions. The maneuvers should always be done lightly, in a supple fashion. If manual treatment is not enough to eliminate the articular and posterior periarticular sensitivity completely at the MID level, injection of minimal quantities of corticosteroid in the facet can be done. This injection is very useful in cases with an inflammatory involvement of capsular structures of posterior joints when only one or two articulations are involved.

It is obvious that these cases constitute a contraindication to manipulation. Besides, in these cases, manipulation cannot be used, because all directions of movement are painful.

Headaches of Cervical Origin

Some headaches of cervical origin frequently can be alleviated by manipulation. When carried out incorrectly, manipulation can aggravate or even trigger the same symptoms. Careful clinical examination of the vertebral area will reveal pain in the upper cervical spine (C2–3).

The only headaches usually considered as cervical are those of the occipital region, for which alternative explanations appear to be lacking, and where x-ray shows advanced lesions of upper cervical arthrosis. Thus, Nick (43) indicates a possible cervical origin of headache in only 50 of more than 2350 headaches evaluated, and confirms this origin in only 12. On the other hand, he considers 52% of the headaches as being of psychogenic origin. Wolff (56) also describes 80% of common headaches as of psychogenic origin. The author's experience (36) is in total contradiction to these statements.

Headaches of purely psychogenic origin surely exist. They are not frequent in current practice, and are easily distinguished from others. On the other hand, there are a large number of headaches of cervical origin which can be triggered by a bad position of the neck, an incident of digestive trouble or gynecologic involvement, or by psychogenic factors. But if the cervical origin of the pain is removed, these same factors will not trigger headaches.

The author has identified a homogeneous clinical picture of these cervical headaches and has described in the supraorbital type (the most frequent) a very constant sign which is "the painful pinch-roll of the eyebrow" (36). An analogous sign, "the painful pinch-roll of the mandibular angle," is present in the auriculotemporal or occipitomandibular form (36). The occipitosupraorbital form (which may be only supraorbital) is the most frequent type (Fig. 4.26). On the other hand, there is the occipital form which radiates to half of the vertex (Fig. 4.26*A*) (topography of the ventral ramus of C2). The scalp of this side is tender to massage.

The occipitomandibular or auriculotemporal occipital form radiates to the angle of the jaw and to the ear lobe and may sometimes mimic otitis (Fig. 4.26*B*)—medial part for the dorsal ramus of C3, lateral part for the dorsal ramus of C2 (Fig. 4.27).

All of the above are, in most cases, unilateral headaches. However, in time they may become bilateral. Sometimes when the pain is very acute, the patient has the impression of diffuse bilateral pain. The examination will always show unilateral signs, and the patient can quite precisely define this unilaterality. The pain is always either on the right or the left for the same patient when the headaches recur.

The occipitosupraorbital or supraorbital headaches (Fig. 4.26*A*) occur in a more or less acute fashion and more or less frequently. In some patients they can be a real handicap. In some cases the involvement appears to have a vasomotor component (somewhat like migraine), with watering eyes and either stuffy nose or rhinorrhea. An essential sign of cervical origin is the

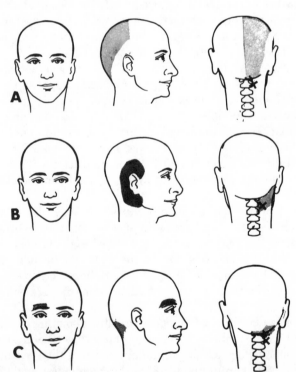

Figure 4.26. (*A*) occipital nerve headache; (*B*) occipitotemporomandibular headache; (*C*) supraorbital headache. (These are described in the text.)

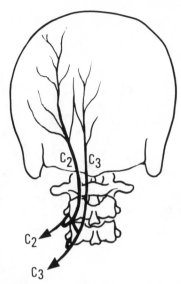

Figure 4.27. Posterior branches of *C2* (great occipital nerve) and of *C3*, and their anterior branches.

repetitive nature of the pain during different crises; it is always right or left. Another important sign is the fact that all clinical and laboratory examinations are negative, including arteriography and air encephalography. The fact that ergotamine tartrate or dihydroergotamine is ineffective is also important.

A very characteristic finding is the pain caused by the pinch-roll of the eyebrow (36). The skin fold which is pinched and rolled between thumb and index finger appears thickened and is painful compared to the opposite side, which remains supple and painless (Fig. 4.28).

The cervical spine, on the same side as the headache and the painful eyebrow pinch-roll, will have great tenderness of the C2–3 articulation. There is frequently tension of the cutaneous regions of the suboccipital area on the same side (Fig. 4.29). Anesthetic injection (Fig.4.30) done at bony contact at the level of the tender articulation (C2–3) will cause the disappearance of this articular sensitivity to palpation and in a few minutes the eyebrow pinch-roll pain will no longer be present. This same result, which will be more lasting, can be obtained by manipulation, when manipulation is possible, if the problem is an MID. This may be a sequela of cervical trauma or possibly the consequence of very old, rather benign, trauma which has been forgotten. Sometimes a bad position at work or during sleep may be responsible.

Three to five sessions of manipulation should generally suffice to rid the patient of these headaches. In some patients, one to three annual sessions may be necessary to maintain this result.

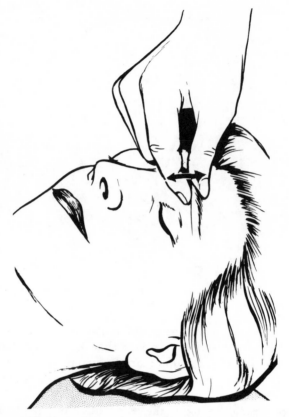

Figure 4.28. Method of evaluating the painful eyebrow pinch-roll.

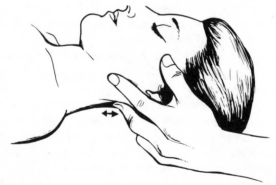

Figure 4.29. Method of determining localized C2–3 sensitivity by palpation.

When manipulation cannot be used because of the status of the spine, the condition of the circulation, or when the rule of no pain is not possible, or when manipulation results in incomplete relief, the injection of longlast-

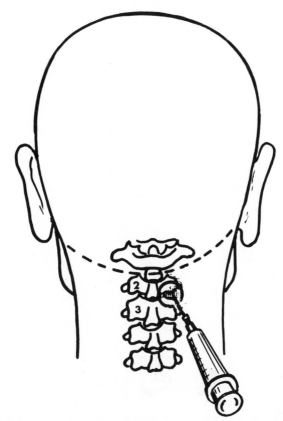

Figure 4.30. The C2–3 interspinous articulation is at the top of the pyramid formed by cervical vertebrae 3–7, and is the most cephalad articulation which can be palpated.

ing corticosteroids into the tender articulation may be useful. The connection between the upper cervical spine and the eyebrow can perhaps be explained by the fact that the spinal nucleus of the trigeminal nerve extends quite caudad. There are some common areas between the lower part of this nerve and the first three spinal segments. The role of the cervical sympathetic system is also possible. Great occipital nerve neuralgia is rare in its typical acute form. However, it is less rare under the form of moderately chronic unilateral headache, with tenderness to scalp massage on the involved side. This can be a valid indication for manipulation. It is the consequence of irritation of the posterior branch of C2 or C3, also tied to posterior articular involvement at C2–3 (36) (Figs. 4.26A and 4.27).

The auriculotemporal or occipitomandibular headache is rare in its acute form but rather frequent in its moderate form (Fig. 4.26B). It is this latter which will be recognized when the characteristic sign is present. This is the painful pinch-roll of the skin of the angle of the mandible (36) compared with the opposite side (Figs. 4.31 and 4.32).

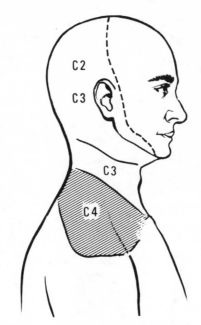

Figure 4.31. Cutaneous territory of C2–3.

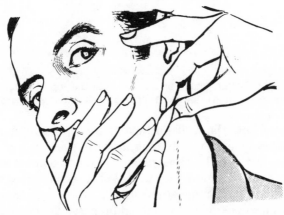

Figure 4.32. Method of evaluating the painful pinch-roll of the mandible, indicating irritation of anterior branch of C3 and C2.

The cutaneous area of the angle of the mandible is supplied by the anterior branches of C2 and C3. In these cases there is articular sensitivity at the level of C2–3 or C3–4 on the involved side. Here this is due to the irritation of the anterior branch of C2 or of C3.

The cervical headache can be triggered by a bad position of the head (using a too high pillow, sleeping prone). In this case the headache is almost always present in the morning. It is triggered when the neck is held in a bad position, for example at work, sitting on badly designed chairs, or backing up an automobile. Sometimes an added factor decreasing the tolerance of the patient (such as digestive, gynecologic, or other involvement) is falsely considered as the entire cause of the headache. The presence of a psychogenic problem or of fatigue can also be a contributing factor.

True migraine, however, often alternates from right to left, has no connection with the spine, and is not influenced by cervical maneuvers. This is not true of the supraorbital headache as described above. The cervical findings noted above are absent in true migraine. If both migraine and supracervical pain are coexistent, the patient usually recognizes the difference between the two types.

The Barré-Lieou Syndrome

The syndrome of Barré (1, 7, 42, 50), although of questionable origin, truly exists clinically. This cervical syndrome includes headaches and otolabyrinthine involvement such as vertigo, nausea, and tinnitus, in addition to visual problems, such as spots before the eyes and burning feeling in the eyes. There are also laryngeal phenomena such as dysphonia, or a lump in the throat. Psychogenic involvement includes anxiety, and loss of memory. These symptoms are rarely all present at the same time. They are most often isolated or diversely grouped.

They are frequently found after incorrect manipulations or after minor cervical trauma (20, 29). Manipulation, correctly done, is one of the best treatments if it is technically possible. However, the whistling or buzzing in the ear is much more rarely helped by manipulation than the headaches or the vertigo. Manipulation can be used only when cervical examination shows that the posterior facets of C2-3, C3-4 have obvious tenderness. Before applying manual treatment, the diagnosis and the mechanical-cervical origin of this involvement must be obvious.

Vertebral or basilar artery involvement completely contraindicates the use of manipulation (26, 50, 51, 53). Although the syndrome of Barré-Lieou is very often considered to be a minor form of vertebral or basilar artery insufficiency, it shows no tendency for progression; this is just the opposite of arterial involvement in which severe paroxysmal accidents can occur, such as the syndrome of Wallenberg, and can result in paralysis and even death (13, 46, 50). There are no objective neurologic signs in the Barré syndrome, and its manifestations are mild and not progressive. Arteriographic investigations in typical Barré syndromes have been found negative by the author.

Decroix and Waghemacker (11) did electronystagmographic examinations on patients with a such cervical syndromes. These were done both before and after manipulation. They were able to demonstrate objective improvements by cervical manipulation. The author has frequently confirmed these findings (20, 36).

It is known that some psychasthenic conditions can give similar manifestations, such as headaches and false vertigo, but in these cases there are none of the clinical cervical signs of MID (36). The clinical picture is also different. When both are present, the psychogenic involvement should be given the first consideration.

Manifestations similar to those described as the Barré syndrome may be sequelae of cranial fractures, where the trauma can cause unrecognized minor cervical sprains. By taking all possible precautions, manipulative cervical treatment, sometimes associated with posterior articular injections, has frequently proved very efficacious.

Cervical Radiculalgia

When these are moderate and not accompanied by any marked antalgic position, they can be helped by manipulation. (The antalgic position might be indicative of a herniated disc.) Manipulation should be carried out every three to five days in the free direction, while localizing as well as possible the effect of the maneuver upon the involved level. It should always be preceded by maneuvers of relaxation and stretching. The use of an immobilizing collar for the neck, at least at night, usually helps the patient (47). He may also benefit from medical treatment such as analgesics and antiinflammatory drugs (7). Two or three manipulations frequently relieve these neuralgias even when they have been present for extended periods. Care should be taken to distinguish some cervical brachial neuralgias from others whose origin is neither mechanical nor benign.

Shoulder and Elbow Pain of Cervical Origin

Shoulder and elbow pain of cervical origin appears to be of tendinous origin whether with or without limited range of motion. These may be in the supraspinous, infraspinous, and bicipital areas especially. They are associated with an MID at C4, C5, or C6. The same is true of some painful lateral epicondylar syndromes (C6 or C7). These painful tendinous conditions are one of the manifestations of the cellulotenomyalgic syndrome (21, 20, 30) caused by minimal chronic irritation of the spinal nerves corresponding to C5–6. Examination will reveal MID present at one of two levels (C4–5 or C5–6). The sensitivity of the facet on the side of the shoulder pain is an invariable sign, easy to demonstrate (Fig. 4.13).

Manipulation causes the disappearance or diminution of the MID and can bring immediate improvement to the shoulder or elbow pain. (See sections on Shoulder and Elbow in Chapter 5.)

DORSAL REGION

Dorsal Pain of Cervical Origin

Interscapular pain is a very common complaint especially in women, where it is very often considered psychogenic. However, although women may perhaps have this type of involvement more often than men, it is seen in both sexes and at all ages. The ensuing disability varies with the profession (e.g., typists). An essential point is for the author the usual cervical origin of these back pains, which have a clinical stereotyped picture of interscapular vertebral pain, mediodorsal, or cervical origin (32, 38).

The examination reveals the same signs in all cases. These include dorsal signs with a very particular localized area that we call the "cervical point of the back" (Maigne), always near T5 or T6 (32, 38), and inferior cervical MID (C5-6, C6-7, or C7-T1) with the tender facet on the same side as the back pain and the dorsal signs. Interscapular pain may be the first manifestation of the sequela of a cervical brachial neuralgia, radicular in character, or may be the only evidence of cervical involvement.

There is one interesting sign which can be seen six or seven times out of ten and which demonstrates the connection between cervical spine involvement and back pain: Pressure with the thumb over the anterolateral portion of the lower cervical spine, maintained for a few seconds at the responsible vertebral level, triggers the patient's dorsal pain. This is the "push button sign" (32, 38) (Fig. 4.33), which simply shows the connection between back pain and cervical spine. Of greater significance is that in some cases cervical discography or irritation of the cervical ligamentous structures can reproduce or increase the painful dorsal radiation when cervical involvement is present (10).

Signs of cervical spine involvement include the presence of a painful unilateral point, precise and constant in the T5 or T6 region about 1 or 2 cm from the median line. This is revealed by light frictional pressure over the involved area, with the symmetrical or neighboring areas having no tenderness. Pressure in the involved area only reproduces the pain described by the patient, although the pain is felt higher or lower, intrathoracic, or even bilaterally. The tender area corresponds to the superficial emergence of the cutaneous branch of T2. The possible mechanism is described below.

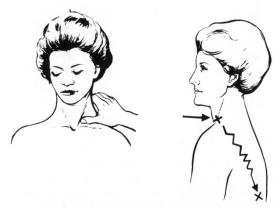

Figure 4.33. The anterior "push-button."

We call this point the "cervical point of the back" (23) (Fig. 4.34A). Another sign is an area of skin more or less thickened, and always extremely sensitive to the pinch-roll maneuver, which includes all or part of the cutaneous territory of the posterior branch of the second thoracic nerve (23) which extends from this point to the acromium (Fig. 4.34B). In addition to these findings, the therapeutic trial is important. Thus, cervical manipulation causes the disappearance of signs of cervical MID and the immediate disappearance of the interscapular point (T5 or T6). The sensitivity of the pinch-roll of the medial dorsal zone clearly decreases. Frequently the back pain may be entirely relieved. This relief may occur instantaneously, while in other cases, three to five sessions may be required, each one immediately causing decreased examination findings. On the other hand, interscapular back pain, having the same character, is a frequent incident in incorrect cervical manipulation and can provoke or aggravate an MID of the lower cervical spine.

The connection between this posterior branch of T2 and the lower cervical spine is quite unclear, but appears to be confirmed by the fact that anesthetizing the posterior branch of T2 in the interspace T2–3 causes the disappearance of tenderness at T5–6, and of the pinch-roll sensitivity described above. It is also true that on the trunk the dermatomes C4 and T2 are neighbors, because during embryologic development the dermatomes C5, C6, C7, T1 are drawn out into the upper extremities. The cutaneous branches of the lowest cervical spinal nerves are described as being quite small or nonexistent (19). It is possible that at the dorsal level the cutaneous branch of T2 represents the sensory supply for the lower cervical levels (C5, C6, C7, T1) (Fig. 4.35). The treatment for this type of back pain is at the

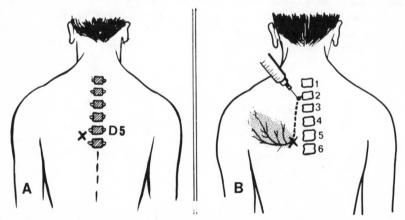

Figure 4.34. (A) the para T5 or T6 interscapulo-vertebral point or the "cervical point of the back", indicating involvement of the lower cervical spine. (B) This point corresponds to the superficial exit area of the posterior branch of spinal root T2. The area of subcutaneous tenderness which the pinch-roll reveals corresponds at least in part to the dermatome corresponding to T2.

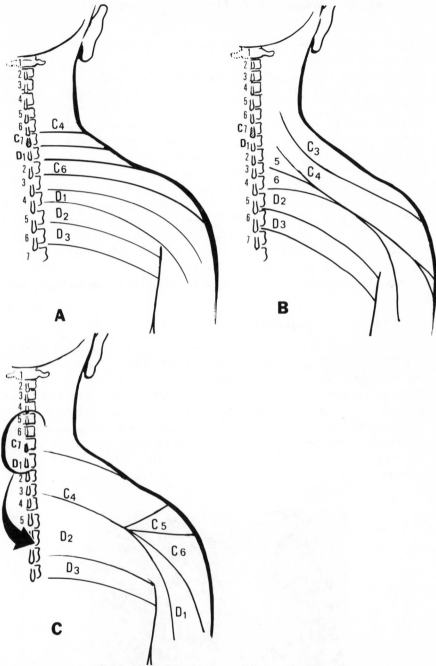

Figure 4.35. Dermatomes of the back: (*A*) according to Keegan and Garrett (18); (*B*) according to Lazorthes (19); (*C*) according to Maigne, the T2 dermatome (*D2*) is very extensive and represents the cutaneous areas of all the lower cervical segments, since the posterior branches of C5, 6, 7, 8, and T1 go to muscles and practically never have cutaneous rami. Thus, dermatome C4 is next to T2, and very extensive.

109

cervical level no matter what the pathogenic mechanism might be. Treatment might be manipulation (Fig. 4.36), injection of the involved cervical facet, or the use of a cervical collar, temporarily or only at night, for patients whose prone sleeping position results in cervical involvement and "morning upper back pain."

In addition to MID, note that isolated interscapular pain with signs similar to those described above (that is, tenderness at T5–6 due to cervical involvement with a nearby area of localized tenderness) may be early signs of any type of disease of the lower cervical spine.

The most frequent form of *acute dorsal pain* is the acute form of this interscapular pain of cervical origin. The same examination signs will be present at the cervical and dorsal levels. Manipulation is not always possible at this stage. The use of a cervical collar and injection of the posterior branch of T2 at its emergence from the spine between T2 and T3 can be useful. This acute interscapular pain is often the first sign of a cervicobrachial neuralgia whose onset may be a few days after the onset of the dorsal pain itself.

Dorsal Pain of Dorsal Origin

Dorsal pain of dorsal origin, while possible, is much more rare than the preceding. Some of these conditions can be helped by manipulative therapy. However, there is always the possibility of nonbenign causes of back pains of visceral origin. These are far from exceptional and may result from involvement of the heart, lungs, stomach, pancreas, gallbladder, etc. Quite frequently back pain may be attributed wrongly to a mechanical cause such as scoliosis or kyphosis, or to a sequela of Scheuermann's aseptic necrosis. These are rarely involved, however, because the pain, as noted above, is usually due to interscapular pain of cervical origin.

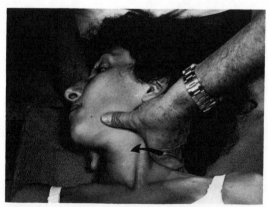

Figure 4.36. An example of lower cervical manipulation, rotation to the right, for back pain of cervical origin. This manipulation usually corresponds to left back pain.

Rib Strains

Some painful thoracic or lumbar conditions are associated with small derangements of the costovertebral or costotransverse articulations. They are always due to trauma, to an effort, or to a false movement, such as turning too rapidly. Some longlasting rib pain due to old fractures of the ribs remain painful for the same reasons. Almost always this is due to a sprain of the floating ribs (T11–12). Failure to recognize the possibility of these small lesions frequently leads to diagnostic errors when lumbar fossa pain is present. This pain can be acute. A history of effort or false movement may be considered by the patient as being the cause, but is not always accepted as the mechanism of onset because examination may reveal a freely movable and supple spine without any paravertebral contracture. There is, however, increased pain upon deep breathing or movements of lateral flexion and rotation of one side of the trunk. The most important sign is that of the "Rib maneuver" (25). With the patient seated, the physician stands behind and has the patient flex the trunk laterally, to the side opposite the pain. The sensitive rib is then "hooked" with the fingers and first pulled up, and then pressed down. One of these movements will be painful and reproduce or increase the spontaneous pain while the other is painless. Manipulation consists of carrying out this maneuver on a relaxed subject, toward the end of expiration, and only in the nonpainful direction (Fig. 4.37).

There are also "anterior chondrocostal sprains" which are usually post-

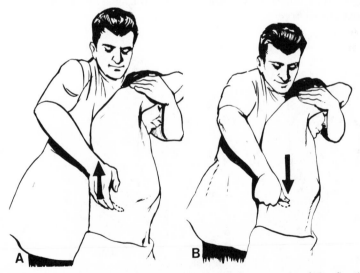

Figure 4.37. Method of evaluation and manipulation for a sprain of the floating ribs. The pain is only in one direction. (*A*) Pull the rib upward; (*B*) push the rib downward (rnanipulation in the direction opposite to the painful direction).

traumatic. The examination should be carried out in a similar fashion, pushing the rib down and then up, using the thumb. The treatment, as above, should be done in the nonpainful direction, while the patient takes a deep breath.

The sprain of the floating ribs can also be associated with a sprain MID of the dorsolumbar area, and occurs much more frequently.

LUMBAR REGION

Low Back Pain

Low back pain due to mechanical vertebral involvement is usually considered as having its origin in the lower lumbar spine (L4–5, or L5–S1).

The classical theories are well known, and will not be described here. But we have drawn attention to low back pain originating in the thoracolumbar junction (T11–12–L1). So we will emphasize this aspect (28).

Low Back Pain of Thoracolumbar Origin. The cutaneous areas of the upper half of the gluteal area and of the sacroiliac region are generally considered to be innervated by posterior branches of L1, L2, L3 (3). However, the essential role of T11, T12, L1, and, to some extent, T10 and L2, has been identified in 25 dissections (39). These nerve roots are related to the corresponding posterior articulation and are closely associated with it (Figs. 4.38 and 4.39). The pain in these cases is low, lumbar, deep, or sacroiliac, and frequently at the level of the iliac crest. There is very rarely spontaneous pain at the T11, T12, or L1 levels. There is sometimes pain in the inguinal or apparently in the abdominal areas, and occasionally pain in the trochanteric region.

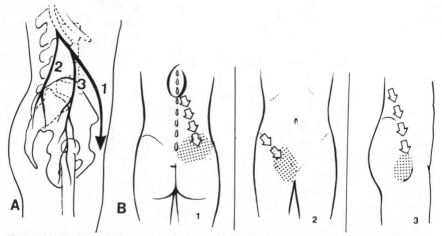

Figure 4.38. (A) Spinal nerves T12 and L1: 1, anterior branch; 2, posterior branch; 3, lateral perforating branch. (B) Irritation of these nerves may be responsible for: 1, low back pain; 2, pseudovisceral pain; 3, pseudo-hip pain.

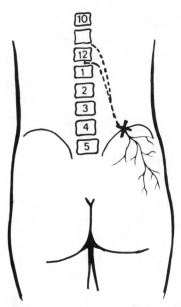

Figure 4.39. Cutaneous innervation of the upper portion of the gluteal area (T11–12–L1). Some cases may even have T10 innervation. Thus, the innervation levels are more proximal than the usual L1–2–3 description.

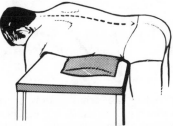

Figure 4.40. Position of patient for the thoracolumbar examination.

In these cases, the examination should be done with the patient prone across the table, a pillow under the abdomen (Fig. 4.40). An iliac crest (crestal) point will be found at the gluteal level, usually situated 8 or 10 cm from the median line, more lateral or more medial. Pressure and friction over the iliac crest, carefully examined in its entirety, will reveal this well-localized and acutely painful point. It corresponds to the pinching of the irritated cutaneous nerve against the iliac crest (Figs. 4.41A and 4.42A). In addition, adjacent to this point, an area of painful subcutaneous tissue can be revealed by the pinch-roll. This area includes all or part of the proximal half of the gluteal area (Figs. 4.41B and 4.42B). Examination of the dorsolumbar area will also reveal the signs of an MID between T10 and L2 (Fig. 4.43). The two most characteristic signs are pain to lateral pressure

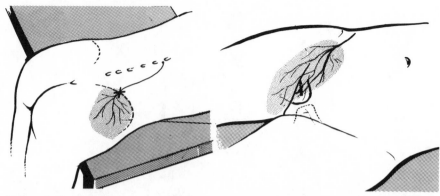

Figure 4.41. (*A, left*) The "crestal point" (*X*), usually at 8 to 10 cm from the midline, occasionally more lateral or more medial, and corresponding to the passage of the cutaneous branch T12 or L1. The painful posterior subcutaneous area is indicated by the *dots*. (*B, right*) The "painful anterior subcutaneous area", which is in the territory of the anterior branch of the same nerve (see text).

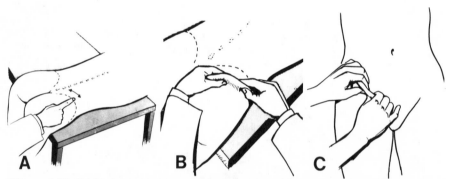

Figure 4.42. (*A*) Method of seeking the crestal point by friction and pressure over the iliac crest. (*B*) Method of seeking painful subcutaneous regions in the gluteal area—by pinching a skin fold and pulling and rolling it. (*C*) Method of seeking painful subcutaneous areas in the lower abdominal region. The anteromedial aspect of the thigh may also be involved proximally.

over the spinous process (usually in a single direction), and posterior articular sensitivity on the same side as the crestal point. Anesthetic injection of the posterior branch of the spinal root related to the articular areas T11-L1 or T11–12 will immediately cause the disappearance of all of the pain and signs described above (Fig. 4.44). X-rays of the involved dorsolumbar level are usually normal. Occasionally there may be minor disc or articular lesions which are unrelated. However, in rare cases the first signs of discitis or metastasis may be found. Sometimes in younger men with somewhat different clinical findings, the early dorsal signs of ankylosing spondylitis may be discovered.

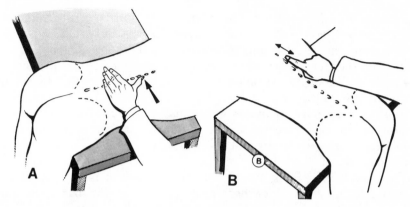

Figure 4.43. Method of determining the thoracolumbar level involved: (*A*) Lateral pressure over the spinous process at the involved level is usually painful in only one direction, left or right; (*B*) seeking the painful posterior articular point by pressure and friction at 1 cm from the midline.

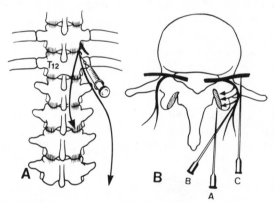

Figure 4.44. (*A and B*) Posterior articular injection, usually T11–12 or T12-L1, sometimes T10–11 or L1–2.

Pain may be acute or chronic. *Acute* lumbago of thoracolumbar junction origin can be seen at all ages. However, it is the usual form of lumbago in the over-40 age group. In this form with involvement at T11, T12, L1, the patient does not assume an antalgic posture. There will be noted only some vertebral stiffness, with severe pain to lateral flexion of the trunk and rotation to one side. On the other hand, *chronic* involvement is the most frequent type. Although noted at all ages, it is also the most frequent type of back pain in those over 40 and very frequent in the aged, where x-rays might suggest other etiologies, such as discopathy, scoliosis, or osteoporosis. There frequently is a crestal point and gluteal tenderness to the pinch-roll maneuver and the signs described above on one segment of the thoracolumbar junction are found. When manipulation is contraindicated because of the condition of the spine or the age of the patient, injection into the painful thoracolumbar facet will bring immediate disappearance of the physical findings, and thus bring complete or partial relief of the symptoms. Manipulation for these conditions should be done with the patient seated, astride the table, with forced rotation applied in the painless direction (Fig. 4.45). Other maneuvers can be used depending on the case in flexion or extension (Fig. 4.46). Two to five treatments are usually adequate. In other cases the treatment can consist of two to four injections with corticosteroids of the involved posterior thoracolumbar articulation which may be associated with the manipulation.

Therapeutic exercise is usually of little value and may frequently be irritating in this form of low back pain. The use of a lumbar brace is not helpful, and may be poorly tolerated unless it extends high (up to T7) and thus helps avoid torsion movements of the trunk.

Low Back Pain of Lumbosacral Origin. Acute lumbago due to disc involvement is a frequent type seen in younger individuals. This involvement includes a characteristic antalgic position with inclination to either the painful side or the other or of kyphosis, and clearly indicates involvement of the disc.

Chronic low back pain may also be of discal origin, and is caused by irritation of the common posterior ligament. Low back pain can also originate in the low lumbar zygoapophysial joints, caused by MID, or by osteoarthritis.

Acute Discal Lumbago. Manipulation can be very helpful when MID is involved. When the acute lumbago is due to disc involvement, a single manipulation may result in complete or marked relief in as many as half

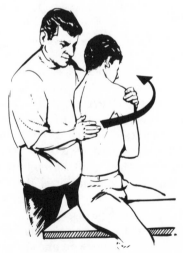

Figure 4.45. Rotary manipulation of the thoracolumbar junction.

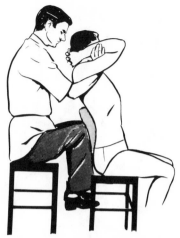

Figure 4.46. Extension manipulations of the thoracolumbar junction.

the cases. A second manipulation three days later should be helpful, in the same manner, in half of those which remain painful. If one continues, the percentage will be near 100% because lumbago frequently cures itself in most cases, when enough time is allowed to pass, and when rest is prescribed. Nevertheless, manipulation shortens the duration of the pain in a manner which is frequently spectacular, and also considerably limits the frequent minimal sequelae. It is of course impossible to determine whether manipulation avoids some sciaticas due to a herniated disc which sometimes follow lumbago, but this does not appear probable. In severe forms, rest must be absolute, using a plaster corset, a frequently very useful method.

Chronic Discal Lumbago. Some of these cases of chronic low back pain, with obvious disc etiology proven by clinical or even myelographic evaluation, can be helped by manipulation without changing the myelographic picture. In low back pain of lower lumbar origin (L3, L4, L5, S1) the use of rehabilitation modalities is essential.

In certain cases in addition to manipulation, epidural, posterior articular, or ligamental injections are complementary treatments, and are often effective. There is usually a cellulomyalgic syndrome present, revealed by the presence of myalgic cordlike structures in the muscles of the external iliac fossa (Fig. 4.47). These are often unilateral, in such muscles as the gluteus medius, tensor fasciae latae, gluteus maximus, or the pyriformis, and are often extremely tender to palpation. The diminution of this tenderness after lumbosacral manipulation is proof of the usefulness of this treatment. However the tenderness of the muscles of the external iliac fossa may not always disappear completely by vertebral treatment, and may be the cause of persistent pain. Treatment by slow and deep massage, and by

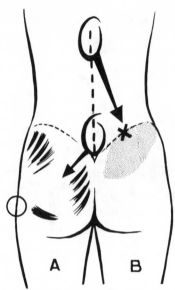

Figure 4.47. The metameric cellulotenomyalgic syndrome involving subcutaneous and tendinous structures, as described in the text. On the left, low back pain having its origin at L4–5 or L5-S1. On the right, low back pain having its origin in the dorsal area (T11–12 or T12-L1). In some patients both forms may be seen together.

maneuvers of long continued manual stretching can be quite helpful; as can procaine injection of trigger points (54).

Frequency of the Different Forms of Lumbago. In a study carried out by the author (37) of 100 cases of chronic low back pain apparently associated with mechanical vertebral problems, a thoracolumbar origin (T11, T12, L1, L2) was found in 38 cases, although in 20, lesions of the disc were present, as shown by x-ray in the L4–5 or L5-S1 areas. In 35 others there was a low lumbar origin (disc or posterior articulation), and in 37 there was a mixed thoracolumbar and low lumbar origin. The 38 cases of low back pain of thoracolumbar junction origin noted above included 10 patients operated on for sciatica L5 or S1 with satisfactory results as far as the sciatic pain was concerned, but in whom the chronic lumbago had either continued or had recurred, and in two of these, recurrence was during rehabilitation. All of these patients were cured or helped by manipulation or by injection of the involved thoracolumbar facet(s). A single patient in this series required surgery.

Besides this series, a few patients had surgery according to the protocol described below (39). These were patients where medical treatment was clearly helpful, but for only very short periods of time. After determining clinically and very precisely which articulations were involved by means of anesthetic injections, capsulectomy of this articulation as well as of the articulations above and below, were carried out by Dr. H. Judet. The results obtained have remained very satisfactory. This is particularly interesting, considering that the patients had previously undergone one or more operations upon the low lumbar and lumbosacral area for persistent low back pain. In these cases, we now prefer percutaneous coagulation of the involved facets.

Discovery of the thoracolumbar junction mechanism of low back pain has been responsible for greatly improving our results in the treatment of low back pain with or without manipulation.

Sciatica

In practice the great majority of true sciaticas are due to disc herniation. When examination reveals that there are three free orientations on the "star diagram", manipulation may be a valid treatment which can shorten the attack and avoid persistent sequelae. However some acute sciaticas are not good indications for manipulation because there are practically never three free orientations in these cases. Moderately acute sciatica or sciatica which has been present for quite some time presents the best indication for manipulation. Particular attention should be paid to mobilization maneuvers and the preparation of the manipulation. These must be carried out in the painfree direction. In these cases three or four maneuvers with various techniques are performed at each session.

For example, in a right sciatica with antalgic scoliosis and convexity to the right, the evaluation of spinal range of motion when the patient is seated on the table will demonstrate that rotation is free to the left, lateral flexion is free to the left, and forward flexion is also free. Other movements are blocked or limited and painful (Figs. 4.8 and 4.48). Useful manipulative movements can only be left rotation, left lateral flexion, and forward flexion, which should be done with the most appropriate technique. The fact that there may be diminished or absent deep tendon reflexes is in no way a contraindication for manipulation, when the mechanical origin is certain. Sciaticas having severe motor nerve involvement should not be manipulated, although experience has shown that even these cases (when manipulation is performed in accordance with the principles stated) have not been aggravated, and in some, very rapid recuperation has been noted after manipulation.

The effect of each manipulation is immediately checked by its effect upon the Lasègue sign. When manipulation has been done correctly there is usually improvement of the Lasègue sign. Sometimes the results are excellent even after the first manipulation; the Lasègue may reveal an increase from 30° to 70° of straight leg raising, and the patient's condition is greatly improved.

The first session may be followed by a painful reaction, 12 to 24 hours after the manipulation, in about one-third of the cases. There is no reaction

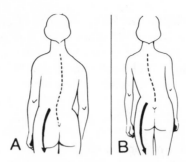

Figure 4.48. The two varieties of antalgic scoliosis in disc herniation with sciatic involvement; treatment outlined in Figure 4.8. (A) Convexity on the side of the root pain; (B) Convexity on the opposite side of the root pain.

after later sessions. Treatment usually includes three to five sessions, three to seven days apart. In successful cases, very clear improvement results from the first two sessions, with the remaining treatments completing the improvement. Some patients are so relieved of pain that they may neglect essential precautions, and symptoms may reappear because of some imprudence a few days after treatment. Patients should be warned concerning the frailty of the results in the early part of the treatment period. Those patients who cannot restrain their activity might benefit from a plaster corset to limit their movements. This should be used for one or two weeks.

Manipulation can result in considerable relief for 60% of sciaticas of medium intensity even after the first two sessions. When combined with other treatments, such as peridural anti-inflammatory injections, results are even better. Manipulation, where possible, even in severe sciatica can be of great help in addition to conservative treatment such as bed rest and the use of anti-inflammatory medication. Manipulation may be very effective even in sciaticas caused by a herniated disc proven by myelography or other x-ray methods. Cases have been noted (20) in which, as mentioned previously for lumbago, clinical signs and pain completely disappeared after manipulation, although the myelogram showed no change in the disc protrusion previously noted. In some of these patients the sciatic pain has never recurred, while others have had a return of pain a few months later and have required operation for the herniated disc. Many cases of sciatica or low back pain recurring after surgery are helped by manipulation. It should be noted that the residual or recurrent low back pain after disc surgery for sciatica is usually the low back pain of T11–12 or T12-L1 origin described previously (27).

Celluloperiosteomyalgic Syndrome of Sciaticas. An L5 or S1 celluloperiosteomyalgic syndrome is very common (20, 32). It can be helped by local treatment. This syndrome can result in pain which is difficult to relieve. Usually the syndrome disappears or diminishes by vertebral treatment alone. In some cases some pain may continue, indicating that the previously present root involvement is still present, but no longer results in any complaints. However, in other cases the condition may be resistant to treatment and cause pain which is more or less disturbing to the patient. This celluloperiosteomyalgic syndrome particularly involves the muscles of the iliac blade, such as the gluteus medius (L5-S1), the gluteus maximus, pyriformis (S1) and the distal portion of the biceps femoris, where a painful myalgic muscular cord resistant to treatment is frequently found. This is especially true in S1 involvements and thus may also involve the lateral portion of the gastrocnemius. The presence of a cellulalgic zone at the posterior aspect of the calf (S1) or the anterolateral aspect of the leg (L5) should always be evaluated by pinch-roll. It is important to note tenderness of the trochanter (L5), often responsible for very persistent pain whose origin is not obvious.

Treatment consists of stretching the muscles manually (41, 54), anesthetic injections into the painful trigger points of the muscles, and massage of the painful cutaneous and subcutaneous areas using superficial petrissage after local anesthesia if this maneuver is too painful. The trochanteric pain almost always disappears after good manipulation of the lumbar spine (L4–5). If it persists, local injection of the corticosteroids is indicated. It should be noted that rehabilitation modalities applied to the lumbar and abdominal areas are the necessary complement to these treatments, once the painful condition has ended.

L3 and L4 Neuralgia

When femoral neuralgia is due to disc or root involvement, manipulation is useful. The results are just about identical to those obtained in sciatica, although they may appear to be somewhat more difficult to obtain. Manipulation should include three to six sessions on the average. It is neither useful nor reasonable, other than in exceptional cases, to go beyond this number. A plaster corset and medical treatment can shorten the necessary and indispensable stay in bed.

COCCYX

Traumatic painful conditions of the coccyx such as those after a fall on the gluteal area or after childbirth can frequently be helped very rapidly by manipulation. The maneuver consists of grasping the coccyx between the index finger (in the rectum) and the thumb. The coccyx is then moved in all directions to free the joint. The author's maneuver is carried out with the patient prone, the index finger is inserted deeply into the rectum in contact with the anterior surface of the coccyx and the lower part of the sacrum. This position will be maintained without pulling the coccyx too much, while with the heel of the other hand a slow firm pressure is exerted on the sacrum for 15 to 20 seconds. A sudden release of muscular tension of the levator ani, which is always tight and painful to examination at least on one side, will occur. After this maneuver, when successful, the painful tension will no longer be present and pressure over the distal portion of the coccyx will be painless. Two to four treatments are required on the average.

PSEUDOVISCERAL PAIN OF SPINAL ORIGIN

A syndrome of pseudovisceral pain may be caused by the radicular cellulomyalgic syndrome of the abdominal wall of vertebral origin (37). Certain kinds of pain, which may be thought to be of visceral origin by the patient (and even by the physician), may sometimes be abdominal-wall pain. These can be areas of skin and subcutaneous tissues painful to the skin rolling technique (Fig 4.41). They will cause deep pain, which can be quite misleading, and can appear to be of intestinal, urologic, or gynecologic origin. The only way to demonstrate them is by using the method of the pinch and roll (Figs. 4.18 and 4.20A). They are caused by chronic irritation of the spinal nerve corresponding to the involved area. The patient is unaware of the existence of these areas. Once found, the corresponding vertebral segment should be examined using the local maneuvers as described previously in addition to routine x-ray examination. So, any minor intervetebral derangement corresponding to a rachidian nerve innervating the anterior part of the trunk may be responsible of a pseudovisceral pain which is referred in the area of the dermatome of its anterior primary ramus. It can mimic cardiac pain, breast pain, abdominal pain, etc. The thoracolumbar junction is very often concerned and may give rise to many errors of diagnosis.

If the diagnosis is MID (5), vertebral treatment should be the first considered when possible. It is usually adequate. Obviously if the treatment is successful, there was no gynecologic or gastrointestinal involvement present. These bands of skin, thickened and tender to the pinch-roll maneuver, and/or these cordlike muscular structures have been noticed and described by many authors (5, 54) under various names. However, none has considered them as having a frequent radicular origin. When radicular origin is present, the treatment should obviously be vertebral first.

PUBALGIA AND TENDONITIS OF THE ADDUCTOR MUSCLES

The periosteum of the anterior part of the pubis is mostly innervated by L1. In case of a chronic L1–2 "minor intervertebral derangement," tenderness to palpation is often found on one side of the pubic bone. It is more often asymptomatic but if the adductors are overstrained (e.g., from soccer, dancing, judo), pain of the pubis (pubalgia) or the tendons of the adductor muscles or the insertion of rectus abdominis may appear. It must be noted that the thoracolumbar junction is overstrained in rotation, especially in hyperextensions which avoid rotation in the lower lumbar spine—very common in these sports. This vertebral source could be the primary one in a large number of pubalgias.

In the early stage of the affection the vertebral treatment may be sufficient to cure the patient.

THE THORACOLUMBAR JUNCTION SYNDROME

The thoracolumbar junction syndrome (Maigne) is due to minor intervertebral derangements of T11–12, T12-L1, or L1–2. It is characterized by low back pain, pseudovisceral pain, pseudo-hip pain, and pubalgia. These manifestations can be either isolated or associated. They have been described in the preceding chapters.

In addition, involvement of the lateral cutaneous branch of L1 also may be observed; it mimics tendonitis of gluteus medius, or sometimes a meralgia paresthetica. In some cases, it may produce an acute pain on the lateral part of the thigh (24, 37).

Accidents Resulting from Manipulations

Indications and contraindications for manipulation have been noted in detail in the preceding pages and will not be repeated. When manipulation is correctly done according to these indications, no danger exists. However, incorrect manipulation can cause accidents; which can result in more or less severe handicaps. In other cases, manipulation may be merely ineffective or result in unimportant changes.

Dramatic accidents are not exceptional, but fortunately are less frequent then one might fear, considering the large number of manipulations done every day, and frequently by inexperienced operators, without diagnosis or consideration of contraindications. The cervical spine is without doubt quite resistant, and the atheromatous vertebral arteries are quite tolerant! It is true that many manipulations are done so gingerly that they avoid any problems. But there are others which unfortunately are more violent and cause dramatic accidents. Most often they occur when the diagnosis has not been made, and with brutal or unappropriate technique. For example, the author knows of a recent case of a mortal accident when a chiropractor manipulated the cervical spine of a young patient for neck pain after a car accident. His physician knew how to manipulate but had refused to do so; in fact, he had advised the use of immobilization in plaster.

Most cases are those of a vascular accident localized to the cord or brainstem. Two quite classical examples in the literature are those of a 35-year-old female, manipulated for hayfever, who died a few hours later because of thrombosis of the basilar artery (13, 46), and a 37-year-old man who was manipulated as a joke by his wife, who rotated the head in not too strong a maneuver. Shortly afterward, this patient became confused and fell, complaining of vertigo, difficulty in seeing and hearing on the right, with loss of sensation in the left upper extremity and sphincter involvement.

His condition progressively worsened and death occurred 3 days later, due to basilar thrombosis with involvement of the cerebellum and brainstem. Sometimes thrombosis of the posterior inferior cerebellar artery can result in a Wallenberg syndrome (50). There can also be quadriplegia or paraplegia after manipulation of the spine, with metastasis, myeloma, osteoporosis, or Pott's disease (45). It is obvious that manipulation of the cervical spine with an unknown odontoid fracture could be dangerous. In other cases a cauda equina syndrome may be present when lumbago or discal sciatica, or even nothing, was present before the trauma caused by the wrong manipulation.

Oger et al. (45) established an interesting list of published accidents before 1964. This work represents only the visible portion of the iceberg. Other accidents may not be as serious as these, but might handicap the patient for a long time or even indefinitely. These are the lumbagos transformed into paralyzing sciatica, the triggering of stubborn vertigo, of tinnitus, or of vertebral pain not previously present, such as cervical pain, lower back pain, cervicobrachial neuralgia, etc. These traumatic accidents are more difficult to treat by manipulation than are those which occur spontaneously or by trauma of another nature. One can also have increased symptomatic pain which should never have been treated by manipulation or which might have been helped by manipulation but where technique was clumsily carried out. One can especially see cases in which manipulation has no place i.e., where manipulation is done in cases of osteoarticular pathology and especially visceral pathology for many unjustified sessions— one or two a week, for months, and even more.

Some Examples of Manipulation Technique

CERVICAL SPINE

Manipulation in Rotation

This is done with the patient supine; for example, for the superior cervical area, in right rotation (Fig. 4.49). Manipulation requires three stages. First, the patient is *placed into position*, supine; the physician, standing at the patient's head, supports the patient's head with his right hand and applies the lateral aspect of his left index to the lateral aspect of the axis. The second stage is the *tension-set* (taking up the slack), done by bringing the upper cervical spine into its maximum right rotation and extension. The physician must, by repeating the end of this movement two or three times, ascertain that the maximum tension has been achieved and that this is painless. Rotation to the left should be painless, because this must be the basis for the decision to manipulate.

The third stage is the thrust, starting from tension maintained at the maximum. The physician then gives a very brief and sudden push with his

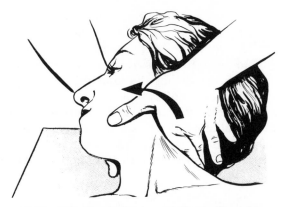

Figure 4.49. Cervical spine rotation to the right.

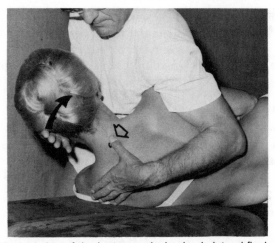

Figure 4.50. Manipulation of the lower cervical spine in lateral flexion to the right.

left index anteriorly and to the left. This should cause the usual cracking sound. Afterward, the right hand holds the head in a good position and allows relaxation.

The entire maneuver is done with both patient and physician relaxed, the physician never wrestling with the patient even when, as in some techniques, the physician uses his body to immobilize the patient.

Manipulation of the Lower Cervical Spine in Right Lateral Flexion (Fig. 4.50)

1. Place in position: The patient should be in left lateral decubitus with the physician facing him, supporting the patient's head with his right hand over the temporomaxillary area. The physician holds the patient's right

shoulder under his own left arm and presses the right portion of the spinous processes T1–2 or C7–T1 (as required) with his left thumb.

2. Tension-set: The physician's right hand, holding the patient's head, brings the neck into right rotation. He modifies the amount of lateral flexion slightly until he feels that the joint to be manipulated is being moved, thus becoming the area of least resistance.

3. Thrust: A brief and limited impulse in an upward direction with the right hand, while maintaining downward counterpressure on the spinous process with the left thumb, completes this treatment.

This maneuver can be associated with flexion or extension, and left or right rotation.

THORACIC SPINE

Mobilization in Extension (Fig. 4.51)

The patient is seated on a table, with his feet on the rungs of a footstool and arms held forward. The operator stands besides him with one foot on the stool and supports the patient's arm with his forearm, which he then places on the lateral aspect of his knee, thus causing stretching of the thoracic spine. These movements are repeated slowly and rhythmically.

Manipulation with Epigastric Counterpressure (Fig. 4.52)

This is one of the easiest manipulative techniques to perform for the thoracic spine, and is therefore one of the most frequently employed (although most vertebral pain of the midthoracic area is of cervical origin).

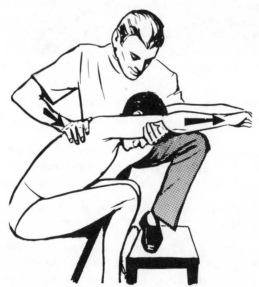

Figure 4.51. Mobilization in extension.

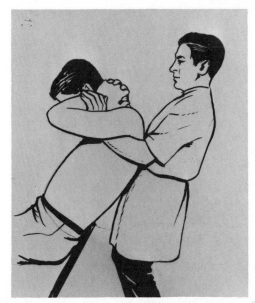

Figure 4.52. Manipulation with epigastric counterpressure.

The method is quite useful for the frequent mechanical involvement of the lower thoracic area, including back pain, pain of apparent gynecologic, urologic, genital, or intestinal origin, and even apparent hip pain.

1. Place in position: Patient is seated on the table, legs hanging, hands crossed behind his neck. The physician stands behind, places his forearms under the patient's arms and takes hold of the patient's wrists, meanwhile pressing his own sternum against the dorsal area to be manipulated.

2. Tension-set: The operator lifts the patient's shoulders and takes a deep breath, while avoiding pressure on the patient's wrists.

3. Thrust: The physician raises the patient's shoulders somewhat more and at the same time presses harder with his sternum and pushes out his chest in a small and brief movement.

Figure 4.53 shows a different technique of thoracic spine manipulation.

THE THORACOLUMBAR SPINE (FIG. 4.54)

Manipulation and Rotation

The following is an example of manipulation in rotation.

1. Place in position: The patient is seated astride the end of the table, with the physician standing behind him. The patient crosses his forearms on his chest and holds his arms with the opposite hands. For left rotation, the physician brings his left arm to the patient's anterior thoracic region and takes hold of the patient's right arm, while placing the heel of the right hand against the transverse process to be manipulated.

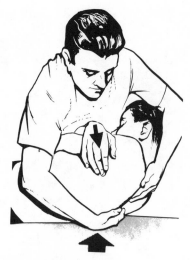

Figure 4.53. Thoracic spine manipulation, patient in supine position.

2. Tension-set: While maintaining this position, the physician turns 90° about the patient, thus bringing the patient's trunk into left rotation, and using simultaneous pressure of his right hand, attains the tension-set.

3. Thrust: This consists of a sudden, brief, and limited rotational movement, with additional pressure of the right hand.

LUMBAR SPINE

Mobilization in Lateral Flexion

Mobilization in lateral flexion (Fig. 4.55) is performed on the patient in right lateral decubitus, with the knees flexed at right angles. The physician stands on the right and presses the patient's left shoulder with his own left elbow. He then takes hold of the patient's ankles, and leans against the patient's knees with his abdomen, maintaining his own hips and knees slightly flexed. The physician then raises the patient's ankles by drawing them toward himself at the same time that he pushes his abdomen forward, thus causing left lateral lumbar flexion. This maneuver is excellent but powerful, and must be carried out prudently and progressively, and repeated slowly.

Manipulation in Rotation with Flexion (Fig. 4.56)

1. Place in position: Patient is in right lateral decubitus (in this example) with his head on a pillow and the left lower extremity flexed at knee and hip. Left rotation will be done in this case. The physician, standing before the patient, pulls the right arm so that the patient's shoulder is at 45° to the table, and then places his own left hand on the patient's left shoulder, holding it firmly; this is the fixed point, and the hand has only to maintain

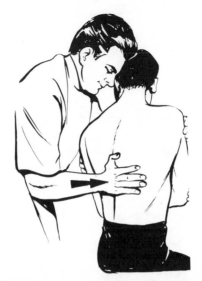

Figure 4.54. Rotational manipulation of the thoracolumbar spine.

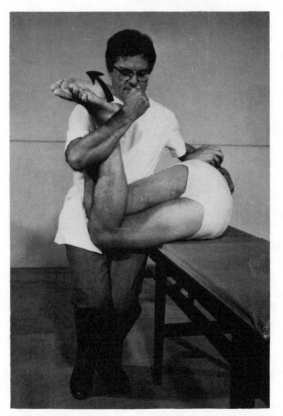

Figure 4.55. Mobilization in lateral flexion of the lumbar spine.

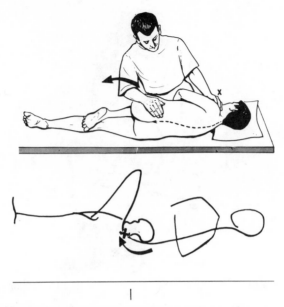

Figure 4.56. Manipulation of the flexed lumbosacral spine.

this position. Then, with the distal portion of his right forearm the physician leans against the patient's ischium.

2. Tension-set: This pressure will now be increased by drawing the patient's pelvis toward the physician and to the right, thus causing some degree of kyphosis and leftward rotation.

3. Thrust: This is accomplished by a small brief movement of the forearm, thus further increasing pelvic rotation.

Manipulation in Rotation with Extension (Fig. 4.57)

This is a similar manipulation which has a quite different effect. Instead of increasing lumbar kyphosis it increases lordosis. The patient's position is the same. The physician again has a hand on the patient's shoulder, but the shoulders remain at right angles to the table. The operator's forearm is not on the ischium in this case, but on the anterosuperior portion of the ilium. This is the most important point of this manipulation, which is to increase lordosis. The operator must be sure that the patient's leg, which is against the table, is pulled backward, thus bringing the patient into lordosis, while the operator's hand remains on the shoulder and the other (active) hand causes pressure toward himself and downward, tangentially toward the ilium, just as if one were trying to rotate the ilium forward, thus increasing lumbar lordosis. The preceding is the tension-set; manipulation consists of suddenly increasing the pressure.

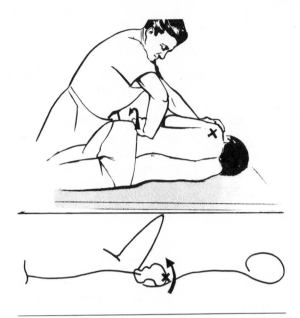

Figure 4.57. Manipulation of the lumbosacral spine in extension or lordosis.

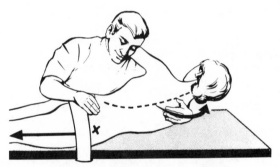

Figure 4.58. The "strap" technique.

Strap Technique

The following is for manipulation in left lateral flexion and rotation:

The patient is prone with a large strap holding him to the table in the sacral area (Fig. 4.58).

The physician holds the patient's right shoulder with his left hand, with the patient's left axilla resting against the operator's left shoulder.

Two variations are possible: Either the manipulator does not increase lateral flexion and rotational manipulation will be essentially applied in the thoracolumbar region (T10-L2), or the operator can pull the patient's shoulder beyond the table, using his left hand, and flex the patient laterally to the left to a greater or lesser degree, and thus affect mainly the lumbo-sacral area.

Tension-set is accomplished by raising the patient's left shoulder with the operator's left shoulder, while rising somewhat from the crouched position. During this time the operator's left hand holds down the patient's right shoulder. At no time must the patient's body rise from the table.

The operator's left shoulder must push upward and forward in a very slow and precise movement, thus placing in tension. The manipulative thrust is accomplished by a small additional movement.

The technique is excellent and permits manipulation of both regions described. This powerful technique should be done only by a trained operator, who alone can properly prescribe it.

REFERENCES

1. Barré, J., and Liéou, Y. C. Syndrome sympathique cervical postérieur. *Paris Med.,* 266–269, 1925.
2. Beal, M. C. Motion sense. *J. Amer. Orthop. Assoc., 53:*151, 1953.
3. Boileau, Grant, J. C. *Grant's Atlas of Anatomy,* Sixth Ed. The Williams & Wilkins Co., Baltimore, 1972.
4. Bourdillon, F. J. *Spinal Manipulation,* Second Ed. William Heinmann Medical Books Limited, London, and Appleton Century-Crofts Educational Division Meredith Corporation, New-York, 1973.
5. Brugger, A. Les syndromes vertébraux, radiculaires et pseudoradiculaires I et II. *Acta Rheumatologica,* 2 Vol., J. R. Geigy, S. A. Basle, 1962.
6. Buerger, A. A., and Tobis J. S. *Approaches to the Validation of Manipulation Therapy.* Charles C Thomas, Springfield, Ill., 1975.
7. Cailliet, R. *Neck and Arm Pain,* Second Ed. F. A. Davis, Philadelphia, 1974.
8. Cailliet, R. *Low Back Pain Syndrome* Third Ed., F. A. Davis, Philadelphia, 1981.
9. Cailliet, R. *Soft Tissue Pain and Disability* F. A. Davis, Philadelphia, 1981.
10. Cloward, R. B. Cervical discography. *Ann. Surg., 150:*1052–1064, 1959.
11. Decroix, G., Waghemacker, R., Nicolas, G., et al. Electronystamographie et cupulométrie, moyen objectif d'evaluation sémiologique et de contrôle d'efficacité des manipulations vertébrales. *Ann. Med. Phys., 8:*3, 1965.
12. Farfan, H. F. *Mechanical Disorders of the Low Back* Lea and Febiger. Philadelphia, 1973.
13. Ford, R. F., and Clark, D..Thrombosis of the basilar artery with softenings in the cerebellum and brain stem due to manipulation of the neck. *Johns Hopkins Hosp. Bull., 98:*37, 1956.
14. Greenman, P. E. Manipulative therapy in relation to total health care. In: *The Neurologic Mechanisms in Manipulative Therapy.* Edited by Korr, I. Plenum Press, London, 1978.
15. Grieve, G. P. *Common Vertebral Joint Problems.* Churchill Livingstone, New York, 1981.
16. Haldeman, S. *Modern Developments in the Principles and Practice of Chiropractic.* Appleton Century Crofts, New York, 1979.
17. Inmann, V. T., and Saunders, J. B. de C. M. Referred pain from skeletal structures. *J. Nerv. Ment. Dis., 99:*660, 1944.
18. Keegan, J. J., and Garrett. *Anat. Rec.,* 102, 409, 1949.
19. Lazorthes, G. *Le Système Nerveux Périphérique.* Masson Ed., Paris, 1971.
20. Maigne, R. *Douleurs d'origine Vertébrale et Traitements par Manipulations (les Dérangements Intervertébraux Mineurs),* Third Ed. Expansion Scientifique, Paris, 1978.
21. Maigne, R. Epicondylalgies, rachis cervical et articulation huméroradiale (à propos de 150 cas). *Ann. Med. Phys.* 3:299, 1960.

22. Maigne, R. Fondamentos fisiopatologicos de la manipulacion vertebral. *Rehabilitacion,* 4:427, 1976.
23. Maigne, R. La dorsalgie interscapulaire, manifestation de la souffrance du rachis cervical inférieur "le point cervical du dos." *Sem. Hôp. Paris, 53*:18, 1067, 1979.
24. Maigne, R. Le syndrome de la charnière dorsolombaire (the thoracolumbar junction syndrome: Low back pain, pseudo-visceral pain, pseudo-hip pain and pubalgia). *Sem. Hôp. Paris, 57*:11, 545, 1981.
25. Maigne, R. Les entorses costales. *Rheumatologie, 9*:35–40, 1955.
26. Maigne, R. *Les Manipulations Vertébrales.* Expansion Scientifique, Paris, 1960.
27. Maigne, R. Les lombalgies après chirurgie discale. Leur origine dorsolombaire tréquente. *Rheumatologie, 30*:329, 1978.
28. Maigne, R. Low back pain from thoracolumbar origin. *Arch. Phys. Med. Rehab., 61*:389, 1980.
29. Maigne, R. *Orthopedic Medicine: A New Approach to Vertebral Manipulations.* Charles C Thomas, Springfield, IL., 1972.
30. Maigne, R. Pseudo tendinites d'épaule et Rachis cervical. *Ann. Med. Phys., 18*:196, 1975.
31. Maigne, R. Pubalgie et tendinite des adducteurs d'origine vertébrale. 7th International Congress of the F.I.M.M. Zûrich, 7–11, 1983.
32. Maigne, R. Semeiologie clinique des dérangements intervertébraux mineurs. *Ann. Med. Phys., 15*:275, 1972.
33. Maigne, R. The concept of painlessness and opposite motion in spinal manipulation. *Am. J. Phys. Med., 44*:55, 1965.
34. Maigne, R. Thoracolumbar facet syndrome and low back pain (T11–T12, L1–L2). Abstracts of the 10th annual meeting of the International Society for the Study of the Lumbar Spine. Cambridge, 1983.
35. Maigne, R. Une origine méconnue et fréquente de lombalgies basses: Les articulations interapophysaires de la charnière dorsolombaire, rôle des posterior rami D11–D12-L1. *Union Med. Canada, 104*:1676, 1975.
36. Maigne, R. Un signe évocateur et inattendu des céphalées cervicales "la douleur au pincéroulé du sourcil." *Ann. Med. Phys., 19*:416, 1976.
37. Maigne, R. Un sindrome neuvo y frecuente: El sindrome D12-L1 (Lumbalgias bajas, dolores seudoviscerales, falsos dolores de la cadera). *Rehabilitacion, 12*:197, 1977.
38. Maigne, R., and Le Corre, F. Sur l'origine cervicale de certaines dorsalgies rebelles et bénignes. *Ann. Med. Phys., 1*:1, 1964.
39. Maigne, R., LeCorre, F., and Judet, H. Premiers resultats d'un traitement chirurgical de la lombalgie basse rebelle d'origine dorsolombaire (D11–D12-L1). *Rev. Rhumatisme, 46*:177, 1979.
40. Maitland, G. D. *Vertebral Manipulation.* Butterworths London, 1973.
41. Mennell, J. M. *Joint Pain.* J. A. Churchill, London, 1964.
42. Neuwirth, E. The vertebral nerve in the posterior cervical syndrome. *J. Med. N. Y., 55*:1380, 1955.
43. Nick, J. Classification, étiologie et fréquence relative des céphalées. A propos d'une série de 2.350 cas. *Presse Med., 76*:359, 1968.
44. N.I.N.C.D.S. Monograph no. 15. The research status of spinal manipulative therapy. National Institutes of Health. US department of Health Education and Welfare, 1975.
45. Oger, J., Brumagne, J., and Margaux, J. Les accidents des manipulations vertébrales. *J. Belge Rhum.—Med. Phys., 19*:56, 1964.
46. Pratt-Thomas, H. R., and Berger, K. E. Cerebellar and spinal injuries after chiropractic manipulation. *J.A.M.A. 133*:600, 1947.
47. Rubin, D. Cervical radiculitis; diagnosis and treatment. *Arch. Phys. Med., 41*:580, 1960.
48. Schmorl, G., and Junghans, H. *Clinique et Radiologie de la Colonne Vertébrale Normale et Pathologique.* Doin Ed., Paris, 1956.

49. Schneider, D. Y. Current concepts of the Barré syndrome or the posterior cervical sympathetic syndrome. *Clin. Orthop., 24:*40, 1962.
50. Schwartz, G. A., Geiger, J. K., and Sapno, A. V. Posterior inferior cerebellar artery syndrome of Wallenberg after chiropractic manipulation. *Arch. Intern. Med., 3:*352, 1956.
51. Sheehan, S. Syndromes of basilar and carotid artery insufficiency; diagnosis and medical therapy. *South. Med. J., 54:*465, 1961.
52. Stark, E. H., McFarlane, T. R. *Osteopathic Medicine.* Publishing Sciences Group, Inc. Acton. MA., 1975.
53. Toole, J. F., and Tucker, S. H. Influence of head position upon cerebral circulation; studies on blood flow in cadavers. *Arch. Neurol., 2:*616, 1960.
54. Travell, J. Referred pain from skeletal muscle. *J. Med., N.Y. State, 55:*331, 1955.
55. Travell, J. G., and Simons, D. G. *Myofascial Pain and Dysfunction. The Trigger Point Manual.* William & Wilkins, Baltimore/London, 1983.
56. Wolff, H. G. *Headache and Other Head Pain.* Oxford University Press, New York, 1963.

5

Manipulations and Mobilizations of the Limbs

ROBERT MAIGNE

Relation between the Cervical Spine and Shoulder Pain

As previously noted, some pain with tenderness occurring particularly in the supra- and infraspinatus and in the biceps brachii may really have its origin in the cervical spine at C4–5, C5–6 levels. The treatment was described in Chapter 4, under Cervical Spine. Manipulation, where possible, can improve even this type of problem (9), which is an example of the celluloperiosteomyalgic syndrome. Pain to the "pinch-roll," and sometimes thickening of the skin, is noted in the territory of the corresponding dermatome. Spontaneous pain, or sensitivity to pressure of the lateral epicondyle on the same side, may be noted when C6 is involved (2, 5, 8) (Figs. 5.1 and 5.2).

GLENOHUMERAL JOINT

Mobilization is useful in sequelae of adhesive capsulitis. The humerus is used as a lever, with the patient in lateral decubitus on the uninvolved side. The head of the humerus should be moved in a sliding manner, laterally, medially, anteriorly, and posteriorly. It is also possible by pulling on the humerus to obtain some separation of the humeral head from the glenoid cavity (Fig. 5.3).

SCAPULOTHORACIC MOBILIZATION

With the patient in lateral decubitus, the operator hooks his hand beneath the vertebral border of the scapula, and then mobilizes the scapula cephalad, caudad, and laterally, thus stretching scapulothoracic muscles (10) (Fig. 5.4).

ACROMIOCLAVICULAR JOINT

Mechanical dysfunction of this articulation can cause shoulder pain. Mobilization is accomplished by moving the lateral extremity of the clavicle

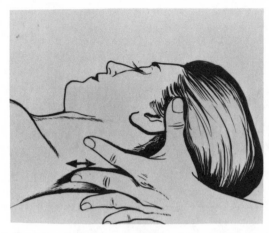

Figure 5.1. How to find the sensitivity of a cervical articulation.

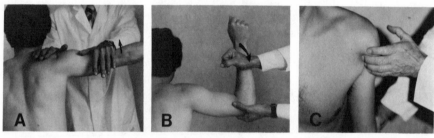

Figure 5.2. Examples of seeking musculotendinous tenderness by movement against resistance. (*A*) supraspinatus; (*B*) infraspinatus; (*C*) by palpation of the infraspinatus or the biceps brachii tendon when the above do not show tenderness.

anteriorly while the operator's other hand moves the patient's arm into internal rotation and adduction, and then abduction and forward flexion. Inversely, to cause pressure posteriorly, the patient's arm is first flexed and abducted and then medially rotated and adducted. Improvement occurs in a moderate number of cases. Steroid injection is quite useful. The combination of manipulation and steroids is even better. Dysfunction of the sternoclavicular joint can also cause shoulder pain. Steroid injection is the treatment.

ADHESIVE CAPSULITIS

In some cases, quite rapid improvement is obtained using the mobilization described above. Excellent results have been described after manipulation of frozen shoulders under anesthesia (1). It is considered dangerous by many (2). The method of "rhythmic stabilization" proposed by Rubin (10)

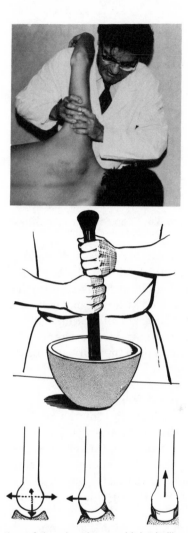

Figure 5.3. Mobilization of the glenohumeral joint is like a mortar and pestle.

may be slower, but is effective and its results are certain. The method can be complementary to the glenohumoral joint mobilization described above.

Elbow

Lateral epicondylar pain is a very frequent involvement at the elbow. Two-thirds of these conditions, like the tendon pain of the shoulder with which they are sometimes associated, are of cervical origin and are frequently accompanied by a minor intervertebral derangement at C5-6-7. The cervical area should be treated first, while in some cases local treatment can also be useful (4, 6, 7).

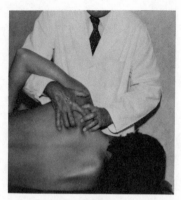

Figure 5.4. Scapulothoracic mobilization.

Pain at the lateral epicondyle can be evaluated by using three evaluation maneuvers in two different positions. The two positions consist of having the forearm either flexed at 90° or fully extended. The three maneuvers are pronation, supination, and dorsiflexion of the hand and fingers, all against manual resistance (Fig. 5.5). For pronation and supination, the patient's hand is grasped in order to give good resistance. The evaluation is graded from 0 (no pain), to 3 when pain prevents any movement. There are thus a maximum total of 18 points. Two points should be added when spontaneous pain is present, thus making a 20-point total.

Cervical origin or cervical facilitation of a painful lateral epicondyle is based on the fact that examination of the neck in these cases reveals a peculiar sensitivity of the articulations C5–6 or C6–7 on the same side; manipulation, when it is possible and effective, immediately brings improvement in the score of the evaluation maneuvers. Cervical treatment is usually sufficient (5, 7, 8). Sometimes lateral mobilization of the elbow, or local intra-articular injection of corticosteroids, may be necessary for any residual pain.

A recent evaluation of 200 painful lateral epicondylar conditions showed that, in 152 cases, cervical sensitivity of C5–6 or C6–7 was present on the same side; 80 were cured by one to five manipulation sessions in the cervical area only; two cases of more than two years' duration which had not been helped by the usual treatments required surgery. In 43 cases the improvement was quite definite but incomplete, while in 29 cases cervical treatment had no effect on either the tests or the pain and disability (Maigne, unpublished).

LATERAL AND MEDIAL MOBILIZATION OF THE ELBOW

Lateral and medial movements of the elbow joint are possible and are illustrated in Figure 5.6. These movements, when compared to the unin-

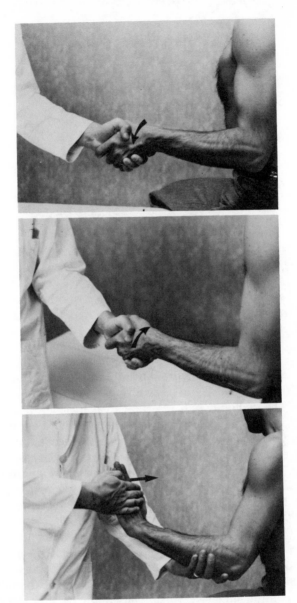

Figure 5.5. Determination of lateral epicondylar tenderness. Pain is evaluated from 0 to 3 for each movement.

volved side, are decreased or disappear in some conditions of lateral epicondylitis, whether the lateral epicondylitis is caused by cervical involvement or not. The decreased range results from a periarticular reaction or a capsulitis of the joint. Repetitive lateral mobilizations can result in a

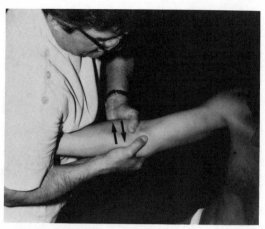

Figure 5.6. Technique for seeking lateral-medial joint play in the elbow, and also for repetitive lateral manipulations in abduction-adduction.

decrease of the pain, which is revealed by a decreased score in the mobilization test. In some cases, intra-articular steroid injection can increase lateral mobilization.

ELBOW MANIPULATION

Some cases of lateral epicondylitis—possibly 10%—occur suddenly during a rapid or false movement. In this form there is always very marked sensitivity of the radiohumeral interline to palpation. This is an inter-radiohumeral derangement, whose causes can be quite varied, but which seem to correspond in most cases to blocking of the inconstant radiohumeral pseudo-meniscus, or to involvement of the synovial fringes. Proof can be obtained only at surgery, which is rarely necessary. In longstanding cases, there is usually a periarticular reaction associated with the involvement, which makes the lateral and medial movements of the elbow limited and painful. There is, however, always one direction which is more painful than the others. This is revealed by small passive movements of the joint. Manipulation of the elbow in the nonpainful direction, opposite to the blocked and painful movement, can bring immediate and rapid improvement. Manipulation is carried out in forced adduction when abduction is blocked and painful, and vice versa, thus applying the rule of opposite movement and no-pain. Manipulation in hyperextension, or a series of mobilizations in flexion-pronation-extension, or on the contrary in flexion-supination-extension, can be used.

Manipulation of the elbow joint is divided into five groups: hyperextension, adduction, abduction, pronation, and supination.

Manipulation in hyperextension is used for anterior or anterolateral blocking of the radiohumeral articulation. It is carried out with the forearm of the patient in extension and in supination. The operator's thumb is held against the posterior portion of the radial head. A brief and short-lasting movement of the operator's wrist results in increased elbow extension.

Manipulation in adduction is used for lateral blocking when abduction is blocked and painful. This is the most frequent case. The forearm is maintained in extension and complete supination. The manipulator holds the wrist of the patient in one hand, while the other hand holds the patient's elbow over its medial aspect. Manipulation consists of a sudden movement, forcing the elbow into abduction.

Abduction manipulation is rarely used and is the inverse of the manipulation in adduction.

Manipulation in pronation is needed when hyperextension is blocked, and when supination is limited and painful. The maneuvers are those of progressive mobilization, but it is possible with patience to perform manipulation. The physician's left hand supports the elbow of the patient whose forearm is relaxed, and he holds the patient's wrist with the other hand between thumb and index finger. The physician then progressively forces pronation, at the same time maximally flexing the elbow. The maneuver is terminated by slowly extending the elbow while maintaining pronation, without returning to the point where the elbow might be painful in extension. This slow movement is repeated 10 to 15 times, with more and more insistence, while the thumb of the left hand presses upon the radial head. When forced pronation is painful, manipulation in supination is used. The operator holds the patient's wrist between his thumb and index finger while supporting the elbow with the other hand. The wrist then undergoes forced progressive supination, while the physician flexes the patient's elbow. The supination is maintained and the elbow is brought into extension again, without reaching the point where the elbow is painful. This movement is repeated several times, five to six sessions being necessary. When a long-standing case with severe periarticular reaction is involved, intra-articular injection of steroids can be added to the manipulation.

Wrist and Hand

DISTAL RADIOULNAR ARTICULATION

When the distal end of the radius is held between the thumb and index finger while the other hand holds the distal end of the ulna, it is possible to note the existence of anteroposterior movement if both hands impart movements in opposite directions (Fig. 5.7). This range of movement can be disturbed in sequelae of trauma to the wrist, and may be responsible for a decrease of the movement, or for pain on movement in pronation or supination.

Manipulation consists of a series of repeated movements, using the same hold as described for the examination. This can rapidly decrease pain and

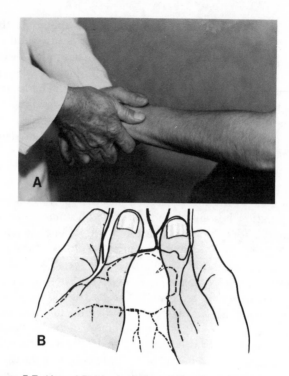

Figure 5.7. (*A and B*) Manipulation of the distal radioulnar joint.

increase movement, when rehabilitation is difficult in spite of good orthopedic results. In addition, a true distal radioulnar subluxation could be present. The same method is used as above. The operator's hand holding the radius pushes the radial head in the direction of supination, while the wrist is maintained in extension. A "click" may be heard during this maneuver. This subluxation can be isolated but it can also be associated (and is frequently unrecognized) with fractures of the distal portion of the radius or ulna.

CARPAL AREA

Some painful conditions of the wrist of a mechanical nature, e.g., sequelae of trauma, with fractures or even slight trauma, can be helped by selective mobilization. (Figure 5.8 shows traction of the radiocarpal joint.) The manipulator examines the mobility of each wrist articulation separately, using the thumb and index finger of each hand. The carpal and metacarpal areas are evaluated for induced pain in various directions. The mobilizing maneuver should always be in the opposite direction to that which causes pain. When the problem is a simple articular stiffness, progressive mobilization in all the various directions is used. A not infrequent situation is

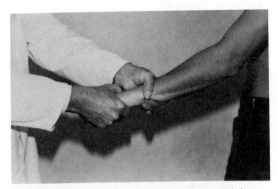

Figure 5.8. Traction on the radiocarpal joint.

that of "capitate navicular blockage," due to mechanical dysfunction between these two bones (7). This results in pain of the carpal area, mainly dorsal, increased by palmar flexion and dorsiflexion of the wrist. The pain frequently follows a fall upon the hand or similar trauma, and responds well to manipulation. Palpation reveals very localized tenderness at the level of the navicular and the capitate, much more intense when the wrist is in marked palmar flexion. X-rays are completely normal. Manipulation is carried out with the patient seated on a high table, or standing, with the arm hanging and the hand relaxed. The carpus is held in both hands, pressing the painful dorsal point with the thumbs, and pressing the anterior aspect of the wrist with both index fingers. The carpal bones are maintained in extension and the relaxed arm is suddenly pulled axially.

METACARPOPHALANGEAL ARTICULATION

This articulation is essential for the mobility of the fingers. Its freedom of movement allows the metacarpophalangeal joints to act in any desired direction. Loss of range here will impair functional use of the hand, even when the interphalangeal joints have full range of motion. This is especially true when there is a dorsiflexion contracture. It is therefore important to have good mobility of these essential joints. The passive range of motion of these articulations should be carefully evaluated, in addition to evaluation of the small degree of articular separation by traction, and also that of axial rotation, lateral-medial flexion, and even of palmar-dorsal sliding movement. Manipulation is carried out using mobilization as described, and maintaining traction (Fig. 5.9). Thumb joints are treated in a similar maneuver. For the hamate-metacarpal joint, axial traction is very useful. The first metacarpophalangeal joint is treated in traction, associated with lateromedial flexion and axial rotation in the nonpainful direction. Intraarticular injections of steroids, added to the manipulation, will help the painful and tenacious sequelae of finger sprains. Contractures should be

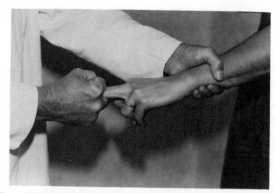

Figure 5.9. Mobilization of a metacarpophalangeal joint.

carefully prevented. The first metacarpophalangeal joint should not be immobilized in extension. Early mobilization is necessary, and should include the passive and active movements described above.

Sometimes severe contractures can be manipulated under general anesthesia, using these same movements. The articulation should then be injected with corticosteroids, and anti-inflammatory and analgesic medications prescribed. Active rehabilitation modalities can be started two or three days later, using splinting between sessions.

Mild finger sprains can be helped by axial traction movements. Post-traumatic sequelae can sometimes be helped by the various movements described.

Painful involvement of the medial epicondyle is much less frequent than that of the lateral. However, the description of painful lateral epicondylar involvement also applies to medial epicondylar pain. Here the flexor muscles should be evaluated. Elbow contracture is frequent and should be treated with passive range of motion, sometimes associated with corticosteroid injections.

"Pulled elbow" or "nursemaid's elbow" is a typical example of mechanical articular involvement, easily treated by simple manipulation. It usually occurs in young children pulled up by the hand to help stair or curb climbing. The pain is sharp and the child can no longer extend the arm. X-rays are normal. Even gentle passive pronation is painful. The operator holds the elbow of the child, using the left hand for the left elbow and vice versa. He then causes a supination movement while pushing the radial head dorsally with the thumb of the other hand. The cure is immediate.

Hip

Manipulation has very little indication in the treatment of painful involvement of the hip; nor is passive mobilization useful. Active mobilization is always better. The only useful modality is axial traction of the limb. This

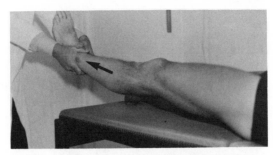

Figure 5.10. Manipulation of the hip (traction).

appears to help in some painful hip conditions, even occasionally resulting in quite spectacular relief when the hip pain is of a benign origin, the mechanism being quite obscure. For this treatment, with the patient supine, the operator holds the patient's leg just above the ankle with both hands. The operator then leans back with his arms extended, using all his weight, to cause progressive traction of the patient's lower extremity. The patient is instructed to relax as much as possible during this maneuver. The operator then gives a few mild jerky movements axially, ascertaining that these movements are painless for the patient; then, after having progressively brought the patient back into tension, the operator applies stronger and suddenly increased axial traction of the limb (Fig. 5.10). The patient is then asked to attempt the previously painful movement, which should now be much less painful.

Mobilization of the hip can be in flexion, extension, rotation, and abduction. During these maneuvers the knee should not be included (Fig. 5.11). Some continuous maneuvers, especially in adduction, also result in stretching of muscles, which can be helpful (Fig. 5.12).

TROCHANTERIC BURSITIS AND TENDONITIS

These involvements often result in pain radiating to the inguinal area or to the anterolateral aspect of the thigh, thus obscuring the diagnosis. The condition is recognized by pain on palpation of the trochanter. Trochanteric bursitis and tendonitis can be associated with hip joint involvement. Injection of corticosteroids is useful treatment. When the involvement is chronic, it may be helpful to also stretch the gluteus medius, using hip adduction.

Painful gluteus medius and pseudotendonitis, having an L4-5 vertebral origin, may have clinical findings similar to trochanteric bursitis or tendonitis. It is frequent after sciatica. Palpation reveals tenderness at the involved spinal level (L4-5). Vertebral manipulation results in immediate reduction or disappearance, both of the tenderness of the tendon to palpation, and of the patient's discomfort.

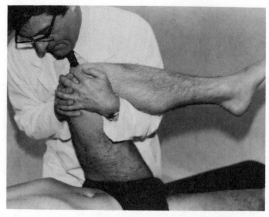

Figure 5.11. Manipulation of the hip in various planes, avoiding stressing the knee.

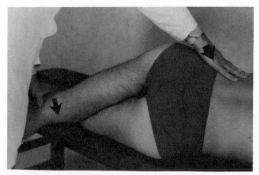

Figure 5.12. Mobilization by muscular stretching of the hip.

PSEUDO-PAIN OF THE HIP OF VERTEBRAL ORIGIN (T12–L1)

In some cases of hip pain where the radiologic examination of the hip may be entirely within normal limits, the possibility of false hip pain, caused by irritation of the 12th thoracic or 1st lumbar nerves, should be considered. Irritation of the anterior root branch can result in inguinal pain, and that of the lateral cutaneous branch can cause pain perceived at the lateral aspect of the hip (Fig. 5.13). The findings include marked tenderness to trochanteric palpation. However, this is not trochanteric pain but pain caused by the pressure of the tender cutaneous tissues against the trochanter. Examination of the corresponding cutaneous zones by the maneuver of pinch-roll will reveal this tenderness. Signs of intervertebral disturbance in the T12-L1 or L1-L2 segments should be sought. Manipulation, where possible, should be done at these levels.

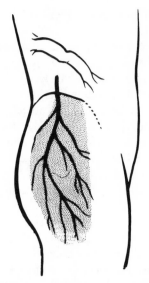

Figure 5.13. Pseudo-pain of the hip of vertebral (T12–L1) origin.

Knee

Manual treatment may be used for knee pain related to mechanical or degenerative problems of the knee itself. Manipulation or manual mobilization may sometimes restore or appear to restore anatomical integrity, for example in meniscal "blocking." It may also be complementary to other treatment, for example, in arthrosis or for sequelae of a sprain. In addition to those cases in which a definite diagnosis can be established, some knee pain may be helped by maneuvers for restoring articular movement, even when the mechanism of this disturbance is not clearly elucidated either by clinical findings or by arthrographic evaluation. These may perhaps include synovial entrapment or minimal meniscal lesions. There also may be knee pain whose origin, in spite of appearances, is not in the knee. The pain may be of vertebral origin (lumbar spine L2–3–4), which can be misleading. Knee pain can also result from involvement of the proximal tibiofibular joint. Meniscal blocking can frequently be reduced by manipulation, affording immediate relief to the patient. When repetitive blocking occurs, many patients learn to do self-manipulation; which may sometimes temporarily avoid but cannot replace necessary surgery. However, for first time involvement and when relief obtained by manipulation is complete, surgery may frequently be avoided. The second block will usually lead to surgery. This second block may not occur in spite of normal use of the knee, and in some cases even when arthrographic evidence of meniscal injury is present. Manipulation should be followed by immobilization in plaster, except in very mild cases with only minimal limitation of range of motion. A bandage to prevent knee flexion, followed by progressive resistive quadriceps exercise may be adequate follow-up.

Manipulation for blocking of the medial meniscus, as elsewhere, must follow the rule of "no-pain and opposite movement." Holding the inferior part of the femur in one hand and the foot in the other, the clinician causes hip and knee flexion. Then he abducts the knee, resulting in gaping of the medial aspect of the joint. At the same time he quickly but smoothly extends the knee with forced medial rotation of the foot (without hurting the patient). When it is successful, free and painless knee hyperextension results. When incomplete relief occurs, the maneuver can be repeated two or three more times. Requesting the patient to contract the quadriceps voluntarily or to extend the leg during the manipulation, is sometimes helpful.

When the lateral meniscus is involved, the maneuver is the inverse of that carried out for the medial meniscus. This consists of flexion and adduction of the knee with forced external rotation of the foot. When manipulation is successful, quadriceps exercises are indicated (3).

Lumbar spine pain with pseudo-blocking of the knee is the "syndrome of the vastus medialis of L4 root origin" (4). Some knee pain occurring even with blocked hyperextension of the knee may have its origin in involvement of the vastus medialis due to chronic irritation of the 4th lumbar root innervating this area (4).

This involvement of the vastus medialis is not perceived by the patient. Careful palpation of the vastus medialis will reveal marked tenderness to palpation of some areas, in addition to the presence of tender indurated myalgic cords. There is always pain over the medial aspect of the knee, more or less annoying, and this is almost always increased by hyperextension and hyperflexion. True blocking of hyperextension may sometimes be present; this sometimes appears to be meniscal blocking, and can vary from annoying to very painful. Arthrography is normal in these cases. Examination by "contrary pressure of the spinous processes" shows that L3–4 are involved. There may have been a previous adductor neuralgia, but in most cases there are no clear abnormalities in the lumbar region, except perhaps some low back pain with vague radiation. Appropriate lumbar manipulation will immediately be helpful, and the patient can immediately extend the knee completely without pain.

Anesthetic injection of the painful cords of the vastus medialis is also useful, and is an excellent test and sometimes adequate treatment by itself. This pseudo-meniscal syndrome has obviously a reflex origin. It appears as though the involvement of the vastus medialis prevents its effective contraction, and the vastus lateralis then predominates. This results in an unstable situation. The blocking mimics a mechanical one, and seems to be caused by something hard or bony. The block could be completely relieved by progressive and continuous extension were the pain not there to prevent it. Corticosteroid injections are of no value when used intra-articularly, although complete relief is obtained when corticosteroids are injected in the tender indurated cords of the vastus medialis, since these are the origin of this defensive reflex. The sensitivity of the vastus medialis, as noted, is frequently of radicular origin and is part of the cellulotenomyalgic syndrome. It is cured immediately by treating the L3–4 vertebral area.

Manual treatment of the arthritic knee, associated with intra-articular injection of steroids and with quadriceps exercise, particularly of the vastus medialis, is quite useful.

Mobilization of the patella is done progressively, the patella being held between the operator's thumb and index finger while the patient's leg is in extension. The movements will include small lateral and medial movements, proximal-distal movements, and rotation of the leg.

Arthrosis of the knee is frequently accompanied by degenerative meniscal lesions. These can cause contractures which contribute to the patient's disability. In the most frequent cases the patient cannot completely extend the knee. This small loss of range of motion, the essential cause of the handicap, may not be noted by the patient. The physician will note this while evaluating passive extension of the knee in the supine patient. When passive extension is not entirely complete, there will be pain on attempted completion of range of motion. The pain is most often at the medial aspect of the knee joint. In this case, the operator should do the maneuvers described above for deblocking the meniscus very gently and may immediately note that hyperextension of the knee is now possible and painless, and that the patient no longer has any complaints.

The proximal tibiofibular joint can also be blocked. The movement of this articulation is entirely dependent upon tibiotarsal movement. When the foot is dorsiflexed, the head of the fibula slides proximally and posteriorly. The inverse movement occurs when the tibiotarsal articulation moves into extension. Frequently, rather diffuse pain of the lateral areas of the knee is present, especially after forced flexion of the knee or after remaining in a crouched position for some time. This pain is severe at the first step, and may reappear again after a long walk. The head of the normal fibula can be moved painlessly. This is not so on the involved side, where range of motion is also quite decreased. Attempts at moving the fibula anteriorly or posteriorly result in sharp pain which is similar to the spontaneous pain. Manipulation is carried out as usual in the nonpainful direction and should move the fibular head anteriorly, as in the example shown in Figure 5.14.

Proximal tibiofibular capsulitis can be present in the course of an L5 sciatica. The joint will have a decreased passive range of motion compared to the opposite knee. The pain will disappear immediately by manipulation of the joint, using the techniques described above, sometimes associated with intraarticular injection of steroids.

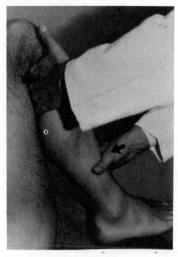

Figure 5.14. Manipulation of the proximal tibiofibular joint.

Ankle and Foot

The tibiotarsal joint (3) can be mobilized in flexion and extension, to restore complete range. It is also possible to improve the lateral and medial movement. The best maneuver is traction, which is carried out with the patient supine and relaxed. (Note position of the hands of the operator, in Figure 5.15.)

The subtalar joint can be manipulated in inversion and eversion. For manipulation in eversion, the patient lies face down and maintains the knee at a right angle. The physician holds the malleolar region firmly with one hand while with the other hand he moves the foot into inversion (Fig. 5.16) or into eversion.

The subtalar joint can also be distracted. Here the operator holds the left calcaneus (for example) in his right hand while leaning against the patient's thigh with his elbow. The operator's left hand is used to steady his right hand. Then the patient's knee flexion is increased; as it is increased, elbow pressure against the thigh also increases and this pressure is transmitted through the operator's forearm to the calcaneus. A powerful distraction movement results (Fig. 5.17).

The midtarsal joints can also be distracted, and brief movements can cause articular sliding. The thrust is applied with a maneuver similar to that used for the subtalar joint, which is also involved. The patient should be supine with the lower extremity relaxed. The hand-hold is different (Fig. 5.18). Both hands, with fingers intertwined, hold the dorsum of the foot somewhat distal to the midtarsal joint, and the foot is moved into pronation and supination.

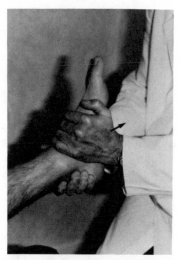

Figure 5.15. Manipulation of the tibiotarsal articulation.

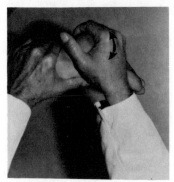

Figure 5.16. Manipulation of the talocalcaneal articulation in lateral flexion.

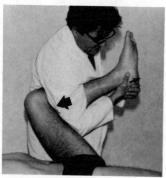

Figure 5.17. Manipulation of the talocalcaneal articulation by stretching.

The cuboid and the navicular can be mobilized as shown in Figure 5.18. The articulations may frequently have contractures or be painful. They can also be manipulated using a "thrust technique." The patient is either prone with thigh and leg beyond the table or, even better, standing, leaning with his hands on the table (Fig. 5.19). The operator holds the foot, pressing on the cuboid with both thumbs superposed. He then extends his arms so that the pressure on the cuboid causes knee flexion and dorsiflexion. Finally, when the foot is well relaxed, he makes a thrusting movement similar to cracking a whip, directing the force distally and laterally at a 45° angle. A characteristic articular separation click will be heard.

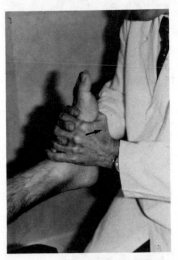

Figure 5.18. Traction on the midtarsal joint.

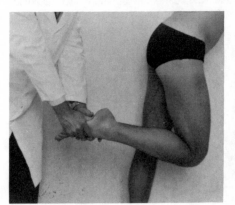 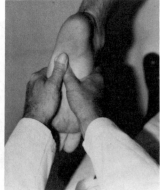

Figure 5.19. Manipulation of the cuboidal and scaphoid joints.

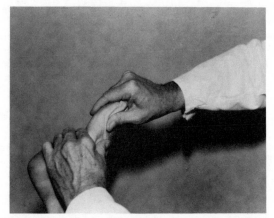

Figure 5.20. Manipulation of the 5th metatarsal joint.

The same maneuver can be performed, using pressure over the navicular or cuneiforms. However the manipulating force in this case is distal and in the axis of the leg.

The tarsometatarsal and metatarsophalangeal joints can be mobilized individually. The maneuver is facilitated by having the patient prone with the knee at right angles. The movement is evaluated or restored by the technique shown in Figure 5.20, for the 5th metatarsal. Movements of rotation and of sliding are possible.

With the foot in the same position, the operator can flex any metatarsophalangeal joint by pressing the metatarsal head in the dorsal direction, using the palm of the other hand as counterpressure on the dorsum of the patient's foot, while maintaining the patient's toes flexed. In a similar manner the tarsometatarsal joints can be manipulated. In the latter case, pressure is maintained over the cuboid or the cuneiforms, and counterpressure is provided over the metatarsals.

The metatarsophalangeal joints can be mobilized in traction and made to slide in the dorsal and plantar direction, or laterally and medially. They can also be rotated or flexed laterally or medially. This is similar to the movements of the fingers.

REFERENCES

1. Bloch, J., and Fischer, F. K. L'enraidissement de l'épaule. *Acta Rheumatol., 15:*53, 1958.
2. Cailliet, R. *Shoulder Pain,* F. A. Davis, Philadelphia, 1967.
3. Cailliet, R. *Knee Pain and Disability,* F. A. Davis, Philadelphia, 1974.
4. Maigne, R. Cotation, diagnostic et traitement d'une épicondylalgie. *Cinésiologie, 56:*113, 1975.
5. Maigne, R. *Douleurs d'Origine Vertébrale et Traitements par Manipulations,* Third Ed. Expansion Scientifique, Paris, 1977.
6. Maigne, R. Epycondylalgies, rachis cervical et articulation huméroradiale. A propos de 150 cas. 1960, *Ann. Med. Phys., 3:*299, 1960.

7. Maigne, R. Manipulations du rachis et des membres. *Encycl. Med. Chir.*, Kinesitherapie, Paris, 1968.
8. Maigne, R. Pseudo-tendinites d'épaule et rachis cervical. *Ann. Med. Phys.*, *18:*196, 1975.
9. Maigne, R. Le syndrome de la charnière dorsolombaire (The thoracolumbar junction syndrome: low back pain, pseudo-hip pain and Pubalgia). *Sem. Hôp.* Paris, *57:*545, 1981.
10. Mennell, J. M. *Joint Pain.* J. A. Churchill, London, 1964.
11. Rubin, D. An exercise program for shoulder disability. *Calif. Med.*, *106:*39, 1967.

Section

II

STRETCHING AND TRACTION

6

Stretching

C. B. WYNN PARRY

Stretching is a therapeutic maneuver to lengthen pathologically shortened structures and thereby to increase range of motion. Structures which may require stretching are: (a) muscle, (b) ligament, (c) connective tissue, and (d) skin. The causes of abnormal shortening of these structures (soft-tissue contractures) may be classified as follows:

1. Pathology resulting in fibrosis
   a. Trauma, as after burn, contusion, crush, effusion, frostbite, hemorrhage, incision, radiation
   b. Inflammation, as after infections
   c. Ischemia, as in Volkmann's ischemic paralysis
   d. Edema
   e. Primary muscle disease, as in muscular dystrophy
2. Connective tissue disease
   a. Systemic, as in scleroderma, dermatomyositis, and other collagen diseases
   b. Local, as in Dupuytren's contracture
3. Restricted mobility
   a. Physiologic, as in failure to move healthy parts through full range, resulting in such conditions as tight heel cord, hamstrings, or iliotibial band
   b. Progressive muscle imbalance, as in postural scoliosis
   c. Prolonged immobility in one position
      (1) Associated with paralysis, spasticity, or spasm
      (2) Immobilization as part of treatment of a systemic disease, such as cardiac or renal disease, with resulting contracture, as in, for example, knee flexion or shoulder adduction
      (3) Immobilization after surgical procedures, for example, after amputation or plaster casting

Pathology of Soft-Tissue Contracture

Both elastic tissue and fibrous tissue are affected singly or together in soft-tissue contractures. Conditions that lead to prolonged immobility in one position always affect elastic tissue. Pathologic conditions resulting in fibrosis and pathologic diseases of the connective tissue always produce fibrous tissue, but either group may involve both elastic and fibrous tissue.

Causes of Soft-Tissue Contracture

PATHOLOGY RESULTING IN FIBROSIS

Trauma

Trauma severe enough to cause a considerable effusion into muscle or other soft tissues, or hemorrhage, may resolve by extensive fibrosis, which in time results in deformity and loss of function. Injuries by direct violence to the limbs or trunk may cause deep and extensive hematomas, especially in the thigh and lower leg, after kicks in sports (without bone damage) and associated with fractures and injuries due to crushing. Fractures of the femur are occasionally associated with adhesion of the quadriceps to the newly formed callus, which causes an extension lag and seriously limits function.

Tendon Adhesions

Tendon adhesions are most often seen in the wrist and hand, especially after multiple severe lesions of the tendons at the wrist where the tendons are inclined to adhere either to the skin or to each other after suture. Examples of such severe trauma are: falling on broken glass or putting the hand through a window, with division of the median and ulnar nerves through a wound of the flexor surface of the wrist. The flexor digitorum superficialis in these circumstances may become adherent to the skin. This causes a 90° flexion deformity of the proximal interphalangeal joints which prevents the fingers from straightening—a very disabling deformity. The diagnosis of this condition depends upon two findings: (a) On attempted passive straightening of the fixed proximal interphalangeal joints, the skin puckers where the tendons are adherent to it (at the wrist) for a distance of 2–3 cm or more. (b) When the metacarpophalangeal joints are fully flexed, the proximal interphalangeal joints automatically extend, indicating that the flexion deformity is caused by adhesion of the tendon rather than by local joint involvement. This condition responds well to massage and stretch splinting (as described under Technique).

Tendons may become adherent in the palm or finger after suture or graft. The development of adhesions depends upon such factors as local infection, hemorrhage, severe tissue destruction at the time of injury, and the patient's propensity to excessive fibrotic response to trauma. We have seen persons with such a tendency, in whom post-traumatic or postoperative fibrosis poses a recurring problem.

Infection

Infection in soft tissue inevitably results in fibrosis. Since the advent of antibiotics, infection has to be widespread and severe before causing disability.

Vascular Involvement

The classical example of soft-tissue contracture after vascular involvement is Volkmann's ischemic contracture. In this condition the brachial vessels are compressed, usually by tissues that continue to swell against ungiving circular plaster casts or by the pressure of bone in supracondylar fractures, resulting in necrosis of the long flexors of the wrist and fingers. The necrotic muscles are repaired by fibrosis; the subsequent contracture causes flexion of the interphalangeal joints of the fingers and the wrist. The blood supply to the extensors is usually affected much less or not at all, so that there is a hyperextension deformity of the metacarpophalangeal joints due to the overaction of the extensor digitorum.

There is another type of ischemic contracture in the hand, which is due to compression of the blood supply of the palmar muscles after use of tight plaster casts or, rarely, because of direct violence at the level of the wrist. The resulting necrosis of the intrinsic muscles causes a deformity that Bunnell (2) called the "intrinsic plus" position. The contracture of the lumbricals and the interossei causes a flexion deformity at the metacarpophalangeal joints and an extension of the interphalangeal joints. This is the reverse of the claw-hand (which is due to intrinsic paralysis after ulnar nerve lesions).

Both types of ischemic contracture, when severe, require surgical correction, but in many cases conservative treatment can either relieve the condition sufficiently to afford useful function or prepare the ground for a subsequent operation, the results of which will be improved by preoperative stretching.

CONNECTIVE TISSUE DISEASE

The cause of scleroderma and dermatomyositis is unknown. Binding occurs between the skin and deep fascia and occasionally between deep fascia and muscle. This appears to be similar to the restricting action of fibrosis.

Dupuytren's Contracture

This is a specific disease in which either the palmar or the plantar fascia—or both—becomes the seat of a contracture causing a flexion deformity of the fingers or toes. It is less common in the foot and requires treatment only when pain interferes with function.

In the hand the first sign is the appearance of a nodule in the palm in line with the ring or little finger. This progresses with gradually increasing tightening of the palmar fascia, which is followed by a flexion of the little finger and, later, of the ring finger. Eventually, in untreated cases, the fingers may be contracted right down into the palm. The disease may be unilateral or bilateral. Much has been written about the effectiveness of massage, stretching, and ultrasound as prophylactics or as reversing agents, but in our opinion no conservative treatment will prevent the advance of contracture in the progressive type of disease.

Surgical excision is the only effective method of treatment. Usually passive physiotherapy is contraindicated after surgery as stretching tends to produce more edema and thus more fibrosis. However, in severe cases when the condition has been present for years, the skin being fibrotic and the surgical wound slow to heal, it may be necessary to prescribe slow gentle stretches to restore movement.

PROLONGED IMMOBILITY IN ONE POSITION

If a healthy joint is immobilized, in a plaster cast for example, a soft-tissue contracture will eventually result, and movement at the joint will be limited.

Tissues that contain the most elastic tissue, in order of importance, are muscle, ligament, connective tissue, and skin. Electron microphotographs have shown that there is a large amount of elastic tissue in the sarcolemma of the muscle fiber. It is probable that there is some elastic component in the sarcoplasm as well. It is also known that the equilibrium length of muscle is shorter than that of the resting length. Thus, if a recently denervated muscle is placed in its most shortened position in the body and its tendon is then cut, it will contract about 20% of its resting length to its equilibrium length. Elastic tissue in living muscle is always under some degree of tension. Placing a joint where the agonist is in its most shortened position and the antagonist is in its most elongated position produces the same effect on the elastic fibers in the sarcolemma, and therefore, after prolonged immobility in this position, the elastic tissue in the agonist will be difficult to stretch while the elastic tissue in the antagonist will have lost most of its elasticity through overstretching.

In the early stages after immobility this condition is reversible by means of simple stretching of the contracted elastic tissue, which produces unfolding of the elastin molecule. Although simple stretching carried out over a prolonged period may restore the range of movement in the joint, surgical division of the contracted structures may be essential before carrying out a stretching routine.

The degree of limitation after immobilization of a joint will also depend on many factors: (a) age (elasticity diminishes with aging), (b) length of period of immobilization, (c) amount of exercise performed (static contractions in a cast diminish limitation of motion), (d) blood supply, and (e) edema.

In certain systemic diseases, particularly in neurologic disorders, the combination of rest in the acute state and the deforming effects of muscle spasm may result in soft tissue contractures.

Three prominent examples may be seen after poliomyelitis: (a) tightening of the clavipectoral fascia with limitation of shoulder abduction, (b) tightening of the hamstrings with limitation of knee extension, and (c) contraction of the muscles of the back, which interferes with proper sitting or standing. In weakness of the lower extremity gravity may rotate the leg laterally, and if there is significant weakness of the lateral rotators there will be severe tightness of the lateral rotators with consequent limitation of hip function, especially when walking is attempted. These contractures are worse in the more seriously afflicted, especially in respirator patients. Other disabling contractures may be seen in inadequately treated sufferers of hemiplegia, paraplegia, and peripheral neuritis.

Immobilization after fracture or amputation is a common cause of contracture. Regardless of how efficiently a fracture has been reduced and immobilized, there is always some tightening of the soft tissues. An example is the tightness of the hamstrings after immobilization for fractures of the femur or tibia and fibula. Similarly, dorsiflexion of the ankle may be severely diminished after immobilization for longer than six weeks due to tightness of the tendo achillis. Fracture dislocations of the shoulder, particularly in the elderly, result in considerable limitation of movement not only because of intra-articular adhesions but because of tightness of the soft tissues around the joint. Here massage and slow stretches with gentle traction can help to mobilize the joint, and are best given after a session in the warm pool.

If amputees are not properly positioned while confined to bed after surgery, tightness will develop in the soft tissues. Patients with above-knee amputations, for example, develop hip flexion and abduction deformity from overaction of the abductors (if most of the adductor insertions are cut). In below-knee amputations knee flexion contracture may result from improper positioning, for example, permitting the knee to rest in flexion on a pillow. Patients with rheumatoid disease if nursed in the acute stage with a pillow under the knees readily develop severe flexion contractures which are extremely difficult to correct. The knees should always be maintained in no more than 10° flexion in splints.

Spasticity

A frequent cause of soft-tissue contracture, as suggested above, is associated with muscle hypertonus. Any lesion of the central nervous system that increases the frequency of discharge from a particular group of anterior horn cells will tend to produce contracture in the muscles whose motor units are supplied by them.

Much can be done to prevent spastic contractures by correct positioning in the early stages as described by Bobath (1). It is imperative to examine the patient's spastic limb in a variety of postures both of the affected limb and of other parts of the body.

Spasticity in an arm may be substantially reduced by placing the arm in medial rotation and extension, or medial rotation and abduction, or by altering the position of the neck, trunk, and in the leg by altering the position of the trunk or other leg. Release of spasticity will suggest that stretching residually tightened structures may be worthwhile for restoring function. If the spasticity is unaffected by positioning then stretching is pointless.

Treatment

The best treatment for tissue contracture is preventive, because, on the whole, most soft-tissue contractures should not be allowed to develop or progress. With proper positioning in bed, careful attention to frequent turning, regularly conducted passive movements (mobilization), elevation of edematous limbs, and a thoroughly cooperative and well-briefed patient, contractures may be kept to a minimum. The rationale of stretching is to improve function and posture. It is wasteful, and indeed harmful, to stretch joints doomed to remain flail.

Therapeutic stretching may be divided into two categories: (a) that used for simple soft-tissue contractures such as those involving elastic tissue and fibrosis, and (b) the contractures associated with muscle spasm.

TYPES OF STRETCHING

Passive

In passive stretching, as the name implies, the patient makes no contribution to the procedure, and the physician or therapist alone is responsible for the stretch (Fig. 6.1). Examples of conditions in which passive stretches are indicated are postfracture adherence of quadriceps to the femur, bound-down patella, contractures of skin and subcutaneous tissues after burns, and adherent tendons.

The therapist stretches the tissues between his fingers, or, in the case of a bound-down patella, the operator uses circular and side-to-side movements as used in frictions.

Active Assisted

In this procedure the patient tries to contract the opposing group of muscles while the therapist gives assistance. For example, when the tendo achillis is tight (postpoliomyelitis) the patient attempts dorsiflexion of the

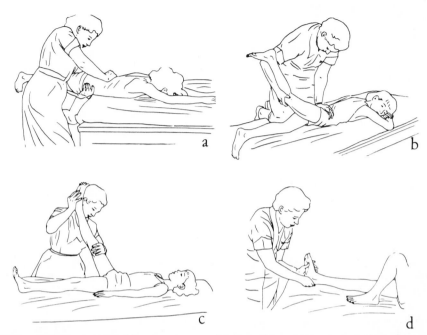

Figure 6.1. Some stretching maneuvers. (a) Stretching the lumbosacral angle; one hand supports the anterior superior spine while the other presses on the lumbar spine toward the opposite side. (b) Stretching of the iliotibial band; it is important to adduct the thigh and keep the foot medially rotated. (c) Stretching of the hamstrings; one hand pushes the heel upward while the other hand prevents the knee from bending. (d) Stretching the heel cord; the thumb supports the arch of the foot. The other hand pulls down on the heel. Avoid pushing the metatarsals.

foot while the therapist stretches the tendo achillis, or, with adherent and contracted flexor tendons, the patient activity extends the wrist and fingers while the therapist forces the palm into extension.

Active

The patient is entirely responsible for the active stretch; for example, when the soft tissues of the back require stretching, the patient can fix his feet in dorsiflexion and then try to touch his toes (Figs. 6.2 and 6.3); or, in sitting, he attempts to touch his knees with his head. Pulleys may be used, but very firm fixation must be secured if the stretch is to be adequate.

TECHNIQUE

Preparation of the Patient

Unless prevented by stiffness, the patient should be seated or lying down and in complete relaxation, inasmuch as apprehension or a strained posture may lessen the efficacy of stretching.

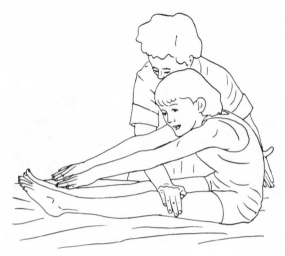

Figure 6.2. Stretching the lower back. Operator presses down on thighs to prevent knees from bending. Close observation is needed to ensure that it is the lower back which is being stretched.

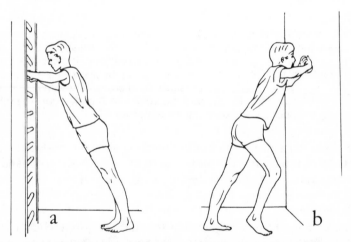

Figure 6.3. Stretching the heel cords without the physical assistance of a therapist. (a) Feet together, heel and toes remain in contact with floor, knees straight. Patient leans as far forward as possible. Stretch is increased as feet are placed farther from wall on successive sessions. (b) One cord can be stretched at a time by keeping the foot on the side to be stretched flat on the floor and allowing the other knee to bend as body leans toward wall.

It used to be taught that heat in the form of infrared, radiant heat, hot packs, wax baths, or hydrotherapy was the most effective preparation for stretching. However, we have learned in recent years that ice packs are often more effective. The local anesthetic effect of ice is very valuable in counteracting the discomfort of the treatment. Moreover, ice is of unquestioned value in reducing spasticity in upper motor neuron lesions through its effect on slowing conduction time and reducing the sensitivity of the muscle spindle. Ultrasonic treatment is often helpful and is always worth trying—it may work by virtue of its direct effect on softening fibrous tissue as well as by its heating properties.

The purpose of the stretching should be explained to the patient, who should be warned that the procedure may be painful. If the explanation is satisfactory the patient will be more cooperative. It is surprising how much fear and ignorance increase pain even in intelligent patients. If stretching is indicated and pain is anticipated, sedation with aspirin or codeine may be tried before treatment sessions.

In most cases the treatment should not cause pain, provided the technique is carefully and gently applied.

Patients must have full confidence in the therapist, and time spent gaining this in the early stages is never wasted, especially when stretching has to be continued over many weeks.

Range Testing

Always assess the range of motion in the contralateral structure or joint on the other side, for it may be that the patient does not have a full range on the unaffected side. It would be fruitless to try to "regain" a range that the patient never had.

Fixation

Stretching of a large joint or the trunk should be attempted only on a firm plinth or on a rubber floor mat. On either of these the patient may roll or crawl to "loosen up" before stretching.

Stretching of large areas requires the use of two operators or therapists: one to stretch and the other to provide fixation; it is important that only one part moves. The same therapist should always perform the stretching on the patient, for only in this way can the rate of progress and the response of the patient be known. Patients, of course, prefer to have the same therapist throughout treatment.

The therapist must never be at a mechanical disadvantage. If you are short-legged and wish to stretch a long-legged patient's leg, you should stand on a small bench, or even kneel on the plinth (Fig. 6.1b). The whole limb must be completely supported by one therapist, while the therapist who is to do the stretching grasps the affected part firmly. For example, when stretching the hamstrings, the patient's leg should rest on the therapist's shoulder while the therapist cups both hands on the knee. The least painful part should be stretched first, and progress should be made toward the most painful part.

Whenever possible, gravity should be used for assistance. For example, when stretching tight structures in the back, the patient is seated on the floor and tries to bring the upper trunk down to the knees. This saves the therapist's energy and allows a more concentrated and efficient stretch.

Maneuvers

Gentle rhythmic movements of the joint are given first to learn the range of motion and the patient's cooperativeness. When the patient is completely relaxed—and not before—an attempt is made to increase the range with gentle but continuous pressure. The pressure is discontinued the moment the patient ceases to cooperate. If the range obtained is unsatisfactory, the therapist holds the part in a position just short of the maximum range gained and then tries to regain the confidence of the patient. When this is achieved, a few more rhythmic movements are given, and these are followed by another prolonged gentle stretch. This procedure is repeated until the therapist is satisfied that the maximum benefit has been obtained in that session. It is always wise to stop if the patient begins to complain of pain and to repeat the stretch later.

The watchwords for all therapeutic stretching are: little and often. It is significant that the best results are obtained in clinics where the patient enjoys a full day's varied treatment and stretches can be given four or six times a day.

Stretches should be given in the midposition of the range. For example, if the lateral rotators of the hip and hamstrings are tight, lateral rotation should be corrected before taking the hip into flexion; otherwise muscles will be overstretched, and that is a serious error.

With children, the therapist should try to make the stretching session seem like play by asking the child to stretch for colored balls or other objects or to stretch mailing cartons into different shapes.

Between stretching sessions the part must be supported in the position of function. We cannot emphasize too strongly the importance of maintaining the stretch gained until the next session. If this precaution is not taken the formal stretching sessions become pointless. Whereas whole limbs or large joints are easily maintained in such stretched positions (as we have learned in the care of poliomyelitis patients) it is less obvious that stretched hands and fingers must also be maintained in the position of stretch between sessions, preferably in plaster splints.

Functional positions for some of the joints are as follows:

Shoulder: 30° forward flexion, 45° abduction, neutral rotation

Elbow: 90° flexion, neutral rotation

Wrist: 30° dorsiflexion, neutral deviation

Metacarpophalangeal: 45° flexion

Proximal interphalangeal: 30° flexion

Terminal interphalangeal: 20° flexion

Thumb: Half opposition
Hip: 10° flexion, neutral rotation (neutral position)
Ankle: Midposition, neutral rotation
Knee: Never more than 10° flexed

Serial Plaster Stretch Splints

We prefer stretch splints to other methods, for example, plaster shells with pulleys and elastics or springs (for gradual extension of flexed fingers) because the latter interfere with circulation and normal posture. They ordinarily do not allow function as offered by lively splints (2), and more often than not they produce a deformity at another set of joints. Attempts to produce continuous traction on proximal interphalangeal joints of the fingers, for example, by a posterior slab and pulleys and elastics, usually result in hyperextension deformity of the metacarpophalangeal joints. Moreover, it is impossible to know what force is being exerted by spring or elastic traction; it is reasonable to assume that it is often too great, as evidenced by the severe pain of which patients wearing such devices often complain.

The principle of serial plaster stretch splints is to apply to the area requiring stretch, in overall uniformly dispersed pressure (as opposed to traction), sufficient support to afford maximum relaxation. Discomfort and circulatory disturbances are thus held to a minimum. These splints are applied when the contractions are due to one or a combination of these factors: (a) shortening of structures around a joint, (b) shortening of a tendon through its entire length, and (c) scar tissue binding down the involved area and preventing full movement of structures in the area.

At each application of a plaster splint the following routine observations must be made: (a) state of circulation and presence of edema, (b) posture, (c) range of motion of all joints, (d) amplitude of tendon excursion, (e) area and extent of adhesions, (f) stretch and spring of contracted joints, and (g) the stretch and spring of tissue adhesions.

If edema or circulatory disturbance is present, the stretches should be applied only if the patient is under constant supervision. The patient should be instructed to report immediately for plaster removal if there is change in skin color or increased swelling. When the patient is returned to his ward the nurse should be impressed with the importance of making such observations and reports. The age and intelligence of the patient are important. A child will have little notion of what is meant by a change of color and may not even notice any swelling.

Whether the area to be treated is large or small, we must remember that during stretching the part should not be allowed to fall into an unnatural position; for example, in the hand, the metacarpal arches must be maintained.

When there are multiple tendon injuries following trauma at the wrist, the flexor tendons are likely to become adherent to the skin, producing flexion deformity at the proximal interphalangeal joints. Attempts to extend the proximal interphalangeal joints show a marked puckering at the site of the adherence. Treatment consists of several sessions of oil massage to loosen scars followed by slow gentle stretches for 5 to 10 minutes. The correction obtained is maintained by the application of a light plaster of Paris splint (four to six layers are usually enough) bandaged onto the hand and forearm which is worn between sessions of physiotherapy and occupational therapy. The most effective way of restoring function is by an integrated program of stretches, exercises, and activities in the occupational therapy department and in games.

Each week the plaster is kept and dated; comparison over some weeks shows progress in a dramatic fashion and is encouraging for both patient and therapist (Figs. 6.4 and 6.5).

Splint Preparation

The following items of equipment will be needed for applying the corrective hand splints: (a) a table about 2 feet (60 cm) wide, covered with waterproof material and padded slightly for comfort, (b) a bench slightly higher than the patient's chair, (c) a table to hold the materials needed, (d) an infrared or radiant heat generator, and (e) a receptacle for waste. The materials required will be: plaster bandages, 3–4 inches (7.5–10 cm) wide, a tube or jar of skin lubricant, crepe bandages, cotton wool padding, and a bowl for warm water.

The patient is placed opposite the operator. The forearm of the patient is laid on the table to obtain complete relaxation. The length of the plaster splint should be determined by measuring the distance from the fingertips to 5 cm (2 inches) below the elbow crease, for if the plaster is shorter than this the weight of the hand will press the plaster into the forearm. About six thicknesses of 4-inch (10 cm) bandage are needed. The skin of the patient's arm is lubricated. The prepared plaster bandages are dipped into water and gently expressed in the usual manner. The plaster slab is then pulled out to its full length and smoothed between the fingers to press out air bubbles (which weaken the plaster) and remove lumps, which might rub the skin. With the patient's forearm and hand lying comfortably (palm up), the plaster is laid along the hand and arm. The forearm piece is molded to shape, the elbow edge being folded back for about 1 cm to form a rounded edge. The wrist is then raised from the table to allow gravity to bring the hand into slight extension. The rest of the bandage is then molded on the hand, and the following procedure is executed: The piece of bandage over the thenar eminence is folded back into the palm so that the thumb can be fully abducted (passively) and rotated into opposition. As the plaster hardens a slow sustained gentle stretch is applied to the tight structures

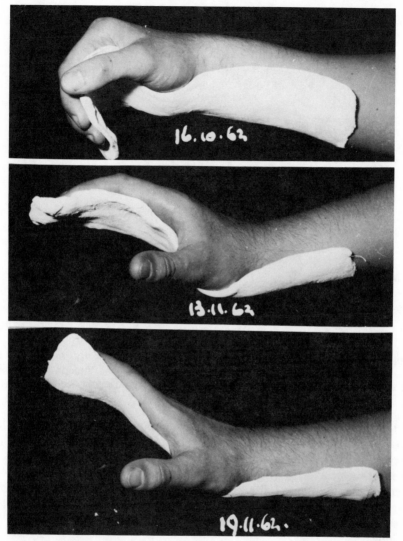

Figure 6.4. Serial correction in a patient with adherence of tendons at the wrist (from Wynn Parry, C. B. [4]).

supporting the wrist and metacarpophalangeal joints throughout. Thus the plaster sets in the position of maximum passive correction. In the early days the metacarpophalangeal joints are kept in flexion but as the deformity yields, so increasing extension can be allowed at these joints.

When, in addition, there is a median nerve lesion, another piece is added to the front of the plaster, about 10 cm (4 inches) above the wrist, covering the posterior aspect of the metacarpal and proceeding up the radial aspect

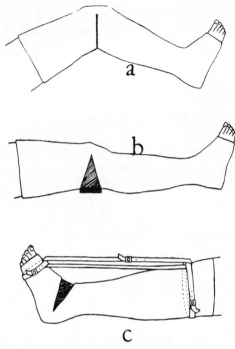

Figure 6.5. Flexion contractures of the knee respond well to serial plasters and are well-recognized treatment in rheumatoid arthritis patients who through neglect have been allowed to develop flexion deformities after prolonged immobilization in bed.

of the thumb so as to hold it gently in abduction and rotation but to allow active flexion. The plaster is then permitted to dry under the heating apparatus and should, when possible, be applied warm to the hand. Plaster conducts heat slowly. The operator must touch the plaster for at least 4 seconds to estimate its full heat before applying it to the patient's arm and hand (directly after exposure to the heating device). It should be applied with only a gentle warmth, especially in the presence of sensory nerve lesions.

A thin woolen lining should be supplied with the splint. Cotton wool batting is not advised because it is difficult to apply evenly and often becomes lumpy, especially if the patient applies the plaster himself at home. Its use may result in incorrect position or pressure points.

A thick layer of cotton wool batting is applied to the posterior aspect of the forearm and the whole is bandaged onto the hand and arm from the fingers to the forearm (leaving the fingertips free for observation). The cotton is not strictly necessary if the bandaging is to be done by the physician or therapist, but, because this type of splint may be applied entirely by the patient, it acts as a safeguard against a too-tight crepe bandage.

At night, a resting plaster that gives about three-quarter correction is applied—a fully correcting plaster splint is too painful and the patient will reject it.

This technique can be modified for individual stiff finger joints after fractures and failed tendon grafts provided that the joint is not involved.

REFERENCES

1. Bobath, B. Motor development, its effect on general development, and application to the treatment of cerebral palsy. *Physiotherapy, 57:*526, 1971.
2. Bunnell, S. *Surgery of the Hand.* W. B. Saunders, Philadelphia, 1956.
3. Smythe, N., and Wynn Parry, C. B. The use of lively splints in upper limb paralysis. *J. Bone Joint Surg., 37B:*591, 1955.
4. Wynn Parry, C. B. *Rehabilitation of the Hand.* Butterworth, London, 1958.

7

Traction

CATHERINE HINTERBUCHNER[1]

Traction is the technique in which a tractive force is applied to a part of the body to stretch soft tissues and to separate joint surfaces or bone fragments.

Traction has been used in the treatment of fractures, dislocations, and spinal disorders since the beginning of recorded history.

Hippocrates advocated use of isometric traction for the treatment of fractures of the femur, and for many centuries this was the accepted method of treatment.

In 1849, Frank Hastings Hamilton published the first of his famous fracture tables for the purpose of evaluating the end results in 136 fractures of all types. Eventually, the tables were expanded to include 579 fractures and showed poor results of treatment. Particularly poor were the results of 83 fractures of the shaft of the femur of which only nine had a perfect outcome.

To improve on these results, better methods of traction had to be devised. Continuous strong isotonic traction was substituted for isometric traction to overcome the powerful contractions of the large muscles of the thigh (64). This method remains to date an essential element in the closed reduction of many fractures.

Sauter in 1812 and Mayor in 1827 introduced the balanced suspension splint in which traction was minimal if at all present. Nathan Smith in 1831 combined both suspension and traction.

Shortly before the Civil War, the application of adhesive plaster to the skin of the leg was introduced for the purpose of applying isotonic traction in the treatment of fractures of the femur.

Josiah Cosby, a student of Nathan Smith, was the first to demonstrate the effectiveness and promote the use of isotonic skin traction for the treatment of fractures of the femur. This form of isotonic skin traction to the leg has become popularly known as Buck's extension after Buck's

---

[1] The author gratefully acknowledges the helpful comments of L. P. Hinterbuchner, M. D., and the technical assistance of Mrs. Marion Fox, senior speech therapist.

publication in 1861 advocating its use in the treatment of fractures of the shaft of the femur.

In 1847, Malgaigne introduced the first device for skeletal traction designed for the treatment of displaced fractures of the patella. It was applied by means of hooks, thus opening a new era in the application of traction for the treatment of fractures.

During World War I, tongs were substituted for hooks, their use spread rapidly, and are still used to date. In 1907, Fritz Steinmann described the application of pin traction for femoral fractures using two pins driven into the femoral condyles. Two years later in 1909, Mark Kirschner introduced skeletal traction utilizing wires of small diameter.

Thus, the last 100 years have seen the development of effective methods of isotonic skeletal traction in the treatment of fractures, their effectiveness established both clinically and radiologically.

In recent times, skeletal traction has also been used in burn patients in conjunction with skeletal suspension during the healing phase of skin grafts in order to maintain joints in proper position and to prevent contractures of granulating burned extremities (50).

The use of traction for the treatment of spinal disorders such as scoliosis and kyphosis also dates back to the time of Hippocrates. Through the centuries it has continued to play an important role in the management of spinal deformities as well as in the treatment of painful disorders of the spine, and it has become increasingly more popular in the last 30 years.

Perry and Nickel (66) in 1959 were the first to describe the halo skull traction in the treatment of scoliosis. Subsequently, Winter and his associates (85) incorporated bilateral femoral traction which led to the development of the halo hoop apparatus by DeWald and Ray (24) in 1970. Direct fixation to the pelvis has eliminated the threat to the hips that exists in the halo femoral traction system (65). Halo pelvic traction has its greatest application in the gradual correction of kyphosis, severe scoliosis, and in the management of the unstable spine in preparation for surgical intervention. The advantages of the technique are the controlled correction of the deformity, the lack of restriction of the chest and therefore no embarassment of respiration, easy access to the anterior and posterior approaches to the spine while the patient remains ambulatory. The complications are numerous and their incidence is high, including pin infections, bowel perforations, delayed onset of paraplegia, degenerative arthritis of the cervical spine, and cranial nerve and brachial plexus palsies (3, 63). The appearance of nerve involvement is influenced greatly by the rate of application of the load, with slow stretching allowing greater increase in length without disturbance of function (8). One other complication which has occurred is dislocation of the first cervical vertebra on the second (40).

The tractive force applied during the surgical correction of scoliosis also carries the risk of serious complications, the most important of which is the development of neurologic deficit secondary to dysfunction of the spinal cord.

Current advances in monitoring the function of the spinal cord during surgery of the spine has greatly improved the safety of these procedures. The neurophysiologic monitoring of the spinal cord is carried out by recording the somatosensory evoked potentials at multiple sites along the conductive pathways (25, 35, 62). Early recognition of alterations or obliteration of somatosensory evoked potentials allows the surgeon to take immediate measures to reduce the deleterious effects of the tractive force on the function of the cord, while still reversible, thus restoring the physiologic integrity of the cord and minimizing the risk of permanent injury with its resultant disability.

Studies in animals have shown that major neurologic deficits result from spinal cord injuries of sufficient severity to produce irreversible obliteration of somatosensory evoked potentials (4, 17, 76). In humans, marked distortion and even complete loss of sensory evoked potentials may be consistent with preservation of neurologic function provided the changes are still reversible (33, 34). The maximum duration of complete obliteration of sensory evoked potentials compatible with functional recovery in humans is not known as of this writing (36).

In this chapter, we shall explore the use of traction as it is applied to the cervical and lumbar spine in the treatment of painful conditions with or without neurologic deficit.

Cyriax (21) in 1950 popularized traction for lumbar disc lesions. Its use occurred to him when pondering the reason for the success of bed rest in lumbago. Realizing that the benefit arose from the avoidance of compression strain on the joint, he thought that the next step should be decompression by traction.

Skeptics, however, have held the view that the benefits of traction were unproven (79) and that there was no evidence that this time-consuming method of treatment yielded significant benefits. They have recommended that this form of therapy as a routine treatment be abandoned (26, 60). Others have maintained that traction is beneficial particularly when root signs are present (7).

Although there is ample experimental evidence that a tractive force of sufficient magnitude and duration applied to the spine produces separation of the vertebrae and of the facets, and increases the size of the foramina, no clear scientific evidence of its therapeutic value has been presented in the few controlled studies that have been reported in the literature to date. Therefore, the effectiveness of traction in the treatment of painful disorders of the spine is still a matter of contention.

Yates (89) wrote that there was no theoretical reason to expect that traction in uncomplicated degenerative spondylosis of the cervical spine would be any more effective than traction to an osteoarthritic hip or knee.

Christie (7) in 1955 was the first to publish the results of a controlled study on the effectiveness of traction in the treatment of acute and chronic lumbar backache with and without root signs. He treated half of a group of about 60 patients with traction, the other half by a bland pill (Dormosan). The patients who received traction were in prone position and received traction of less than 150 pounds. Traction was exerted until the patient was either relieved of pain or the pain was aggravated. In those patients for whom relief of pain was obtained, the same degree of traction was maintained for 20 minutes, and the treatment was repeated three times a week for four weeks. Christie's findings are summarized in Tables 7.1 and 7.2. Table 7.1 compares the results of treatment of all patients in the two series and shows similar improvement for traction and bland pill. Table 7.2 compares the results between traction and a bland pill in chronic backache with and without root signs and shows that traction, when effective, was most effective in chronic backache with root signs, bringing about improvement in 30%, worsening in 10%, and no change in 60% of the patients.

Goldie and Landquist (31) in 1970 carried out a blind study in a group of 73 patients suffering from cervical pain with radiation into the upper extremity. The patients were divided into three groups at random: one receiving isometric muscle training; the second receiving traction; and the third receiving neither exercise therapy nor traction. All received analgesics and muscle relaxants. The tractive force ranged from 25 to 40 pounds and was applied intermittently for 8 seconds followed by 8 seconds of rest for a total of 20 minutes, repeated three times a week for three weeks. Those evaluating the results were not aware of the type of treatment each patient received. The study showed no significant difference in the results among

Table 7.1.
Comparison of Results of Treatment in the Two Series

	% better	% worse	% same
Traction	30	18	52
Dormosan	30	5	65

Table 7.2.
Comparison of Results in Chronic Backache

	Dormosan			Traction		
	% better	% worse	% same	% better	% worse	% same
With root signs	17	0	83	30	10	60
Without root signs	30	10	60	24	29	47

the three groups, although there was a somewhat larger number of improved patients among those who were subjected to traction.

Weber (82) in 1973 conducted a double-blind control study with 72 patients suffering from sciatica due to prolapsed disc. The treated group received modulated intermittent traction with a tractive force corresponding to one-third of the body weight for 20 minutes a day for five to seven days. In the control group, he simulated traction by applying a force of 7 kg, which had no other effect than merely to tighten the harness. Weber concluded that comparison between the treated group and control group failed to show any significant difference in pain, mobility of the lumbar spine, or the presence of neurologic signs such as weakness, reflex changes, or sensory deficit.

Mathews and Hickling (60) in 1975 published the results of a double-blind control study of lumbar traction for sciatica. They defined sciatica as a well delineated pain posteriorly in the leg which radiates distally to the knee. They excluded subjects who had neurologic deficit, "twinging" leg pain, were pregnant, had radiologic evidence of sacroiliitis or osteoporosis, or had evidence of psychologic disturbances. The patients were allocated at random either to the treatment or control groups. Treatment consisted of traction on a plain couch using a force of 80 to 135 pounds applied through a pelvic harness while the trunk was restrained by a thoracic harness, given for 30 minutes daily, five days a week for three consecutive weeks. The control group underwent the same routine except that the traction force applied did not exceed 20 pounds, an amount insufficient to overcome the inherent friction in the system. The two groups were comparable in age, sex, and duration of symptoms. Traction produced improvement of pain in 28.8% in the group of treated patients, as compared to 18.9% of controls. The average improvement in straight leg raising was 3.1° in the treated group and 0.7° in the controls. The authors did not consider the differences to be of statistical significance.

Thus, we see that controlled studies have failed to establish the therapeutic efficacy of traction beyond a reasonable doubt. In spite of this, traction continues to enjoy widespread use, and informal accolades from many clinicians abound (55). However, some authors believe that traction not only is not therapeutic but is harmful to the tissues to which it is applied.

Weinberger (83) in 1976 wrote that traction is "irrational counterproductive, nonphysiological and traumatic." He likens the stretching or over-stretching of muscles from traction to sprains and strain of the fine muscle fibers, elastic reticulum, and intermuscular fascicles with tears of small blood vessels and states that "traction perpetuates new and aggravates already present skeletal abnormalities." He cites statistical data from insurance companies that showed no decline in cervical injury claims in the six years after the headrests had become mandatory equipment for automobiles, suggesting that the post-trauma treatment may have ensured the persistence of complaints in whiplash injury patients, and that furthermore, the traction aggravated the condition it was supposed to have treated.

It must be pointed out that although there is a paucity of hard data about the therapeutic value of traction, there is an equal lack of scientific proof that traction is not physiologically sound. In addition, Weinberger's reasoning does not take into account the psychologic factors of "compensation neurosis."

Principles of Traction

To achieve separation of spinal segments by traction, a force of sufficient magnitude and duration must be exerted. Traction may be delivered manually, by weights and a pulley system, or by mechanical devices. The direction of the tractive force may be vertical, horizontal, or at an angle. During traction, the patient may be standing, sitting, or lying on a horizontal or inclined plane either prone or supine.

The magnitude of the tractive force is dependent on the frictional or surface resistance to traction, and the resistance to stretch of the musculature and the soft tissues which account for most of the required force. A small additional force only is needed to bring about the separation of the vertebrae.

During traction, movement of the body by the tractive force must be resisted by an equal and opposite force. In vertical traction, the weight of the patient acts as the countertractive force, whereas in horizontal traction, the frictional force between the patient's body surface and the couch acts as such.

Surface resistance to traction is dependent on the weight of the body or body segment undergoing traction and the size, quality, contour, and texture of the two surfaces in contact (46). It is approximately equal to half the weight of the body or body segment (45). Therefore, a force equal to half the body weight is needed to overcome its friction. Gravity may either assist or resist traction, thereby increasing or decreasing the force, respectively.

When frictional resistance is not sufficient to prevent movement of the patient, additional countertraction of suitable magnitude must be applied. However, a force which opposes traction will be also responsible for the dissipation of energy and, proportionately, the diminution of the effectiveness of traction. Therefore, the part of the force which is lost as a stretch force must be made up by applying heavier traction unless frictional resistance can be eliminated. This latter effect may be accomplished by the use of the split traction table, the use of devices for the application of traction in the upright position, or other devices that permit the positioning of the patient in ways calculated to reduce frictional resistance.

Separation of the joint surfaces is also resisted by the muscles and other soft tissues surrounding the joints. Therefore, the tractive force must be increased by a force sufficient to overcome this additional resistance to stretch before distraction of joint surfaces can take place. These consider-ations must be taken into account in calculating the minimum effective force required to accomplish vertebral separation. In clinical practice, however, the patient's tolerance and response to stretch must be the ultimate guide in the therapeutic use of traction.

The traction force may be delivered as continuous, sustained, intermit-tent, or intermittent pulsed. In continuous traction, low tractive forces are employed to prevent discomfort of the patient because of the prolonged duration of traction, usually for 20 to 40 hours. Judovich and Nobel (47) found that most patients could not tolerate the necessary force to relieve pain when administered as constant pull. Cyriax (20), on the other hand, states that traction must be constant so that the muscles may tire and the strain fall on the joints. He also points out that it takes 2 minutes of sustained traction before the intervertebral space begins to widen (18). He therefore believes intermittent traction to be ineffective.

In sustained traction, which is usually given for 20 minutes to 1 hour, somewhat larger forces may be used.

Based on the observation that many intractably painful cases obtain rapid relief with application of adequate load, traction has been adminis-tered intermittently. In intermittent traction, and in intermittent pulsed traction which provides for a gradual increase and decrease of the tractive force, the brief periodic nature of the application permits the use of larger loads without significant discomfort to the patient. No form of traction is entirely without discomfort.

Cervical Spine

MOTION OF CERVICAL SPINE

The range of motion of the cervical spine is dependent on the ability of the intervertebral discs to respond to the movement of the cervical spine, the shape and inclination of the articular facets, the laxity of the ligaments, and the integrity of the capsular structures. The cervical spine in the normal resting position[2] exhibits mild lordosis which is primarily due to the in-creased height of the intervertebral discs anteriorly and decreased height posteriorly.

Colachis and Strohm (13) found the mean total cervical intervetebral disc height in 10 normal male subjects in neutral position to be 31 mm anteriorly and 21.5 mm posteriorly. The mean total depth of the vertebral bodies, on the other hand, was 79.6 mm anteriorly and 85 mm posteriorly. The difference therefore in the total intervertebral disc height between the

---

[2] Some authors prefer to use "neutral" position instead of resting position. The latter is more adequate because this position varies from time to time in the same individual, and it varies in different subjects depending on body build and habits.

anterior and posterior measurements in the resting position was twice that of the vertebral bodies.

Fielding (27) demonstrated by cineroentgenography of the cervical spine that the intervertebral discs narrow anteriorly and widen posteriorly in flexion, the reverse occurring in extension. At the same time, the foramina enlarged in flexion and narrowed in extension.

He also demonstrated that below C1, each vertebra shifts over the lower vertebra anteriorly in flexion and posteriorly in extension. The sliding motion of the vertebrae is greatest in the upper region with little sliding taking place at the two lowest cervical segments. The forward and backward shift of the vertebral bodies during flexion and extension is due to the inclination of the facets, the superior pointing backward and upward, the inferior pointing downward. In flexion, the superior facets glide upward and forward in relation to the ones below, and the vertebral body shifts forward a corresponding amount, the opposite occurring in extension. In full flexion, the facets are almost at the point of subluxation in the area of greatest motion.

The cervical spine shows a greater motion in flexion than in hyperextension, and individuals with long slender necks show greater overall neck motion than those with short necks.

Colachis and Strohm (13) measured the ratio of anterior disc compression to posterior disc elongation in the cervical spine. As the spine moved from the hyperextended to the fully flexed position, the ratio was 2:1, but when measured from the resting or neutral position to the fully flexed position, it was 1.5:1. On the other hand, the ratio of anterior elongation to posterior compression measured from the resting position to the fully hyperextended position was 2.5:1.

They also found that the greatest intervertebral motion in the cervical spine occurred at C5–6 interspace, both anteriorly and posteriorly in flexion and hyperextension followed by C4–5 and C6–7, the least motion taking place at C7–T1 interspace. They superimposed radiographs of the cervical spine taken in the neutral, fully flexed, and hyperextended positions in seated subjects, measuring from the second cervical vertebra to the first thoracic vertebra in all three positions. These findings are in agreement with those of Kottke and Mundale (48), who reported that the greatest range of flexion and extension occurred between the fifth and sixth cervical vertebrae, the C4–5 and C6–7 showing almost as much motion. Jones (43), however, reported the greatest motion taking place at C4–5, and Jackson (42) at C4–5 in hyperextension and C5–6 in flexion.

This variation in the site of maximum flexion and extension may be due to anatomical variations, soft-tissue differences in flexibility, and habits (5). However, it is safe to say that below C2, maximum movement, whether in flexion or extension, occurs in the region of C4 to C6, and that this part of the cervical spine undergoes the most wear and tear. During flexion and extension of the spine, the cord within the canal does not ascend or descend, but it merely folds and unfolds as the spine moves (5). The roots in the foramina on the other hand become taut and slack alternately as the dura folds and unfolds during spine movement.

Parameters of Traction

MAGNITUDE AND DURATION OF TRACTIVE FORCE

Clinicians and investigators have been trying for many years to ascertain the minimum amount and time that a tractive force must be applied in order to be effective. In reviewing the literature, one finds a great deal of variation in the magnitude and duration of the tractive force required to achieve optimal results with a minimum discomfort to the patient.

In the cervical spine, Lawson and Godfrey (52) applied 40 to 60 pounds of traction for 20 minutes. De Sèze and Levernieux (23) applied a tractive force of 260 pounds in order to obtain total separation of 2 mm between C5 and C7 vertebrae. In one patient, they applied a tractive force of 440 pounds and obtained a 10-mm lengthening measured in the anterior/posterior view of radiographs of the cervical spine between the top surface of C4 and the top surface of T1. Cyriax (20) claimed to have been able to apply a force of approximately 300 pounds by manual traction, almost doubling the total cervical interspace distances. Measurements were taken by superimposing anterior/posterior radiographs, and he reported that the distance between the upper surface of T1 and the upper surface of C4 increased during traction by 1 cm, from 7 to 8 cm.

Judovich (44) was the first to attempt to define the minimum required force to achieve separation of vertebrae. He applied continuous cervical traction of 5, 10, 15, 20, 25, 35, and 45 pounds to seven patients and noted that the earliest measurable separation occurred at approximately 25 pounds of traction. He recommended 25 pounds of traction as the minimal amount of adequate traction to bring about relief of pain in herniated disc. At 45 pounds of traction, the maximum separation was 14 mm, the minimum 3 mm, and the average elongation 5 mm. Measurements were taken from the inferior surface of C2 to the superior surface of C7. He also reported that the normal lordotic curve of the cervical spine appeared to straighten at about 20 to 25 pounds of traction but he could not obtain accurate measurements because of the variations in the degree of curvature that existed in individual patients.

Lawson and Godfrey (52) measured vertebral separation in a group of 22 patients by the use of radiographs taken before and during cervical traction, and by measuring the patient's height before and after traction. Forty to sixty pounds of traction for 20 minutes was applied by a head sling of the Sayre's type, then, in some cases, 100 pounds was applied for 1 minute. Two of the patients received traction while in horizontal position, one 6 pounds for 8 hours and the other 16 pounds for 8 hours.

Height measurements showed that there was usually an increase in measured height of an average of 3.43 mm per treatment. All patients' heights except two returned to normal by the afternoon of the day of the treatment. The two exceptions showed a residual increase in height the following day and a gradual increase in height of 8 mm over a 4-week period. The authors believed that variations in measurement of less than 2 mm could not be regarded as significant.

The x-ray measurements were taken by arcs drawn through the centers of the vertebral body from the tip of the odontoid process of C2 to the inferior border of the body of C7. The results showed that the cervical traction produced an increase of 1 or 2 mm in the arc length of the cervical spine.

Similar results were reported by Wramner (88) in 63 patients with complaints referable to the cervical spine. He used 10 to 20 pounds of traction for 10 to 30 minutes and found that the cervical spine lengthened by 1.8 to 2 mm.

McFarland and Krusen (61) applied traction of 45 to 100 pounds to six normal adults and three patients (ages 55 to 56 years) with osteoarthritis of the cervical spine. They took measurements along the tips of the spinous processes and the posterior and anterior margins of the vertebral bodies. They found an increase of 10.9 mm along the spinous processes, 6.5 mm along the posterior margins, and 2.8 mm along the anterior margins of the vertebral bodies.

Jackson (42) studied the cervical spine cineradiographically during intermittent traction and found that 10 pounds of traction was required to lift just the weight of the head but produced no visible distraction of the vertebrae until about 20 to 25 pounds of traction. Measurements in the oblique view showed increase in the size of the intervertebral foramina.

Bard and Jones (1) confirmed cineradiographically that under traction there is separation of the vertebrae and the facets. However, they found that occasionally the facet separation was unilateral or with one side predominating. They also found that the influence of traction on degenerative disc disease was unpredictable, with both increased and decreased distractions recorded. However, they gave no actual figures of the changes observed.

Taylor (77) found that in cadavers when the cervical spine was hyperextended, the ligamenta flava became compressed between the adjacent laminae and bulged into the spinal canal. This may be of considerable clinical significance in the presence of anterior wall protrusions such as osteophytes which could compress the cord as it moves anteriorly or in the presence of congenital narrowing of the canal.

Colachis and Strohm (10) studied the relationship of traction time to a varied tractive force with a constant angle of pull. Tractive forces of 30 and 50 pounds were applied to the cervical spine for 7, 30, and 60 seconds. The mean total separation of the vertebrae was measured from the lower surface of the second cervical vertebra to the top surface of the first thoracic vertebra. They found that a tractive force of 50 pounds can produce greater separation of the vertebrae than a 30-pound force applied for the same length of time. There was separation both anteriorly and posteriorly, which increased with the tractive force.

The anterior intervertebral changes, however, were less consistent than the posterior and related more to the angle of traction. There was anterior intervertebral elongation in seven of the ten subjects and compression in three. However, the mean values in the ten subjects showed elongation for every increase of tractive force and duration.

The ratio of mean anterior to posterior elongation showed a relationship of 1:5 for both 30 and 50 pounds of tractive force. Stated in another way, under traction, the posterior intervertebral surfaces separated five times more than the anterior surfaces. Traction, therefore, produced both posterior and anterior elongation unlike simple flexion of the normal neck where the movement from the hyperextended position to the fully flexed position produces anterior compression of twice the magnitude of the posterior elongation, a ratio of 2:1.

They also administered intermittent traction for 25 minutes at a constant angle of rope pull and tractive force and found that the mean separation both anteriorly and posteriorly increased, with the duration of traction reaching maximum at 25 minutes (11). Under traction, the greatest vertebral separation occurred anteriorly at C4–5 and reached maximum at 25 minutes. Posteriorly, the greatest separation occurred at the C6–7 level and increased during the application of traction to a maximum at 20 minutes. The next segmental level showing the greatest vertebral separation both anteriorly and posteriorly was the C5–6 interspace with the least amount of separation noted at C2–3 and C7–T1 interspaces.

After cessation of traction, there was residual separation after 5 and 10 minutes which was statistically significant at the 1% level both anteriorly and posteriorly when compared to the initial position. The greatest residual vertebral separation was present at C5–6 interspace anteriorly and C6–7 posteriorly. The least residual was seen at C7–T1 interspace. At the end of 20 minutes after cessation of traction, the residual effects posteriorly were no longer evident, but the vertebral separation anteriorly was still significant at the 1% level. In other words, after cessation of traction, there was a gradual decrease in the posterior but not in the anterior elongation. At 25 minutes after cessation of traction, residual anterior separation was still present, but no further observations were made past this time. The prolonged anterior residual separation after cessation of traction may be due to the relatively inelastic nature of the anterior longitudinal ligament which when stretched may require longer time to return to normal.

During traction, the mean angle of displacement which represents the total movement of the cervical spine from a specified initial position was 4°, but at the end of 20 minutes after cessation of traction, it was −1.3°. This negative value of mean displacement reflected the residual increase in total height of the anterior intervertebral discs from their initial position. This means that, at this point, there was an increased cervical lordosis. They thought this to be of clinical significance because it might be possible to reverse a pre-existing "straightened spine" with the use of traction.

ANGLE OF PULL

Crue (15, 16) was the first to call attention to the fact that the position of the cervical spine, and therefore the angle of pull, during traction could have a profound effect on the effectiveness of traction. He studied 20 patients with a history of neck pain who showed no relief with cervical traction in the supine position. He reported that when traction was applied with the cervical spine in about 20° to 30° of flexion, 19 of the 20 patients showed moderate to complete relief.

In one normal subject, the vertical diameter of the C5–6 intervertebral foramen increased by 1.5 mm when the neck moved from 10° of extension to 20° of flexion without traction. This happens because the foramina are anterior to the midline of the spinal canal and the fulcrum of motion lies not at the facets but anteriorly at the vertebral bodies. Therefore, relief of pain may be achieved by flexion of the neck alone where pain is due to compression of the root as it passes through the foramen.

Colachis and Strohm (9) found that with a constant tractive force, the mean separation of the vertebrae posteriorly increased as the angle of rope pull increased, reaching maximum at 24°. The separation of the vertebral bodies increased also with the tractive force at a given angle or rope pull. Thirty pounds of traction was applied to 10 medical students (ages 22 to 33 years) in the supine position for 7 seconds at 6°, 15°, 20°, and 24° of flexion, and 50 pounds of traction for 7 seconds were applied in a single application at 24° of flexion. A one-piece cervical halter was used. The mean separation of the vertebrae posteriorly at 30 pounds of traction was 1.6 mm, 2.7 mm, and 3.4 mm at 6°, 20°, and 24° of rope pull, respectively. At 50 pounds of traction given at 24° the mean posterior separation was 3.8 mm.

The changes that occurred anteriorly were less consistent, with some subjects showing compression and others elongation at the lower angles of rope pull. However, the mean values at angle of rope pull exceeding 15° were negative, indicating anterior compression of the disc. The anterior compression appeared to be an expression of the function of neck flexion alone since increase in tractive force from 30 to 50 pounds at 24° of flexion did not produce any difference in the amount of anterior compression achieved.

Lumbar Spine

MOTION OF LUMBAR SPINE

The site of greatest motion in the lumbar spine was reported by some authors to be at L4–5 followed by L3–4 and L2–3, the least movement taking place at L5–S1 (12). Others, however, have found L5–S1 to be the site of greatest motion (53).

The normal lordosis of the lumbar spine is due to the increased height of the intervertebral discs anteriorly, as is the case in the cervical spine.

Measurements of the mean height of the lumbar intervertebral discs in the resting supine position showed a significant difference between the anterior and posterior values: 55.5 mm anteriorly, and 25.5 mm posteriorly (12). The height of the vertebral bodies, on the other hand, showed no significant difference between anterior and posterior measurements, which were 139.5 mm and 145.5 mm, respectively.

MAGNITUDE, DURATION OF TRACTIVE FORCE, AND ANGLE OF PULL

The traction load necessary to produce vertebral separation in the lumbar spine is much greater than that required to produce vertebral separation in the cervical spine. Judovich (46) showed this to be due to the larger muscle mass and the greater frictional resistance that must be overcome in the lumbar spine and calculated that a force equal to about 26% of the body weight was required to overcome just the surface resistance of the lower half of the body. This means that only weight in excess of this amount has a stretch effect upon the lumbar spine. It follows that if one would reduce the frictional resistance to traction, one could also reduce the magnitude of the tractive force needed to produce vertebral distraction. Toward this end, various devices such as the split traction bed (23, 46) were developed to reduce frictional resistance while others applied traction in an upright position (53). In addition, elimination of lumbar lordosis or flattening of the lumbar spine before the application of traction allowed further reduction of the tractive force required to produce vertebral distraction, because flexion of the lumbar spine is known to separate the vertebral bodies posteriorly. It has been reported that pain subsides more rapidly under traction when the lumbar spine is in slight flexion (45). Therefore, in lumbar traction as in cervical traction, the proper positioning of the patient or, stated in another way, the proper angle of pull, is essential in reducing the tractive force required for optimal results, thus making traction more tolerable for the patient.

Some investigators have used several hundred pounds of traction to bring about minimal vertebral separation in the lumbar spine. De Sèze and Levernieux (23) estimated that a tractive force of 730 pounds was required to obtain a separation of 1.5 mm at L4–5 vertebral level and that 810 pounds were required to obtain a separation of 2 mm at L3–4 level. They estimated that 400 pounds of this force was required to overcome the mechanical resistance of the apparatus.

In postmortem specimens consisting of segments of spine with muscles removed, a traction force of 9 kg was sufficient to overcome the resistance of the fibroligamentous structures producing 1.5 mm of elongation between two lumbar vertebrae (23). In living tissues, however, high forces are necessary to achieve the same degree of separation because of the resistance to stretch offered by the musculature.

Frazer (30) considered the amounts recommended by de Sèze and Levernieux excessive and used 300 to 400 pounds for 4 to 5 minutes, while Cyriax (21) advocated the use of 100 to 200 pounds for ½ to 1 hour. Crisp (14) was able to use effectively a force of only 40 to 80 pounds applied for 15 to 20 minutes by eliminating friction between the body and the traction table.

The massive tractive forces recommended by some authors are of no practical value in a clinical setting and are difficult for the patient to endure. Furthermore, when large tractive forces are applied, it is necessary to stabilize the patient through the application of countertraction with a harness in the lower thorax which causes discomfort, makes breathing difficult, and, in obese persons, produces a tendency to faint, probably from decreased venous return. More than half of the volunteers in the Lehman and Brunner (53) experiments felt an uncomfortable stretch in the lumbar area at traction levels between 300 and 400 pounds. In addition, the use of forces above the range of 50 to 100 pounds requires specialized mechanized equipment which may not be readily available to the practicing physician.

Lehman and Brunner (53) delivered 100, 200, and 300 pounds of lumbar traction with a hydraulic device to 19 healthy subjects, ages 18 to 30 years, in an upright position with a buildup and release of the traction each within 30 seconds. It was found that significant widening of the intervertebral spaces occurred at traction of 200 to 300 pounds.

In another group of 19 volunteers, traction of 300 pounds was applied for 5 minutes. The results monitored by x-rays taken at rest during traction and 30 minutes after traction showed an intervertebral separation of 2.6 mm at L5–S1 interspace, 1.5 mm at L4–5 interspace, and 1.3 mm at L3–4 interspace. The widening occurred mainly between the posterior aspects of the vertebrae but some widening was also present anteriorly. This is important in clinical practice, because posterior elongation may not be effective unless there is either some anterior separation or at least there is no significant anterior compression. The mechanical effects of the traction could not be demonstrated 30 minutes after cessation of traction. Colachis and Strohm (12), on the other hand, found residual separation still present 10 minutes after traction, at which time they terminated their observations.

Lehman and Brunner (53) selected a series of 10 patients with the diagnosis of a degnerative L5–S1 intervertebral disc and gave them 5 to 11 treatments, each consisting of 5 to 15 minutes of traction up to 300 pounds applied intermittently as tolerated. The diagnosis was based on clinical examination and x-ray findings. All patients had "objective" signs of backache before treatment was started. All patients were on bedrest and received radiant heat and massage. After the treatment, five patients had lost part or all of the "objective" signs of backache while the other five still had them. All 10 patients improved subjectively. The nature of the "objective" signs of backache was not specified.

Lawson and Godfrey (52) applied lumbar traction of 100 or 150 pounds to six subjects in a Scott traction frame through a thoracic girdle while a pelvic girdle was anchored to the bed. Although the authors believed that there was no statistically significant change, they reported an average increase in body height up to 4 mm after traction.

Worden and Humphrey (87) applied tractive forces up to 132 pounds for approximately 60 minutes in five normal subjects. The forces were divided between the head and thorax, the pelvis and ankles. Increases in standing height before and after traction were recorded ranging from 1 to 30 mm, with an average increase of 8 mm in the relaxed standing position and 11.5 mm in the "tall" standing position.

Colachis and Strohm (12) studied the effects of pelvic traction on vertebral separation in the lumbar spine. Ten subjects, ages 22 to 25 years, were positioned supine on a split table with their legs elevated on a stool parallel to the split table, the thighs at 70° of flexion. This position reduced the frictional resistance and made the application of 50 and 100 pounds an effective tractive force. In a series of successive applications of traction, they first applied 50 pounds of intermittent traction for 15 minutes followed by 10 minutes of rest, then 100 pounds of intermittent traction for 15 minutes followed by 5 minutes of rest, followed immediately by the application of 100 pounds of continuous traction for 5 minutes. The angle of pull in all subjects was approximately 18°. Three lateral radiographs were taken before, during, and after traction of all subjects in the supine, the Thomas, and the curl position with both hips and legs completely flexed and measurements taken from the anterior-superior apex of S1 to the same point of L1.

The results showed that the mean total posterior separation along the lumbar vertebrae increased as the tractive force increased, while the mean total anterior separation decreased minimally during traction. Also during traction, the posterior elongation was much greater than the anterior compression. When 50 pounds of intermittent force was applied, there was a ratio of anterior compression to posterior elongation of 1:3; when 100 pounds of intermittent force was exerted, the ratio was 1:4.5; and when 100 pounds of continuous force was employed, it was 1:3. This represents a reversal in the normal relationship of the vertebral movement in the lumbar spine brought about by traction. During normal movement without traction, the ratio of anterior compression to posterior elongation was 1.4:1. Ten minutes after traction ceased, there was residual posterior separation of the vertebrae measuring 1.75 mm, which was statistically significant at the 5% level.

Therefore, the increase in posterior separation reported in this study may represent the effects of each tractive force plus the residual separation from the preceding application inasmuch as the rest period between each application did not exceed the period in which residual separation is still present, namely, 10 minutes. Lehman and Brunner (53), as already noted, found no statistically significant residual separation 30 minutes after cessation of traction.

Masturzo (57) carried out discograms to study the resistance of the disc to compressive and tractive forces. He applied forces up to 200 pounds to produce both distraction and compression of the lumbar spine in normal subjects and patients suffering from disc syndrome. He found that in normal subjects there was little or no modification in the size and shape of the intervertebral space, whereas in the presence of rupture of the annulus fibrosus there were changes which were greater during compression than during traction. This is in accord with the findings of Hirsch and Nachemson (38) who showed that degenerative discs in fresh autopsy specimens of lumbar spines were more sensitive to compression than normal discs. Masturzo also found that in the presence of osteophytes there was little increase in the intervertebral space under traction, but there was a remarkable decrease of the space under compression. He concluded that variations exceeding 10% of the disc area under the influence of traction or compression are an indication of pathology of the disc.

In epidural injections of contrast medium used to outline the posterior aspects of the lumbar discs, separation of lumbar vertebrae by traction was demonstrated, the extent of which was only significant when a disc prolapse was present (58). During traction, there was flow of contrast medium beyond the line of the posterior longitudinal ligament into the disc spaces, suggesting the presence of a suction force (59). Traction reduced the extent of lumbar disc prolapse, but shortly after release of traction the filling defects reappeared. Nevertheless, in clinical practice, the therapeutic use of traction may bring about lasting relief of symptoms.

Clinical Application of Traction

Traction has long been in use in the management of painful disorders of the neck and back. Used judiciously, the results may be beneficial, but the clinician must be aware of its potential dangers.

Traction as a rule should not be administered until complete workup has been carried out, a definitive diagnosis has been made, and specific indications for traction have been established.

Complete workup consists of a careful history, physical examination, and diagnostic radiographies of the spine, with anterior/posterior, lateral, and oblique views. Minimal laboratory workup should include a complete blood count, sedimentation rate, urinalysis, serum calcium and inorganic phosphate, serum alkaline phosphatase, and acid phosphatase in men, blood urea nitrogen, 2-hour postprandial blood sugar, and plasma protein electrophoresis.

In clinical practice, traction is usually administered in conjunction with heat, massage, and immobilization. Exercises and manipulations (32) may also be used if indicated.

PATHOGENESIS OF PAIN

The pathogenesis of pain in painful disorders of the neck and back is poorly understood. It is well accepted that irritation or compression of a nerve root will cause pain, but its exact mechanism has not been established.

It is believed that compression of the root alone may not be sufficient to cause pain, but that movement and entrapment of the nerve are essential elements in the causation of pain (5). It is also considered possible that pain may be due to impaired circulation associated with stretching of the root and its dural sheath (5).

However, pain in the cervical and lumbar area may be present without evidence of root involvement. This pain presents even a greater challenge to the practicing physician because of its frequency and the uncertainty of its causes.

Crisp (14) believes that the source of pain is the osteoarthritis and capsulitis resulting from the erosion of the articular cartilage in the vertebral joints. He suggests that pain may also arise from subluxation of the facets or locking of the facets due to a loose body, or it may be caused by a "nipped" synovial membrane (14, 72). The latter may happen when the synovial membrane prolapses between the facets and becomes impacted, giving rise to pain.

Cyriax (18) discards this theory, believing that the synovial membrane is devoid of nerves and that pain cannot arise from it; Bauer and his associates (2), however, state that the existence of nerve elements in the synovial tissue has been reported with great unanimity. They quote a study by Gerneck in which he reported the presence of a "myelinated ground plexus" and a "superficial plexus of nonmyelinated fibres." Both vasomotor and sensory functions were postulated on the basis of the type of end organs found.

Pain may also arise in the anterior or posterior longitudinal ligament, or the capsular tissue. Finally, it may originate in the muscles themselves, either from direct causes or by reflex mechanism.

According to Frazer (30), it was Covalt's opinion that the principal factor in backache was psychologic. This opinion has been voiced by others at various forums. Unfortunately, it is not uncommon to suggest psychogenic origin of a symptom complex when there is paucity of objective findings on physical or radiologic examination. In the low back, this becomes reinforced by the fact that gross degenerative changes of the spine may be present radiologically in patients who have little or no symptoms.

Nevertheless, considering our present state of knowledge, it is accurate to say that the whole story about pain and of backache in particular is not yet known, even though the influence of psychologic factors in the origin of pain and in the reactivity of the individual patient to pain cannot be minimized.

The difficulty is further compounded by a plethora of theories and opinions and by the indiscriminate use of terminology the medical practioners apply to description of abnormalities leading to painful syndromes of the cervical and lumbar spine. Some speak of osteoarthritis of the spine as being sharply different from spondylosis (74). Others use the terms interchangeably or simply refer to "changes" which may consist from a simple stiff neck without objective or radiologic abnormalities to changes in the posterior articular facets, the joints of Luschka, narrowing of the intervertebral spaces, and spurring along the anterior or posterior borders of the vertebral bodies. Irritation or compression of nerve roots may also be present associated with weakness, atrophy, or sensory impairment, and in very severe cases the "changes" may cause direct pressure on the spinal cord posteriorly, leading to a central spinal cord syndrome (69).

Still others prefer to use the general term of cervical or low back syndrome to signify a group of symptoms and clinical findings that occur as a result of involvement of the roots in the intervertebral foramina, the pathology consisting of narrowing and protrusion of the intervertebral discs, osteophyte formation at the margins of adjacent vertebral bodies, osteoarthritis and periarthritis of the posterior intervertebral joints, inflammation and fibrosis of the meningeal sleeve investing the nerve roots, and local interference with the blood supply of the roots caused by osteophytes (81). Frazer (30) states that backache often falls into the category of nonarticular rheumatism.

INDICATIONS FOR TRACTION

From the available evidence, it is apparent that the main effects of traction on the vertebral articulations are mechanical and consist of (a) distraction of the vertebral bodies with enlargement of the intervertebral space producing a suction effect; (b) stretching of muscles and ligaments, with the tautening of the posterior longitudinal ligament exerting a centripetal force on the adjacent annulus fibrosus; (c) separation of the apophysial joints; and (d) enlargement of the foramina. Therefore, the therapeutic use of traction should be limited to those painful conditions of the spine where the mechanical effects of traction would be expected to produce improvement. These are generally conceded to be painful conditions due to irritation or compression of nerve roots whether from trauma, degenerative process, or disc protrusion.

In disc lesions, Cyriax (20) recommends the use of traction only in "pulpy" protrusions and in indeterminate protrusions where manipulation has failed to produce relief. Masturzo (57), on the other hand, believes that traction can be successful only during the early stages of disc pathology. He describes three stages of intervertebral disc involvement, the first showing dehydration and loss of elasticity of the nucleus pulposus with fibrillary degeneration, the second showing rupture of the annulus fibrosus, and the third showing production of osteophytes. He believes that traction can be successful only during the first two stages, because in the third stage the osteophytes do not permit the vertebral space to enlarge. This differs from the recommendations of other investigators who believe that traction is contraindicated in purely annular displacements (21). By and large, however, most clinicians apply traction in the presence of discogenic abnormalities regardless of their specific nature, except in midline protrusions of cervical herniated discs because of the possibility of cord damage (19, 44).

In low back pain, some authors recommend traction in all cases except in the presence of malignancies and infectious diseases (37). Others disagree.

In fact, there is a great deal of contradiction in the literature regarding the value of traction in lumbago, and in sciatica with neurologic deficit. The disagreement arises partly from the lack of precise definition of terms and even more so from the lack of precise etiology of these two symptoms. Cyriax (19) emphasizes the absolute contraindication of traction in acute lumbago and the lack of any value of the use of traction in sciatica with neurologic deficit. Christie (7), on the other hand, has shown that in chronic backache, when effective, traction was most effective in the presence of neurologic signs. Hood and Chrisman (41) reported good results in 57.5% of a group of 40 patients with low back pain, all of whom, except one, had radiation of pain to the leg. De Sèze and Levernieux (23) gave traction to patients with lumbago and sciatica and reported good results in 71% and 68%, respectively. The group of patients treated included both acute and chronic cases with 89% of the cases with acute lumbago and 70% of those with chronic lumbago showing improvement. In sciatica, 93% showed improvement if the symptoms were of less than one month's duration, but only 60% if the symptoms were of one year's duration or longer. Based on this, they recommended early application of traction. Other investigators found no correlation between the duration of the symptoms and the results of the treatment (81).

Traction has also been used for recurrent pain after laminectomy although this is not universally recommended. Judovich and Nobel (47) failed to obtain relief by traction in one patient, whereas Cyriax (20) reported traction to have been effective; Cyriax has also used traction in spondylolisthesis with secondary disc lesion in a small number of patients, with relief of pain.

Traction in the form of Buck's extension has been used frequently for immobilization with the full knowledge that no effects other than those attributed to immobilization are to be expected.

Finally, traction may be used for diagnostic purposes in rare cases when the diagnosis cannot be established in spite of thorough investigation.

CONTRAINDICATIONS FOR TRACTION

Traction is not indicated in all painful conditions of the neck or low back; it is contraindicated in some and dangerous in others (37).

The main contraindications for traction are:

1. Malignancy, either primary or metastatic. LaBan and Meerschaert (49) reported two patients presenting with marked paravertebral cervical and shoulder pain associated with radiographic evidence of severe cervical degenerative disc disease who were rendered quadriplegic when treated with intermittent heavy, overhead cervical traction. They were subsequently shown to have had extradural metastasis from a previously unrecognized prostatic adenocarcinoma. The clinician should be alert to this possibility in elderly males.

2. Cord compression. Traction should never be applied in the presence of signs of compression of the cord. Instead the patient should be referred for neurologic evaluation and possible neurosurgical intervention.

3. Infectious diseases of the spine, such as tuberculosis.

4. Osteoporosis.

5. Hypertension or cardiovascular disease.

6. Rheumatoid arthritis because of the instability, subluxation, and damage of the ligamentous structures seen in rheumatoid arthritis.

7. Old age.

8. Pregnancy.

Cyriax (19) cautions against the indiscriminate use of traction in the presence of compression of the fourth sacral root from a disc, because paralysis of the bladder may develop. Similarly, traction should be applied with great caution or not at all in midline protrusions of herniated discs in the cervical spine because of the possibility of cord damage under traction (19, 44). In the cervical spine, traction is also contraindicated in the presence of atherosclerotic obstruction of the carotid or vertebral arteries which may be exacerbated by pressure on the neck with disastrous results.

In lumbar traction, further contraindications cited are the presence of active peptic ulcers, hiatus hernia or other hernias, aortic aneurysm, and gross hemorrhoids.

Frazer (30) quoted the European literature in which, out of 25,000 tractions reported, only six untoward sequelae resulted. One was an apophysial articulation dislocation, one a cardiovascular reaction in mitral disease, one a paresis of the leg after the disappearance of sciatica, and three were "hyperalgic" reactions.

Technique of Application of Traction

CERVICAL SPINE

Traction of the cervical spine may be applied manually or by a head halter. Manual traction is usually given in combination with manipulation of the cervical spine. The patient may lie prone but usually lies supine with the physician standing at the side of the patient's head. The operator's hands are placed on the head of the patient, the right hand holding the occiput, the left placed under the chin and traction applied in flexion, extension, or rotation.

Although manual traction has the advantage of greater control of the position of the head, in this country traction is rarely given manually. Instead, a head halter or head sling is used (Fig. 7.1).

The head halter is connected to a crossbar which is then attached to a weight by a cord running over a pulley (37), or may be connected to a mechanical device.

There are several types of head halters, the most common being the Sayre or modified Sayre sling. Disposable types have appeared on the market in the last few years (71).

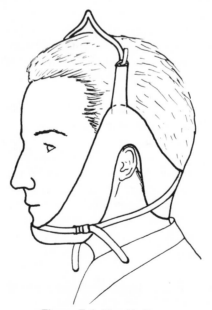

Figure 7.1. Head halter.

Traction by a head halter may be exerted either in the horizontal or inclined position or in vertical position, usually sitting. Some authors prefer the sitting position because the patient may be more relaxed and because there is no contact of the head with the couch, thus eliminating frictional resistance. However, this position, if totally unsupported, may be less stable, permitting the patient to move, altering the line of pull, and interfering with the effectiveness of traction. Because of this, others prefer the patient in the supine position in which he is fully supported. When cervical traction is given on an inclined plane, the body weight is used as the tractive force (Fig. 7.2). As the angle of inclination increases, so does the amount of weight applied to the cervical spine.

The angle of rope pull in cervical traction should be at about 20° to 25° of forward flexion. This requires that greater pull be applied to the occipital part of the halter rather than the part under the chin. There should be no pressure along the large vessels of the neck or over the ears, and the side straps should be so attached as to prevent slippage of the halter. However, no head halter is entirely effective or comfortable even when properly fitted because the occipital protuberance is not adequate for the secure attachment of the posterior piece of the halter.

In the beginning, light traction is used until the patient becomes accustomed to it, and then the force is slowly increased. The progressive increase of the duration of traction may prevent development of dizziness or nausea (78). Effective cervical traction is achieved at the range of 20 to 35 pounds. No traction of the cervical spine takes place until the weight used exceeds that of the weight of the head.

During traction, the temporomandibular joint becomes a weight-bearing joint because force is transmitted to the joint through the chin portion of the head halter, the mandible, and the teeth. This effect becomes exacerbated when the halter is so fitted as to cause extension of the neck. When

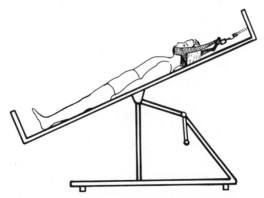

Figure 7.2. Cervical traction on an inclined plane.

dental occlusion is normal and traction is delivered at a proper angle, this stress produces no discomfort to the patient. However, in the absence of the posterior teeth, the temporomandibular joint dysfunctions and pain results. Restoration of the dentition by partial dentures or use of bite splints should serve to deflect the stress forces away from the temporomandibular joint (28, 29, 75).

Traction is usually administered in a series of treatments given daily for seven to ten days or three times a week for three to four weeks. Treatment may be given daily only during the initial phase followed by treatment on alternate days or three times a week for a total period of treatment of three to four weeks. If relief of pain is not achieved by the end of this period, traction is usually discontinued.

In most series reported in the literature, patients underwent traction for 10 to 12 sessions within a period of three to four weeks.

Cyriax (20) has recommended daily treatments for two months in long-standing backache in "youngish" persons who show marked limitation of straight leg raising on both sides while all other movements of the lumbar spine are painless and of full range.

In painful syndromes of the neck and low back, recurrence of symptoms is not unusual. Upon recurrence of symptoms, traction may be repeated and a new series of treatments given as described above. Levernieux (54) recommends the preventive use of traction two to three times a year in cases of recurrent low back pain of long standing.

Cervical traction may also be delivered by mechanical devices activated hydraulically (23, 68) or by a motor. The reader is referred to the Chapter 8 for a description of these devices.

Cervical traction may be given in the hospital on an inpatient or outpatient basis, in the office, or in the patient's home (68).

The apparatus for home use is similar to the one described for hospital use, consisting of a head halter attached to a bar with a rope going over a pulley with a weight at the end of the rope. It may be used over a door with the patient sitting in a chair facing the frame of the door (Fig. 7.3). Special instructions must be given to the patient as to the optimal position which grossly is one that permits the patient to read a book while traction is applied (51). Should the patient sit improperly, for example, with his back to the door, the cervical spine will be pulled in extension during traction; this defeats the purpose of the traction (67). Poor technique may lead not only to poor results but to aggravation of the condition for which traction is applied. Instructions should also be given as to the amount of tractive force to be used as well as the frequency of the treatment sessions. Usually home traction is given for 5 to 20 minutes, either daily for one week or three times a week for three weeks, using a tractive force which is at first sufficient to condition the patient to traction, then slowly increasing the weights and reaching approximately 15 to 25 pounds of weight. Traction

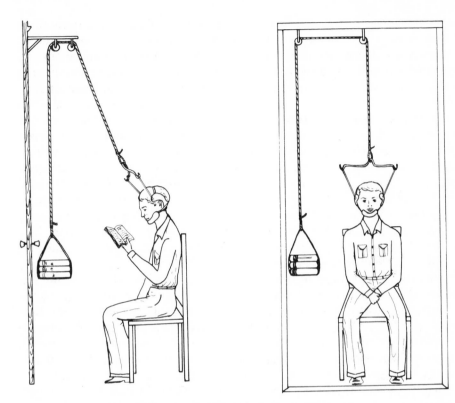

Figure 7.3. Cervical traction at home.

may be maintained for 15 to 20 minutes continuously if tolerated, but may be interrupted from time to time if the patient experiences discomfort. This is done by having the patient lift the weight for a few minutes and then reapplying it.

During the period of home traction, the patient should return regularly to the physician for reevaluation. In the series of Martin and Corbin (56), none of the patients who used the traction at home reported any untoward effect even though some of the patients continued to use traction intermittently for many months after discharge. Caldwell and Krusen (6), on the other hand, in a comparative study of the use of different methods of traction in the treatment of neck problems, state that constant traction at home had not been found satisfactory.

LUMBAR SPINE

Traction to the lumbar spine may be delivered in the upright position, the horizontal position, or at an inclined level. The simplest way is having the patient hang from an overhead bar or beam by his arms, using the body weight as the tractive force (37). In the lumbar spine, manual traction is not practical because large tractive forces are required. Traction, therefore, is applied either by weights and a pulley system, or by mechanical devices. The weight and pulley system usually delivers continuous traction, but the heavy traction required in lumbar spine is better tolerated when administered intermittently (47) by motorized devices which are described in Chapter 8. However traction is delivered, purchase on the body must be well secured, usually by straps or corsets. Care should be taken, however, not to apply the corsets more tightly than necessary and not without adequate padding to avoid discomfort (39). The pelvic corset or pelvic harness is attached by cords or straps to a spreader bar from which the cord goes over a large pulley mounted to a bracket which in turn is attached to the frame of the bed. Countertraction for stabilization of the body and prevention of movement is applied through the use of a thoracic corset. The thoracic harness may embarrass respiration and, in obese individuals, it may be difficult to keep in place.

To reduce frictional resistance, various split traction tables have been devised enabling the delivery of effective traction with lesser loads and the better localization of traction to a particular segmental level of the spine (23, 46) (Fig. 7.4). A simple split traction table consists of two sections: one fixed, the other mobile. The lower part of the body is placed on the mobile section with the segment of the spine upon which traction is to be applied placed at the junction of the two sections. When the lower section of the table is moved, the lower part of the body moves with it and no longer offers resistance to traction. Therefore, the dissipation of the tractive force from the surface resistance is eliminated.

Sheffield (73) adapted a tilt table which utilizes the element of gravity by suspending the body to produce lumbar traction which increases as the angle of tilt increases. The top of the table is highly polished to eliminate friction. The patient may be positioned on this table either in a normal position with head up and feet down, or in reverse, feet up and head down. In addition, special tables were designed to deliver simultaneously other modalities of treatment. Worden's table (86) includes a built-in heating pad, a soft rubber roller that applies an upward thrust to the spinal column plus mechanical oscillations if desired. Weinstein and Gordon (84) designed

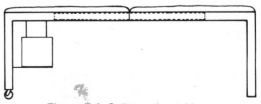

Figure 7.4. Split traction table.

a therapeutic traction table so that specific exercises can be performed while the patient receives traction.

A spinal traction treatment table for home use was described by Turner (80) but has not received acceptance. Overtreatment is easily possible and the patient should be cautioned against it.

Conclusion

Traction properly administered by experienced physicians and therapists can provide dramatic relief of pain. It is recommended that traction be used with prudence and rarely before a definitive diagnosis has been established.

REFERENCES

1. Bard, G., and Jones, M. D. Cineradiographic recording of traction of the cervical spine. *Arch. Phys. Med. Rehabil., 45*:403, 1964.
2. Bauer, W., Ropes, M. W., and Waine, H. The physiology of articular structures. *Physiol. Rev., 20*:1940, 272, 1940.
3. Bradford, D. S., Moe, J. H., and Winter, R. B. Scoliosis. In *The Spine.* vol. 1. Edited by Rothman R. H., and Simeone F. A. W. B. Saunders Co., Philadelphia, 1975, p. 302.
4. Brodkey, J. S., Richards, D. E., Blasingame, J. P., et al. Reversible spinal cord trauma in cats: Additive effects of direct pressure and ischemia. *J. Neurosurg., 37*:591, 1972.
5. Cailliet, R. *Neck and Arm Pain.* F. A. Davis Co., Philadelphia, 1964.
6. Caldwell, J. W., and Krusen, E. M. Effectiveness of cervical traction in treatment of neck problems; evaluation of various methods. *Arch. Phys. Med. Rehabil., 43*:214, 1962.
7. Christie, B. G. B. Discussion on the treatment of backache by traction. *Proc. R. Soc. Med. (Section of Physical Medicine), 48*:811, 1955.
8. Clark, J. A., Hsu, L. C. S., and Yau, A. C. M. C. Viscoelastic behavior of deformed spines under correction with halo pelvic distraction. *Clin. Orthop., 110*:90, 1975.
9. Colachis, S. C., Jr., and Strohm, B. R. A study of tractive force and angle of pull on vertebral interspaces in the cervical spine. *Arch. Phys. Med. Rehabil., 46*:820, 1965.
10. Colachis, S. C., Jr., and Strohm, B. R. Cervical traction; relationship of time to varied tractive force with constant angle of pull. *Arch. Phys. Med. Rehabil., 46*:815, 1965.
11. Colachis, S. C., Jr., and Strohm, B. R. Effect of duration of intermittent cervical traction on vertebral separation. *Arch. Phys. Med. Rehabil., 47*:353, 1966.
12. Colachis, S. C., Jr., and Strohm, B. R. Effects of intermittent traction on separation of lumbar vertebrae. *Arch. Phys. Med. Rehabil., 50*:251, 1969.
13. Colachis, S. C., Jr., and Strohm, B. R. Radiographic studies of cervical spine motion in normal subjects; flexion and hypertension. *Arch. Phys. Med. Rehabil., 46*:753, 1965.
14. Crisp, E. J. Discussion on the treatment of backache by traction. *Proc. R. Soc. Med. (Section of Physical Medicine), 48*:805, 1955.
15. Crue, B. L. Importance of flexion in cervical halter traction. *Bull. Los Angeles Neurol. Soc., 30*:95, 1965.
16. Crue, B. L. Importance of flexion in cervical traction for radiculitis. *U.S. Air Force Med. J., 8*:374, 1957.
17. Cusick, J. F., Myklebust, J., Zyvoloski, M., et al. Effects of vertebral column distraction in the monkey. *J. Neurosurg.,.57*:651, 1982.
18. Cyriax, J. Trial by traction (letter). *Br. Med. J., 1*:522, 1976.
19. Cyriax, J. H. Conservative treatment of lumbar disc lesions. *Physiotherapy, 50*:300, 1964.
20. Cyriax, J. H. Diagnosis of soft tissue lesions. In: *Textbook of Orthopedic Medicine.* vol. 1. Hoeber and Row, Great Britain, 1962.

21. Cyriax, J. H. Discussion on the treatment of backache by traction. *Proc. R. Soc. Med. (Section of Physical Medicine and Rehabilitation), 45:*808, 1955.
22. de Sèze, S., and Levernieux, J. Physio-pathologie de la traction. *Bull. Soc. Med. Hop. Paris, 68:*1089, 1952.
23. de Sèze, S., and Levernieux, J. Pratique rhumatologie des tractions vertebrales. *Sem. Hop. Paris, 27:*2085, 1951.
24. DeWald, R. L., and Ray R. D. Skeletal traction for treatment of severe scoliosis; the University of Illinois halo-hoop apparatus. *J. Bone Joint Surg., 52A:*233, 1970.
25. Engler, G. L., Spielholz, N. I., Bernhard, W. N., et al. Somatosensory evoked potentials during Harrington instrumentation for scoliosis. *J. Bone Joint Surg., 60A:*528, 1978.
26. Editorial: Trial by Traction. *Br. Med. J., 1:*2, 1976.
27. Fielding, J. W. Cineroentgenography of the normal cervical spine. *J. Bone Joint Surg., 39:*1280, 1957.
28. Frankel, V. H., Shore, N. A., and Hoppenfeld, S. Stress distribution in cervical traction; prevention of temporomandibular joint pain syndrome. *Clin. Orthop., 32:*114, 1964.
29. Franks, A. S. T. Temporomandibular joint dysfunction associated with cervical traction. *Ann. Phys. Med., 8:*38, 1965.
30. Frazer, E. H. The use of traction in backache. *Med. J. Aust., 41:*694, 1954.
31. Goldie, I., and Landquist, A. Evaluation of the effects of different forms of physiotherapy in cervical pain. *Scand. J. Rehabil. Med., 2–3:*117, 1970.
32. Gray, F. J. Combination of traction and manipulation for the lumbar disc syndrome. *Med. J. Aust., 54:*958, 1967.
33. Grundy, B. I., Heros, R. C. Tung, A. S. et al. Intraoperative hypoxia detected by evoked potential monitoring. *Anesth Analg (Cleve), 60:*437, 1981.
34. Grundy, B. L., Lins, A., Procopio, P. T. et al. Reversible evoked potential changes with retraction of the eighth cranial nerve. *Anesth Analg (Cleve), 60:*835, 1981.
35. Grundy, B. I., Nash, C. I., Brown, R. H. Arterial pressure manipulation alters spinal cord function during correction of scoliosis. *Anesthesiology, 54:*249, 1981.
36. Grundy, B. L., Nelson, P. B., Doyle, E., et al. Intraoperative loss of somatosensory-evoked potentials predicts loss of spinal cord function. *Anesthesiology, 57:*321, 1982.
37. Harris, R. Traction. In: *Massage, Manipulation and Traction.* Edited by S. Licht. Elizabeth Licht, Publisher, New Haven, 1960, pp. 223–251.
38. Hirsch, C., and Nachemson, A. New observations on the mechanical behavior of lumbar discs. *Acta Orthop. Scand., 23:*254, 1954.
39. Hickling, J. Spinal traction technique. *Physiotherapy, 58:*58, 1972.
40. Hodgson, A. R. Halo-pelvic traction in scoliosis. *Israel J. Med. Sci., 9:*767, 1973.
41. Hood, L. B., and Chrisman, D. Intermittent pelvic traction in the treatment of the ruptured intervertebral disk. *Phys. Ther., 48:*21, 1968.
42. Jackson, R. *The Cervical Syndrome.* Second Ed., Charles C Thomas, Springfield, IL., 1958.
43. Jones, M. D. Cineradiographic studies of the normal cervical spine. *Calif. Med., 93:*293, 1960.
44. Judovich, B. D. Herniated cervical disc; a new form of traction therapy. *Am. J. Surg., 84:*646, 1952.
45. Judovich, B. D. Lumbar traction therapy and dissipated force factors. *Lancet, 74:*411, 1954.
46. Judovich, B. D. Lumbar traction therapy—elimination of physical factors that prevent lumbar stretch. *J.A.M.A., 159:*549, 1955.
47. Judovich, B. D., and Nobel, G. R. Traction therapy; a study of resistance forces. *Am. J. Surg., 93:*108, 1957.
48. Kottke, F. J., and Mundale, M. O. Range of mobility of the cervical spine *Arch. Phys. Med., 40:*379, 1959.
49. LaBan, M. M., and Meerschaert, J. R. Quadriplegia following cervical traction in patients with occult epidural prostatic metastasis. *Arch. Phys. Med. Rehabil., 56:*455, 1975.

50. Larson, D. L., Evans, E. B., et al. Skeletal suspension and traction in the treatment of burns. *Ann. Surg., 168:*981, 1968.
51. Laurin, C. A. Cervical traction in the home. *Can. Med. Assoc. J., 94:*36, 1966.
52. Lawson, G. A., and Godfrey, C. M. A report on studies of spinal-traction. *Med. Services J. Can., 14:*762, 1958.
53. Lehmann, J. F., and Brunner, G. D. A device for the application of heavy lumbar traction; its mechanical effects. *Arch. Phys. Med. Rehabil., 39:*696, 1958.
54. Levernieux, M. J. A propos de tractions vertebrales. *Rhumatologie, 16:*453, 1964.
55. Longton, E. Traction therapy of the lumbar spine. *Excerpta Medical Rehabil. Phys. Med., 18:*139, 1975.
56. Martin, G. M., and Corbin, K. B. An evaluation of conservative treatment for patients with cervical disk syndrome. *Arch. Phys. Med. Rehabil., 35:*87, 1954.
57. Masturzo, A. Vertebral traction for the treatment of sciatica. *Rheumatism, 11:*62, 1955.
58. Mathews, J. A. Dynamic discography; a study of lumbar traction. *Ann. Phys. Med., 9:*275, 1968.
59. Mathews, J. A. The effects of spinal traction. *Physiotherapy, 58:*64, 1972.
60. Mathews, J. A., and Hickling, J. Lumbar traction; a double-blind controlled study for scaitica. *Rheumatol. Rehabil., 14:*222, 1975.
61. McFarland, J. W., and Krusen, F. H. Use of the Sayre head sling in osteoarthritis of cervical portion of spinal column. *Arch. Phys. Ther., 24:*263, 1943.
62. Nash, C. L., Lorig, R. A., Schatzinger, L. A. et al. Spinal cord monitoring during operative treatment of the spine. *Clin. Orthop., 126:*100, 1977.
63. O'Brien, J. P., Yau, A. C. M. C., and Hodgson, A. R. Halo pelvic traction; a technique for severe spinal deformities. *Clin. Orthop., 93:*179, 1973.
64. Peltier, L. F. A brief history of traction. *J. Bone Joint Surg. (Am.), 50:*1603, 1968.
65. Perry, J. The halo in spinal abnormalities; practical factors and avoidance of complications. *Othop. Clin. North Am., 3:*69, 1972.
66. Perry, J., and Nickel, V. L. Total cervical spine fusion for neck paralysis. *J. Bone Joint Surg. (Am.), 41:*37, 1959.
67. Richardson, P. F. Traction in Cervical Arthritis. *Md. State Med. J., 21:*19, 1972.
68. Rowe, C. R. Current changes in therapy. II. Cervical osteoarthritis. *N. Engl. J. Med., 268:*1351, 1963.
69. Rowe, C. R. Current concepts in therapy. I. Cervical osteoarthritis. *N. Engl. J. Med., 268:*1178, 1963.
70. Rudd, J. L. Hydraulic lift for cervical traction. *Arch. Phys. Med. Rehabil., 43:*120, 1962.
71. Rudd, J. L. Need for better cervical (neck) traction. *Med. Trial Tech. Q., 11:*51, 1965.
72. Scott, B. O. Trial by traction (letter). *Br. Med. J., 1:*284, 1976.
73. Sheffield, F. J. Adaptation of tilt table for lumbar traction. *Arch. Phys. Med. Rehabil., 45:*469, 1964.
74. Shields, C. Cervical spondylosis. *Rheumatism, 19:*50, 1963.
75. Shore, N. A., Frankel, V. H., and Hoppenfeld, S. Cervical traction and temporomandibular joint dysfunction. *J. Am. Dent. Assoc., 68:*4, 1964.
76. Schramm, J., Hashizume, K., Fukushima, T. et al. Experimental spinal cord injury produced by slow, graded compression: Alterations of cortical and spinal evoked potentials. *J. Neurosurg., 50:*48, 1979.
77. Taylor, A. R. Mechanism and treatment of spinal-cord disorders associated with cervical spondylosis. *Lancet, 1:*717, 1953.
78. Toubeau, M. C. Tractions cervicales et reeducation. *Rhumatologie, 14:*53, 1962.
79. Traction for neck and low back disorders. *Med. Lett. Drugs Ther., 17:*16, 1975.
80. Turner, D. New apparatus; a spinal traction treatment table. *Br. J. Phys. Med., 20:*259, 1957.
81. Valtonen, E. J., and Kiuru, E. Cervical traction as a therapeutic tool. *Scand. J. Rehabil. Med., 2:*29, 1970.

82. Weber, H. Traction therapy in sciatica due to disc prolapse. *J. Oslo City Hosp., 23:*167, 1973.
83. Weinberger, L. M. Trauma or treatment? The role of intermittent traction in the treatment of cervical soft tissue injuries. *J. Trauma, 16:*377, 1976.
84. Weinstein, M. V., and Gordon, A. H. Traction-exercise table. *Arch. Phys. Med. Rehabil., 52:*389, 1971.
85. Winter, R. B., Moe, J. H., and Eilers, V. E. Congenital scoliosis; a study of 234 patients treated and untreated. *J. Bone Joint Surg. (Am.), 50:*1, 1968.
86. Worden, R. E. A new spinal traction table. *Arch. Phys. Med. Rehabil., 44:*605, 1963.
87. Worden, R. E., and Humphrey, T. L. Effect of spinal traction on the length of the body. *Arch. Phys. Med. Rehabil., 45:*318, 1964.
88. Wramner, T. Observations on the symptoms and diagnosis of cervical rhizopathia and experience with vertebral traction. *Acta Rheumatol. Scand., 3:*108, 1957.
89. Yates, D. A. H. Indications and contra-indications for spinal traction. *Physiotherapy, 54:*55, 1972.

8

Motorized Intermittent Traction

JOSEPH B. ROGOFF[1]

As we can read earlier in this section, traction was a widely accepted procedure as long ago as in the time of Hippocrates. Petit (16) tells us that Glisson resurrected it in 1669 for spinal deformities and that Nuck used continuous cervical traction in 1692 for wryneck. He applied a chin-occiput suspension device to the head and used the body weight of the patient for countertraction. In the late 19th century Sayre (17) popularized the treatment of vertebral deformities by suspension of the body followed by plaster cast immobilization of the correction thus obtained. Since the end of World War II, increasing stress has been placed on greater tractive forces and periodic or intermittent application of them.

Judovich (12–14) demonstrated that cervical traction, to be effective, requires forces of from 35 to 45 pounds, while effective lumbar traction requires 75 to 100 pounds. De Sèze and Levernieux (9) feel that a pull of at least 200 pounds must be used in lumbar traction; Cyriax (7) claims 200 to 300 pounds are necessary. The discomfort experienced by the patient from such large forces led to the development of methods of applying intermittent traction. Cyriax, however, believes that constant traction is necessary to fatigue the muscle countertraction (spasm) to traction and that intermittent traction is unrewarding. Although most writers on the subject of traction believe that it is useful in some conditions, in a discussion of a paper given by Crisp (6), Christie described a one-year study of more than 60 patients with backache (with and without radiation of pain from the lumbar region), half of whom were treated with traction and the other half with placebo pills, with almost no difference in the final results.

There are several methods of giving intermittent traction. In the first, the patient is anchored by straps or gravity and, through a mechanical

---

[1] Dr. Rogoff died in September, 1984 after a lengthy illness which earlier had forced him to relinquish the editing of this edition.

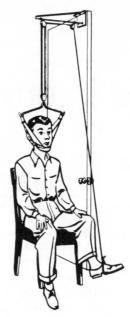

Figure 8.1. A simple method of applying intermittent traction. (Courtesy of the Tru-Eze Manufacturing Company.)

system, exerts a force on a rope or lever, which is transmitted to a belt or halter. The force may be exerted by a hanging weight, by a hand pull or, as in Figure 8.1, with foot power. A more sophisticated device, and one with which a greater force may be applied, is shown in Figure 8.2. Intermittency and force are patient-controlled and can only be given with accuracy if a strain gauge and metronome are used. A second method would be to have the therapist apply the pressure. In such a case there could be better control of the timing and in some instances, at least, the possibility of applying greater forces. The therapist could also use a mechanical traction device similar to that pictured in Figure 8.3. A modification of this idea could be designed to give shorter periods of traction than would be practical with the device pictured. The third method uses motor-driven apparatus.

Judovich (12–14) was probably the first to apply motor-driven traction with automatic timing. His original apparatus utilized a bed built in two sections, each fitted with its own half-mattress. The upper half of the bed was fixed, while the lower portion could be separated periodically by motor power. Traction forces of up to 50 pounds could be obtained from the friction of the body on the mattress sections. Much greater forces could be obtained with specially designed slings or harnesses.

The apparatus generally available in the United States at the time of this

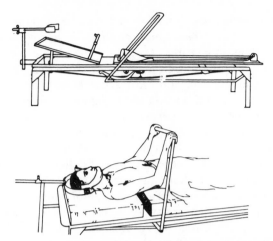

Figure 8.2. A mechanized traction treatment table designed by Dr. Donald Turner of London. Above, a diagrammatic representation of a split table in the extended position with ratchet in operation, headboard fitted and the head traction attachment at its highest position (cushions removed). Below, patient has applied head halter and by pulling on crossbar can apply tractive force, which will pull his head upward with a force and intermittency under his own control. (Drawn from photographs supplied by Dr. Turner.)

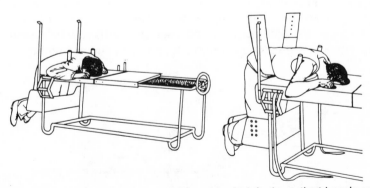

Figure 8.3. Drawing of the Vaquette traction table. At *left*, the patient kneels on knee support with head lowered into opening in table top. Other half of table top is also furnished with an opening for the head (not shown). By turning the handwheel, a physician or therapist can separate the two halves of the table and thus obtain a tractive force. At *right*, patient is shown in a harness that will permit traction on different structures in the body.

writing utilizes a cabinet that houses a motor and a method of transmitting a variable tractive force. Because most emphasis is being placed on cervical traction, American manufacturers are not paying too much attention to the split bed, but in our opinion such a device can give more effective lumbar traction. One of the simplest and most accurate ways to supply a pulling force is through the use of a pivoted lever. Figure 8.4 shows a motor-driven cam that, as it rotates, applies periodic pressure on a lever, from the other end of which the patient is suspended by halter or belt. Through the simple application of leverage principles, the force is increased by lengthening the lever, that is, attaching the patient support further from the fulcrum. Of course, any movement, even slumping, on the part of the patient will change the characteristics of the mechanical system, and alter the pull. In order to compensate for patient movement with respect to the apparatus, more complicated devices are available. At least one apparatus incorporates a feedback mechanism that changes the range of movement to compensate for patient movement and in this way keeps the predetermined maximum tension at a constant level. Almost all companies make devices that can be used in the upright or horizontal positions, with attachments for door frames or bed frames. Figure 8.5 shows a method of developing a hydraulic force transmitted through a metal cable. It is possible to vary the duration of the pull and of the relaxation periods on many machines.

The position of the patient for traction is the subject of much controversy, especially as regards cervical traction. It would seem that the arguments given in favor of one or the other methods are based more on subjective preferences than upon controlled studies. Braaf and Rosner (2, 3) state that, after continuous experimentation, it has been demonstrated conclusively that head traction, to be effective, must be carried out in the supine position. Traction in the upright position, either sitting or standing, usually tends to make the patient more apprehensive; upright traction cannot be carried out for as long as horizontal traction. In supine traction, the pull

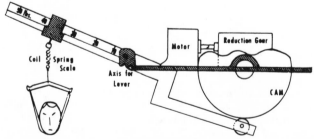

Figure 8.4. A simple method of developing rhythmic traction. The faster the motor turns the cam, the shorter will be the cycle of pull and relaxation. As the attachment for the patient connection is moved to the left, the amount of force exerted increases.

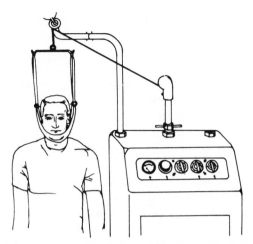

Figure 8.5. Drawing of a hydraulic pressure device with automatic feedback compensation for patient movement and cable transmission. (Drawn from a photograph supplied by the Hausted Manufacturing Company.)

can be adjusted more easily, and the position of the head can be varied according to the angulation of the cervical spine found on x-rays.

Gartland (11) quotes Frazer as stating that, in vertical traction, the resistance of the body against the table is overcome and the patient's own body weight is utilized in treatment. Frazer advocates the vertical position for lumbar as well as cervical traction. Gartland also quotes Krusen as listing the following advantages of vertical over horizontal traction: (a) convenience of application, (b) elimination of friction, (c) accuracy of measurement, and (d) facilitation of certain types of manipulation. We agree with Krusen's conclusion that there is a place for both horizontal and vertical traction in treatment.

Where horizontal traction is used in the lumbar region, we must consider the findings of Judovich and associates (13, 14), who showed that surface traction resistance due to the area, shape, and manner of surface contact of the body on the bed, the weight of the body or body segments, and the quality, contour, and texture of the contacting surfaces may amount to from one-fourth to one-third of the total body weight. In other words, because in a 170-pound patient, the dissipated-force factor is 44 pounds, the first 44 pounds of applied force exert virtually no influence on the lumbar spine and may be considered as the level from which to start calculating the force to apply. It is for this reason that a split bed is more useful in applying effective lumbar traction.

Application

The consensus of many physicians who have used traction is that relief of pain and sometimes of other neurologic manifestations is possible, at least in the cervical region, but the amount of tractive force applied must be adequate. If the treatment is uncomfortable it defeats the purpose (relief of pain) and should be discontinued.

Traction of the cervical region may be applied with the patient sitting or lying down. We prefer when possible to give the treatment in the sitting position because maximum countertraction is thus provided. Care should be exercised in the application of the head halter in relation to padding and the avoidance of creases or contact between the skin and mechanical annoyances. Whether the head should be placed in flexion or extension will depend on the direction in which we hope to influence the curve of the cervical spine. The aim is to obtain comfort, and for most patients this will occur when traction is applied with the use of slight flexion. The use of heat before or during treatment has been suggested by some, but in our hands it has not made a significant difference in the relief experienced by the patient. In most instances we start with a pressure of about 15 pounds, which we increase progressively to a maximum of 40 to 50 pounds after about five treatments for from 20 to 30 minutes applied daily or at least three times weekly. If the relief is apparent after four to five treatments we recommend a discontinuance, because we do not believe in exceeding a force of 50 pounds. It is probable that intermittent traction produces about the same ultimate results as does constant traction, provided that the patient can tolerate the required forces. However, we have been impressed by the increased amount of traction a patient will tolerate, with comfort, when the force is applied intermittently.

Traction of the lumbar region is more difficult, and its effects are less clear. As mentioned above, a force of 100 or more pounds is required if the lumbar area is to be influenced. For this purpose a special traction table and countertractive harnesses are necessary. When smaller forces are used, traction does little more than ensure absolute bed rest, which, in some instances, is all that the physician desires in the treatment of some types of low back pain.

REFERENCES

1. Barbor, R. Spinal traction. *Lancet, 1:*437, 1954.
2. Braaf, M. M., and Rosner, S. Symptomatology and treatment of injuries to neck. *N.Y. St. J. Med., 55:*237, 1955.
3. Braaf, M. M., and Rosner, S. The treatment of headaches. *N.Y. St. J. Med., 53:*414, 1953.
4. Coste, F., and Galmiche, P. Table de vertebrotherapie. *Rev. Rhumatisme, 17:*301, 1950.
5. Coste, F., and Pajault, L. Valeur du traitement non sanglant des lombo-sciatiques. *Rev. Rhumatisme, 17:*295, 1950.
6. Crisp, E. J. Discussion of the treatment of backache by traction. *Proc. R. Soc. Med., 43:*805, 1955.
7. Cyriax, J. Treatment of lumbar disc lesions. *Br. Med. J., 2L:*1434, 1954.
8. De Sèze, M., and Levernieux, J. Physiopathologie de la traction. *Bull. Mem. Soc. Med. Hop. Paris, 30:*1089, 1952.

9. De Sèze, M., and Levernieux, J. Prècision sur l'emploi des tractions vertèbrales. *Rev. Rhumatisme, 17:*303, 1950.
10. Erickson, D. J. Cervical traction and other physical therapeutic procedures for pain about the neck and shoulders. *Minn. Med., 39:*373, 1956.
11. Gartland, G. J. A survey of spinal traction. *Br. J. Phys. Med., 20:*253, 1957.
12. Judovich, B. D. Herniated cervical disc—a new form of traction therapy. *Am. J. Surg., 84:*646, 1952.
13. Judovich, B. D. Lumbar traction therapy and dissipated force factors. *Journal-Lancet, 74:*411, 1954.
14. Judovich, B. D., and Nobel, G. R. Traction therapy, a study of resistance forces. *Am. J. Surg., 93:*108, 1957.
15. Parsons, W. B., and Cumming, J. D. A. Mechanical traction in lumbar disc syndrome. *Can. Med. Assoc. J., 77:*7, 1957.
16. Petit, J. Contribution à l'Etude de l'Orthopédie. Thesis, Paris, 1940.
17. Sayre, L. A. History and treatment of spondylitis and scoliosis by partial suspension and retention by means of plaster of Paris bandages. *N.Y. Med. J.,* March, 1985.
18. Shenkin, H. A. Motorized intermittent traction for treatment of herniated cervical disc. *J.A.M.A., 156:*1067, 1954.
19. Turner, D. New apparatus: a spinal traction treatment table. *Br. J. Phys. Med., 20:*259, 1957.

Section

MASSAGE

9

History of Massage

HERMAN L. KAMENETZ

The application of a soothing hand can be considered the prototype of any treatment. Pressing a hand to an aching head, rubbing a cold foot, squeezing and tapping a numb area are instinctive reactions, and analogous gestures are observed in animals (174). The act of laying hands on the sick person developed along either magic or religious lines into folkloric and modern medicine. The role the hand had played originally in the art of healing in general is still recognized in terms used to designate therapeutics, such as the German *Behandlung*, the Danish *Behandling*, the Dutch *behandeling*. Although less specific, the English term "handling" may also be defined as *"treatment"*, and the same can be said of "management", a term which derives from the Latin *manus*, hand.

From intuitive gestures developed the therapeutic manipulations of the soft tissues that today we call massage. Primitive reactions are still recognized in the basic maneuvers of palpation, stroking, and kneading. Palpation and kneading are also terms which seem to vie for the origin of the word massage.

Etymology

The controversy about the etymology of the word "massage" deals mainly with two possible derivations, one Semitic, the other Greek. To the first belongs the Arabic verb *mass*, to touch. This origin was proposed by Savary (202) as early as 1785 in his report on Egypt where he observed massage.[1] The Greek origin from the word *massein*, to knead, was suggested in 1819 by Piorry (178).[2] Littré, in 1873, held the Arabic origin more likely than the Greek, because of the widespread use of massage in the East.[3] However,

---

[1] Akin to the Arabic *mass* is the Hebrew *mashesh*, to feel, touch, grope. This derivation was suggested by Zabludowski (240). The term was used as feeling the darkness, in Exodus 10:21.

[2] This verb is akin to *maza*, barley bread or barley cake. Homer used a word with the same root, *epimassetein*, to indicate a direct action by the hand of the physician, as pointed out by Daremberg (59, p. 78).

[3] Emile Littré, *Dictionnaire de la Langue Française*, Paris, 1873, 1957. Discussing the Arabic term, Littré recalls Pihan but gives no reference.

most lexicographers today favor the Greek etymology. Graham (85) suggested the Sanskrit term *makch* (*mar* in modern Hindi), to strike, press, or condense, as a possible origin.

The first use of the word seems to come from French colonists in India. Guillaume Joseph Le Gentil (129), who went to India in 1761 and 1769, wrote: "I mention here the art of massaging, which is practiced by women as well as by men. . . . Here, along the Coromandel Coast, they call it *macer* or *masser* (having oneself massaged), and there are *masseurs* and *masseuses*." He reports that *massement* (he does not use the noun *massage* itself) "renders the limbs more supple and more agile."

One year after Le Gentil's report appeared, Joseph-Clément Tissot (223) published his classic on exercise, in which he devoted the last 25 pages to massage, yet without using the name a single time—evidence that it was not as yet adopted by the medical profession. Tissot repeatedly uses terms such as friction, rubbing, kneading, and alternate compression.

When, a few years later, Savary (202) in 1785 proposed the Arabic origin of the term, he also mentioned only the verb (the French *masser*). Describing the way the procedure was administered by a servant, he wrote: "He massages, seemingly kneading the flesh without producing the slightest discomfort." Another example of the use of the verb in the same year is an advertisement in the *Journal de Paris* of May 6, 1785. A Monsieur Albert boasted of his medicinal baths and the *usage de masser*, explaining that this "consists in softly kneading the flesh" (140).

The noun massage must have been hardly known when it appeared, possibly for the first time in print, in a French-German Dictionary, in 1812.[4] However, seven years later, in 1819, appeared volume 31 of the 60-volume French *Dictionary of Medical Sciences* (178) with an 8-page article entitled "Masage."

The term was still little used until the latter part of the 19th century, even in France. Its entrance into the English language is dated 1876 by *The Oxford English Dictionary*,[5] 1933.

Writers, especially outside of France, continued to use mainly the Greek *tripsis*, the Latin *frictio*, or national equivalents such as the English *rubbing*. In 1866, Johnson (103) in England called his book on massage *The Anatriptic Art*. Rossbach (196), in Germany, as late as 1882, avoided the use of the word massage in his book on physical medicine by entitling the respective chapter "Stroking and Kneading." Mendelson, in the United States,

---

[4] D. J. Mozin. *Dictionnaire Français-Allemand,* Paris, 1811–1812. In Albert Dauzat, *Dictionnaire Etymologique de la Langue Française,* Paris, 1938. Also in *Lexis: Dictionnaire de la Langue Française,* edited by Jean Dubois, Paris, 1975.

[5] Also *The Oxford Universal Dictionary,* ed. 3, 1955. This dictionary considers next to the French origin of the term a possible adoption from the Portuguese *amassar,* to knead, from *massa,* dough. This could of course in turn derive from the Greek *massein* (*cf.* Footnote 2).

publishing in 1887 his translation of a German book by Schreiber (206) and using the term massage in its title, added the following comment in discussing it: "It is perhaps hardly necessary to note that the word *movement-cure* is the term most frequently used by English-speaking authors."

While older terms continued to be used until the turn of the century, the new French terms were naturalized by many countries of the Western world, either in the original or with some variations. French authors named also the individual maneuvers, adding to the ancient term of friction the new ones of *effleurage*, *pétrissage*, *tapotement*, and *vibration*, all of which were widely accepted in France and elsewhere; they are still used universally.

Ancient Usage

Not only was massage called by many names, it was at times not named at all but understood when therapeutic manipulations, passive exercises, kinesitherapy or—notably in older writings—simply external measures were mentioned. We found particularly in ancient literature that exercise and massage were mentioned without sufficient differentiation between the two. In fact, we know of no history of massage of any importance which excludes the subject of exercise. In our attempt to limit our discussion to the history of massage, we were often obliged to disregard information which was not clearly limited to our subject. The problem of terminology will unavoidably accompany us throughout our history.

BABYLONIA AND ASSYRIA

The evolution of medicine from magic to religion to empiricism to science is recognized in the history of massage. The phases are often difficult to distinguish, notably in ancient cultures. Characteristic is the following reference to Babylonian-Assyrian medicine: "If a man has cramps, . . . place his head downwards and his feet [under him?], manipulate his back with the thumb, saying 'be good', manipulate his arms 14 times, manipulate his head 14 times, rolling him on the ground. . . ." Jastrow (102), who reported this, comments: "Massage must have been recognized as beneficial in certain cases, but the point of view necessarily was that what was good for the patient was bad for the demon. The drugs, the poultices, the hot and cold douches and the massage all were supposed to act not on the patient but on the demon who was in this way to be forced out or to be coaxed out."[6]

The oldest city of the Assyrian Empire was Nineveh, which achieved

---

[6] Throughout history, many travelers in primitive and more or less developed countries have observed similar mixtures of the naive and the reasonable in the domain of manual treatment, as in all other aspects of medicine (213). Particularly amusing is an example in which the rational seems to have preceded the magical. Rivers (192) was indeed reported by Garrison (79) as saying that Polynesian castaways brought their massage, an apparently rational therapeutic measure, to Melanesia, where it acquired the status of a superimposed magic rite.

magnificence as its capital under King Sennacherib of biblical fame. Before his death in 681 B.C., the monarch built a palace which among many other reliefs shows one of alabaster, representing a scene of massage or similar manipulation, as reported by Kirchberg (115).

CHINA

Possibly the oldest extant medical work is *The Yellow Emperor's Classic of Internal Medicine*, usually referred to as the *Nei Ching*. Attributed to Huang Ti, the Yellow Emperor, who died in 2598 B.C., the book dates probably back to about 1000 B.C. We find in Chapter 12 of Veith's book (225) mention of "complete paralysis and chills and fever . . . most fittingly treated with breathing exercises, massage of the skin and flesh, and exercises of hands and feet." The book discusses in Chapter 24 the cessation of the circulation in the arteries and the veins for which "one uses massage and medicines prepared from the lees of wine." In Chapter 27 a question is posed about what to do when supplementing is insufficient. "Ch'i Po answered: 'One must first feel with the hand and trace the system of the body. One should interrupt the sufficiencies and distribute them evenly, one should apply binding and massage.'"

The difficulties of separating massage from exercise, on the one hand, and of the dating of certain practices, on the other hand, have probably led to the belief of several authors (58, 85, 113, 206, 226, 230, and others) that massage was mentioned in a Chinese work said to have been written about 2700 B.C. This refers to the Kung-fu, a system of physical and religious-philosophic discipline. This system, together with many other observations (a total of 15 folio-volumes, published 1776–1789), was brought to the attention of the Western world by missionaries upon their return to France from Peking (6). Pierre Martial Cibot, the interpreter of the "Cong-Fou," did not translate the entire system. His 11 pages (in volume IV), including 20 figures, deal only with postures, exercises, and the schooling of respiration. No mention is made of massage. Massage is, however, briefly mentioned in a later volume (XIII, p. 373) as having been directly observed by the reporting missionaries. It may also be considered part of Kung-fu, albeit of a later date than the mentioned 3rd millenium B.C. Kung-fu has always been associated with Taoism, a religion and philosophy based on the doctrine of Lao-tse of the 6th century B.C. Multifaceted from the beginning, Taoism has changed over the centuries and must have at one time or other incorporated Kung-fu, which in turn might have expanded to include massage.[7]

Wylie (237), a scholar of Chinese literature, confirms that Taoism has

---

[7] We may find an analogy in another addition to the ancient system in its development as a martial art, a development which became quite apparent in the United States in the 1960s and 1970s.

"changed its aspects with almost every age, . . . [and] subjects in the course of time were super-added. . . ." John Dudgeon (65), a British physician living in China, who also quoted Wylie, believed, however, that the Taoists have always practiced medical gymnastics; he emphasized that Kung-fu embraces massage.

In the 3rd century B.C., massage was mentioned by Mencius, the Confucianist, and Pien Ch'iao, the physician (235).[8]

The *Annals of Art*, the official history of the Early (or Western) Han dynasty (202 B.C.–9 A.D.), mentions a treatise in 10 chapters on massage (*an mo* in old Chinese, literally "press rub"), entitled *Huang Ti Ch'i Pai An Mo*. Like the *Nei Ching*, it was ascribed to Huang Ti as a matter of honoring the Emperor, not of indicating its authorship or age.

During the T'ang dynasty (619–907 A.D.) four kinds of medical practitioners were recognized: physicians, acupuncturists, masseurs, and exorcists. "Special chairs were established with a 'Po Shih,' or professor, in charge of each department. The *Official Repertory of the New T'ang Annals* described the organization of the Imperial Medical Bureau as follows: . . . The Department of Massage had one Professor of Massage and four masseurs. . . . They gave lessons in physical exercise and treated cases of fractures, injuries and wounds" (235).

According to Yabuuchi (238), there were doctors of massage and students who prepared for their degree during three years of study. Massage was often combined with breathing and postural exercises and was used in various diseases and after injuries.

After the Sung dynasty (960–1279 A.D.), massage seems to have declined in esteem and it became the province of barbers (235). First in China, later also in Japan, it was delegated to the blind (79).

INDIA

Long before French colonists gave massage its present name, its usage was well known in India, as reported by many travelers. British writers spoke of it usually as *shampooing* (probably an adoption from the Hindi *champna* [*chapna* in modern Hindi], to press), a term often used in the 19th century, while it now refers to washing. Mac-Auliffe (140) reported on massage as "a custom of long standing in India under the name of *samvahana*." Massage is mentioned in Sanskrit literature under the name of *mardan*. Dally (58) tells us that in ancient India, "the laws of Manoo, collected around the 13th century A.D., made religious duties of diet, bathing, friction, and unction."

---

[8] The book of Mencius, or Meng-tzu, is one of the famous Four Books of the Confucianists and contains his conversations with the princes and grandees of his time. Mencius died about 289 B.C. (237). Pien Ch'iao probably lived about 255 B.C. According to Major (144), his name eventually was applied to all famous physicians.

To Buddhism, massage is no stranger either, as witnessed by a relief on the Borobudur temple built about 800 A.D. (Fig. 9.1). It shows Buddha being treated by a masseuse.[9]

To Sudraka, a legendary figure, poet, and king, who may have lived in the 1st century B.C. or A.D., is attributed a most famous Indian play, *The Little Clay Cart* (218). One of its characters is a masseur who later takes the Buddhist cloth and becomes chief abbott.[10]

Going still further back in history, to the 3rd century B.C., Megasthenes, the Greek historian, reported that "among the Brahmans there is an order of physicians who rely particularly on diet and regimen as well as external procedures."[11] We might assume with Dally (58) that massage was part of these external procedures.

Describing the Indians of the time of Alexander the Great, in the 4th century B.C., Strabo[12] (217) wrote: "In the way of exercise, they think most highly of friction, and they polish their bodies smooth with ebony staves."[13]

Having thus gone back in history, we come to the sacred writings of India, the Atharvaveda. Its medical part, the Ayurveda, is indeed the earliest medical writing known of India, dating from the 2nd millenium B.C.[14] As reported by Wise (234), who in 1845 published his studies on this ancient Hindu system of medicine, it included massage, which he names, in the fashion of the day, shampooing and rubbing.

GREECE

Of all ancient cultures, none has left us so much of its literature as the Greek. The Greeks were also more interested in physical beauty and physical education than their predecessors and contemporaries. In Greece—and later in Rome—massage in some form or other was desired by all classes, from wealthy patricians to impoverished slaves, and for the most diverse purposes. For some, massage served as a luxury that followed the bath; for

---

[9] *Encyclopaedia Britannica* of 1974 qualifies Borobudor "one of the most impressive monuments ever created by man. It is both a temple and a complete exposition of doctrine. . . ." Located in central Java, it was excavated and restored by the Dutch in 1907 and thereafter.

[10] The author's name is also spelled Shudraka; the masseur is, depending upon the translator, a shampooer or a barber-masseur; the historical events described are of the 5th century B.C. The play may have been written in the 5th century A.D.; it is also known as *The Toy Cart*, and this "rambunctious comedy", that was shown in New York in 1924, runs "from farce to tragedy, from satire to pathos." (Notes from the program.)

[11] Strabo (217), Vol. II, Chapter 15, p. 1044; in Mac-Auliffe (140), p. 390.

[12] Strabo, the Greek geographer, lived three centuries after Alexander. We are quoting here from Graham (85, p. 30).

[13] A stave is an elongated strigil or scraper, similar to the metal objects used by the Greeks and Romans for the same purpose. See Figure 9.4.

[14] According to *Encyclopaedia Britannica*, 1974, no definite date can be ascribed to these compositions of sacred literature, but a period *ca.* 1500–1200 B.C. would be acceptable to most scholars.

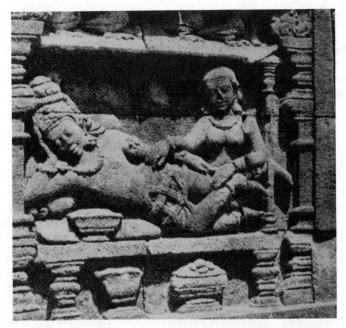

Figure 9.1. The Lord Buddha receives treatment at the hand of his masseuse. Relief on the wall of one of the terraces of the temple in Borobudur, 9th century. (From Sir John Alexander Hammerton, editor, *Wonders of the Past*, New York, 1937.)

others, its purpose was to hasten convalescence; and for still others it was applied to render their tissues more supple before and after undergoing severe tests of strength, so that strains and ruptures would be less likely. It was also used by gladiators after the games to stroke away ecchymoses and to relieve pains and bruises as well as to reinvigorate the body. Sometimes massage was applied by the medical practitioners, sometimes by the priests, at other times by slaves, but probably most often by *aliptae* (anointers), whose duty was to anoint the wrestlers before and after their exercises (85). *Iatrolipts* were physician-anointers, but most practitioners were slave-alipts (140). Gymnastics and physical therapy were practiced in gymnasia and palestrae, to which were often annexed rooms for baths, massage, and inunction.

It is usually reported that early Greek writers did not mention massage, but Graham (85) refers to a passage from Homer's *Odyssey* (? 8th century B.C.) in which "beautiful women rubbed and anointed warworn heroes to rest and refresh them." Beard (18) writes of a bas-relief "showing massage for returned soldiers, as described in Homer's *Odyssey*, [that] depicts massage given to Ulysses. He is seated and the masseuse is giving massage to his leg."

Daremberg (60) quoted Solon (640–558 B.C.) as saying, "The physicians do the work of Apollo, versed in the knowledge of remedies, but the result does not always correspond to their efforts. From a little pain a great ill grows which does not yield to soothing remedies but at other times, laying on of hands reestablishes promptly the health of a man sunk in dangerous and painful diseases." Graham (85) found a passage in Herodotus (5th century B.C.) describing friction performed with the help of a greasy mixture, beginning slowly and gently, becoming more rapid and vigorous, and ending again gently.

Herodicus, one of the teachers of Hippocrates, made exercise and massage a part of medicine. "To such an extent did he carry his ideas that he compelled his patients to exercise and to have their bodies rubbed, and by this method he had the good fortune to lengthen for several years the lives of so many enfeebled persons that Plato reproached him for protracting that existence of which they would have less and less enjoyment" (Hufeland, in [85]).

Hippocrates (*ca.* 460–*ca.* 375 B.C.) was the first to discuss the qualities and contraindications of massage. In his book *On Articulations*, he wrote (92): "The physician must be experienced in many things, and among others, in friction.[15] Friction can bind a joint that is too loose and loosen a joint that is too rigid." In another passage he states, "Rubbing can bind and loosen, can make flesh and cause parts to waste; moderate rubbing makes them grow." Elsewhere, Hippocrates wrote, "At Elis, a gardener's wife had a continuous fever which was not relieved by drinking or evacuating remedies. In her abdomen below the umbilicus, there was a hardness which was elevated and caused violent pain. This hardness was vigorously kneaded with the hands which were anointed with oil. Then blood was evacuated abundantly downward. . . . The woman recovered and was cured."

Among the successors of Hippocrates was Praxagoras, who followed his master's practice in the treatment of occlusive ileus. "Where the caecum filled with fecal matter has become a pocket, Praxagoras pressed with his hands" (14).

Although massage, recognized as an important therapeutic agent by Hippocrates, was well used by his followers, it received its great impetus by another Greek physician who strongly opposed the school of humoralism. Born in Bithynia (Asia Minor) in 124 B.C., Asclepiades studied in Alexandria, traveled extensively, and developed a school of his own which earned him, in the opinion of some, the title of father of physical medicine.

ROME

Like many other Greek physicians, Asclepiades of Bithynia settled in Rome. In his treatment, he relied mainly on diet, massage, wine, pleasant

---

[15] Hippocrates and other Greek writers used the term *anatripsis*, literally "rubbing upwards," which we have translated as "rubbing" or "friction" interchangeably, avoiding as often as possible the word "massage," which was not in common use until the 19th century.

drugs, and bathing (144). Pliny (179), who lived in the century after him, reported that Asclepiades had recommended massage as the third most important measure of treatment, after hydrotherapy and exercise. As noted by Aurelianus (14), for abdominal pains Asclepiades said that the suffering parts should be rubbed with oil long and energetically to tolerance. To dispel the frigid torpor, he advised that the parts be massaged with warm hands and then wrapped in cloth. For convulsions, he rubbed the vertebral column day and night in the hope of dissipating spasms. He did not advise massage in fever except during its remission, but he prescribed it in dropsy and leucophlegmasia.

One form of massage Asclepiades recommended was to strike the parts with inflated skins. Another type of mechanical treatment he advocated was gestation.[16] Also called transportation, it was indeed made famous by him. It was, according to Pliny, one of the mainstays of Asclepiades' therapeutics.[17] As reported by Cumston (53), Asclepiades "considers the three principal means of cure that he speaks of as gestation, friction and wine."

Gestation was prescribed for a variety of diseases for its virtues of "dissolving the stagnations of the body", "opening its passages", and promoting sleep. In treating certain mental disturbances, which he called "phrenitis", it was said of Asclepiades (11):

"...But if the signs of fever should remain without remission, immediately at evening he anoints the entire body with oil, but the head and neck with oil of roses, and gives liquid food; then, if he employs a sitting transportation, the motion will be sufficient for bestowing sleep, for it soon makes the sick soft and gentle."

Gestation has been called passive exercise but may be likened to shaking or vibration, one type of massage, more than to exercise. The patient can use it, as said Asclepiades, "even if he is so infirm that he cannot move himself." Depending on the condition of the patient a choice was made between a great variety of means of therapeutic gestation, from the gentlest by boat in a harbor to the strenuous of a ship on the sea, to the roughest of a litter or a carriage (11). To these Asclepiades added another variety, swinging beds (Fig. 9.2).[18]

Celsus (41), a medical encyclopedist of the 1st century A.D., but probably not a practitioner, wrote:

"Asclepiades speaks of friction as if he were the inventor of it. According to him there are only three therapeutic agents: first is

---

[16] Now meaning pregnancy, the term derives from the Latin *gestare*, to bear or to carry.

[17] Pliny's *Natural History*, Book XXVI, Chapter 3 (180).

[18] There is no agreement about what these swinging beds really were. Descriptions (and suppositions) vary from cradles to litters suspended by ropes. But Asclepiades is generally considered to be their principal proponent if not their inventor (see Fig. 9.2).

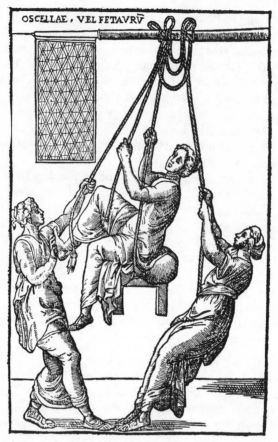

Figure 9.2. Swinging as passive motion (gestation), after Asclepiades. (From Mercurialis, *De Arte Gymnastica*, Second Ed., Venice, 1573.)

friction, to which he devotes most space, then water and gestation. No doubt we should not take away from the young the glory of their discoveries, but that is no reason for not leaving to the older what they have established in their writings. Assuredly, no one has presented more precisely and clearly than Asclepiades how and at which parts of the body frictions are to be applied. However, in this respect he has added nothing to what Hippocrates expressed as follows: 'Vigorous frictions harden the fiber, light frictions loosen it. When pursued a long time, weight is lost; applied with moderation they increase weight.' Consequently, frictions are indicated to strengthen relaxed organs, to relax those which are too tense, to dissipate detrimental plethora or to add weight to lean subjects without strength. If we try to determine how these different results are produced (which is beyond the physician's realm) we see that they all consist in the removal of the noxious principle. Indeed, tightening occurs with elimination of the cause of relaxation. Relaxation of the parts results after what made them hard is removed. Gain of weight does not result directly from frictions but with the help of friction the skin, which becomes more supple, becomes more permeable to nutritious substances. The difference among these results depends upon the procedure used. Both inunction and light friction may be used in acute disease of recent onset provided they be applied during the remission and with an empty stomach. However, prolonged frictions are contraindicated in acute diseases, particularly during their *anabasis*, except as a soporific for a madman. By contrast they are useful in chronic diseases during remission.... Frictions are as favorable when the disease is beginning to decline as they are detrimental when fever is increasing. Thus, as far as is possible we should, before using them, wait for the fever to subside or at least for a moment of remission. Frictions are applied either to the whole body, as when we wish to invigorate a debilitated person, or only to a part, in order to remedy the weakness of a limb or some other local condition. Frictions may alleviate inveterate headaches, provided that the treatment is not applied at the acme. Frictions also give strength to the palsied limb. Most often, however, we should apply frictions at a distance from the painful region; thus, when we wish to draw matter from the upper or middle parts of the body we rub the lower limbs.

"It is difficult to determine the exact number of frictions to apply to a person since this will depend upon the strength of the individual. A weakened subject might not stand more than fifty, while a more vigorous one might take two hundred.... Thus, we must be more careful in applying them to women than to men and to children and older people more than to young adults.

"Finally, if we rub certain limbs, we proceed vigorously for a long time, for, acting on one of its parts, we do not fear to weaken the body soon, and the noxious matter should be resolved as much as possible, be it to remove it from the limb we treat or to divert it from another area. However, if a weak constitution necessitates frictions of the entire body, we rub for a shorter time and less vigorously with the thought of softening the skin so that it can draw new material from the nutrients taken more easily. I have already noted as untoward signs the chilling of the surface while heat and thirst are experienced internally. The only thing to do in such a case is to rub the patient, and, after having succeeded in producing warmth exteriorly, we can then apply other therapeutic agents."

Themison of Laodicea, in the 1st century B.C., a pupil of Asclepiades, prescribed exercise and frictions.[19] "At the beginning of the disease he does not permit the abdomen to be touched or rubbed with ointments, but in

---

[19] It was Themison who founded the Methodist school of medicine which carried his master's tradition over the following centuries.

case there is a widespread suffusion of fluid he has the other parts of the body rubbed down at the beginning of the disease, the massage proceeding outward from the ends of the abdomen with increasing force. But, in order to bring the body back to normal, it is necessary to subject the whole of it to the treatment by massage" (14).

A physician of the 2nd century A.D., who used the teachings of Hippocrates as well as those of Asclepiades, Aretaeus of Cappadocia (9) mentioned anointment, friction, rubbing, and other forms of physical therapy after hematemesis and heart disease to preserve the remaining spark of life. Along with many other ancient writers he recommended massage as an aid in supportive therapy and thus in conditions as varied as muscle strain, melancholy, and asthma. For *cholera morbus* he recommended that the feet be anointed and rubbed gently as high as the knees. He advised massage for the spasms that are characteristic of the disease, stating, "If the feet and muscles are convulsed, anoint them . . . [as well as] the spine, tendons, muscles and maxillae. . . ." He recommended rubbing the legs for headache and vertigo. "The head and hands should be rubbed gently to excite heat in order that the strength of the body might be increased. Later, let friction be performed on the head in an erect position and continued for some length of time." Aretaeus also suggested massage for epilepsy, affections of the stomach, and for phthisis, although in the latter the rubbing was apparently a method of introducing drugs into the body through the skin.

During the flourishing age of ancient Rome many persons other than physicians spoke in favor of massage. Graham (85) relates several examples. Cicero said that he owed as much of his health to his anointer as he did to his physician; Caesar had himself pinched daily by an especially trained slave to alleviate his neuralgic pains; Pliny, writing the emperor that his life had been in danger but was saved by a physician who cured many of his patients with rubbing and anointing, asked him to grant that medical practitioner—a foreigner—the freedom of the city and the privileges of Roman citizenship. Perhaps the most amusing anecdote is told of Emperor Hadrian. One day he saw a veteran soldier rubbing himself against the marble wall at the Roman public baths and asked him why he did so. The veteran answered that he was too poor to have a slave rub him and this was the best substitute he could find, whereupon the Emperor gave him two slaves and enough money to maintain them. A few days later several old men rubbed themselves against the wall in the Emperor's presence, hoping for similar good fortune, but the shrewd Hadrian, perceiving their object, ordered them to rub one another. Massage had indeed entered the daily life of Romans rich and poor[20]; it was practiced to a large extent in the famous baths built by Romans at home and abroad (Fig. 9.3).

---

[20] Plautus (*The Boastful Soldier*) and Terence (*Andria*) wrote of massage practitioners in their comedies, and Martial described a banquet at which a masseuse massaged the host, as related by Mac-Auliffe (140).

After Hippocrates the most renowned physician was another Greek, Galen (*ca.* 129–199 A.D.), a native of Pergamum in Asia Minor, who settled in Rome and became physician to Marcus Aurelius. According to Jüthner (107), he wrote at least 16 books related to exercise and massage, but of these only fragments remain. In the second book of his work on hygiene (77) he discusses massage at length: "And the rubbings should be of many sorts, with strokes and circuits of the hands, carrying them not only from above down and from below up, but also subvertically, obliquely, transversely and subtransversely. . . . But I direct that the strokes and circuits of the hands should be made of many sorts, in order that so far as possible all the muscle fibers should be rubbed in every direction." Galen classified

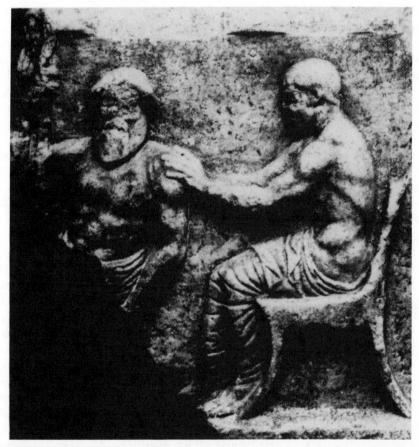

Figure 9.3. Massage of the shoulder. Fragment of a relief found in Cyrene, an ancient Greek colony on the northern coast of Africa. It may have decorated the Roman baths built in 98 A.D. (Photograph by permission of the Museum of Antiquities, Cyrene, Libyan Arab Republic.)

massage into three qualities (firm, gentle, and moderate) and three quantities (little, much, and moderate). By different combinations he arrived at nine forms of massage, each of which had its own indications.[21]

Flavius Philostratos, who lived in the middle of the 3rd century A.D., wrote a treatise on gymnastics in which massage is also discussed (107).

Oribasius (168), who lived during the 4th century A.D., preserved many fragments of ancient medical writings. In discussing preparatory frictions, he reminds the reader of the danger of rupture or sprain by violent movements of those parts not prepared for them. He advised moderate rubbing with a piece of cotton cloth by a few sweeps of the hands at moderate speed without much pressure; this serves to warm the skin and make it ready to receive the oil as indicated by the appearance of redness.

At the end of the exercise period, most of the ancients recommended *apotherapy*. Oribasius describes this as a method of evacuating the superfluities which remain after exercise. Evacuation is effected by frictions in which the hands are used alternately with as much speed as possible. During the friction the treated parts should be stretched. Large quantities of oil are spread on the skin to speed the motions and to diminish the tension of the parts which have tired from too strenuous exercise. An intermediate form of massage is recommended with the hands applied firmly, approaching hard friction.

Caelius Aurelianus, a physician of the Methodist sect, lived in the 5th century in the northern part of Africa. To this outstanding medical writer we are indebted for the preservation of many statements from predecessors whose work exists for us in no other form. Drabkin, who translated his books on acute and chronic diseases (14), summarized the philosophy expounded:

> "A few technical terms may also be noted in connection with the Methodist treatment of chronic diseases. When an attack has declined, the treatment in the interval of remission is divided into two parts: (a) A treatment designed to restore the patient's strength. This treatment is called κύκλος ἀναληπτικός or merely ἀνάληψις, terms which Caelius translates by *cyclus resumptivus* and *resumptio*, that is, 'the restorative cycle' or 'restorative treatment.' It generally includes rest, passive and active exercise, vocal exercise, anointing and massage, and a series of dietary changes leading to a normal regimen. (b) A treatment designed to alter the bodily state so that the disease itself may be overcome. This treatment, called 'metasyncrisis', . . . may include drastic dietary measures . . . vigorous cupping, sun-bathing and more intense applications of heat, massage, various kinds of exercise and bathing, the use of mineral waters, as well as such milder measures as travel and cruising and mental diversion generally."

---

[21] Galen classified movements in active, passive, and mixed.

Drabkin found almost 50 references to massage in the works of Caelius Aurelianus. Sometimes the indications make modern sense, as for example paralysis and cold extremities, but the ancients used massage, as they did so many other agents, for conditions in which we would now consider them inappropriate, for example, in intestinal obstruction.

Aetius of Amida (2), who lived in the 6th century, devoted the seventh of his sixteen books to ophthalmology. In discussing the management of eye diseases, he advises a general hygiene in which exercise and massage play an important role; he often refers to this as a "mode of living." This way of life includes anointment and frictions three times a day. Aetius prescribed massage of the entire body for glaucoma and massage of the lower extremities for ulceration of the eyes and paralysis of the eyelids. In his last book, devoted to gynecology and obstetrics (3), his instructions for the pregnant woman with swelling of the feet, were to "massage or rub with rose water and vinegar and a modicum of salt." In "strangulation of the uterus" he advised the midwife to "rub the part gently and for a long time, so that the thick and irritated humor which clings to the uterus may come out. . . ." For leukorrhea (white flux) he recommended massage of the upper parts of the body, not of the lower abdomen and back. He also ordered massage for "those who do not conceive on account of humidity of the uterus."

Paul of Aegina (Paulus Aegineta) of the 7th century has left us only a small part of his writings. He mentioned in his *Medical Compendium*, according to Verleysen (226), the use of frictions in certain chronic conditions. "He advised bending, stretching and rubbing of paralyzed limbs", as reported by Coulter (50).

ANCIENT MASSAGE INSTRUMENTS

Massage was administered in ancient times either with bare hands, with pieces of cloth of various textures, or with instruments. Very frequent was the use of oil, be it for its medicinal value or be it as a lubricant. Medications were also occasionally administered by inunction, but this is beyond the scope of this chapter. Rough cloth was used to produce warmth; it drew blood to the treated area. The instruments were mostly long and thin, made of bone, wood, or metal. Staves, or ferules, were straight; strigils were curved.

Strabo (217) reported on ebony staves used in India in the 4th century B.C., as we mentioned above, for smooth "polishing" of the skin. The ferule was probably used for tapping. Mac-Auliffe (140) quotes Galen as applying it to the buttocks of dehydrated children and as saying that slave merchants made their subjects look fresher and fatter by this method. The therapeutic fustigation that Galen applied to children was still used by wet nurses in 1795.

The strigil (Fig. 9.4) is a curved scraper, usually made of bronze or iron,

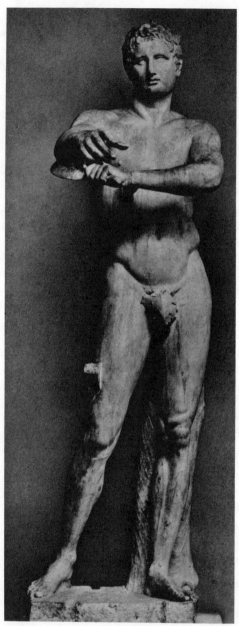

Figure 9.4. Apoxyomenos. "The Scraper." Roman marble copy after a probably even more beautiful lost bronze original of the Greek sculptor Lysippos of Sikyon of the 4th century B.C. (By permission of Vatican Museums.)

about 20 cm long and 3 cm wide, the blade being slightly hollowed so as to collect the oil from the skin.[22]

Dally (58) believed that the strigil was of Indian origin and that it appeared at about the time of the Olympic games (i.e., 776 B.C.). It was an indispensable instrument for removing the oil that had been applied before exercise, especially because it collected the dust of the arena during the exercise period. In the baths, the rubbers used the strigil to scrape the skin after inunction. Though obviously an instrument of cleansing, the strigil was probably also considered an adjuvant to massage. Estradère (69) quotes Oribasius as saying: "After that, one produces a rubefaction by intense friction with pieces of rough cloth ... after that, one reddens the body by scraping it vigorously with strigils which should not be too blunt."

In Finland and other northern countries, since time immemorial, twigs, with or without leaves, have been used after the bath, particularly in connection with the sauna bath. The skin of the whole body was whipped with the twigs, either by the bather, by a companion bather, or an attendant. Mac-Auliffe said that during the Roman period and up to the 17th century physicians used such flagellation with twigs against atrophy and emaciation of certain parts of the body. Patients were flogged until redness, warmth, and swelling of the skin resulted. We will see flagellations preserved by the French surgeon de Chauliac in the 14th century and his commentator two centuries later (43). Meibomius (146) dedicated in 1629 a monograph to the subject of flagellation, writing: "Everybody knows that flagellation with green nettles is most successful in hardening the limbs and in drawing warmth and blood into deprived regions." His book is rich in history but he dwells much on the erotogenic effects of flagellation as well as on its use in the treatment of erotomania. It was indeed used for centuries in the management of manic states, whereby the motive may have been one of punishment, purification, exorcism, or therapy.

Middle Ages

The concern for physical care and physical beauty, so evident during Greek and Roman times, declined over the following centuries. The Olympic games were banned as pagan by a Roman Christian emperor in 393 A.D. The gymnasia were abandoned. Gymnic culture[23] and Roman libertinism were followed by a widespread decadence which, under the influence of religious teaching, changed to a disdain of nakedness and of all preoccupa-

---

[22] Strigils can be seen in several antique collections. There are several statues, mostly Greek, and many grave-steles showing a youth with a strigil. The best known sculpture is shown in Figure 9.4. Another beautiful statue, found at Ephesos, is shown and other sculptures and steles are listed in Franklin P. Johnson: Lysippos, Durham, N.C., 1927, and New York, 1968.

[23] Both gymnasium and gymnastics are terms derived from the Greek *gymnos*, nude.

tion with body health and welfare. Medicine and its literature declined, as did medical gymnastics and massage which probably fell rapidly to its former level of folk medicine. There is virtually no mention of massage in the medical literature for centuries after the fall of Rome; it was considered too commonplace to qualify for therapeutic mention.

For the most part, ancient medical literature was kept alive during that period in the Arabic countries largely through translations of the classics into Arabic and other Semitic languages. Coulter (50) quotes Avicenna (980–1037) as having written: "As a sequel to athletics, restorative friction produces repose. Its object is to disperse the effete matters formed in the muscles and not expelled by exercise. It causes them to disperse and so remove fatigue, the feeling of lassitude. Such friction is soft and gentle and is best done with oil. It must not be hard or heavy or rough, because that would roughen the members."

Maimonides (1135–1204), the renowned Jewish philosopher and physician of the Middle Ages, recommended to his older patients: "Massage with oil in the morning, after sleep, followed by walking or slow riding."[24]

As reported by Licht (132), Arnold of Villanova (ca. 1235–ca. 1312), a Catalan physician, used massage as a form of heat for colic, and Guy de Chauliac (1300–1368), a French surgeon, combined massage with the heat of the sun in the treatment of dropsy: "The patient should be rubbed in the sun, while protecting the head and liver" (43). Chauliac was the most important physician of his time and a precursor of the renaissance in medicine. His treatise on surgery, published in 1363, instantly became a classic and remained a standard work for the next 200 years. He discussed massage in a chapter treating of "steam, baths, frictions, inunctions and similar agents",[25] prescribing it in various conditions. In the management of coldness and dehydration he cited three aims: to produce blood by a good diet, exercise, and moderate friction; to draw the blood to the flesh by flagellation or rubbing until the skin is red; and to strengthen the "nutritious virtue" by frictions, fomentations, and flagellations.

Renaissance

The renaissance in medicine started in southern and western Europe, following a long period of poverty in medical writings and lack in the mention of massage. Toward the end of the 15th century, Antonius Gazius of Padua (80) published his *Florida Corona*, in which he gathered a "crown of flowers" from ancient writings. In it he repeats the recommendations for massage made by Hippocrates, Galen, and Avicenna (104). Symphorien Champier (42), borrowing one of the flowers from the crown of Gazius,

---

[24] *Regimen Sanitatis,* Book V, in Rosner (143), Vol. 2, p. 46.

[25] We are quoting from the 1641 edition with commentary by Laurent Joubert (43), Part VI, pp. 372 *ff.*

called his book *Rosa Gallica*. In this work he mentions that in the weak, the elderly, and children health can be maintained with friction. According to Graham (85), Paracelsus (1493–1541) also found friction indispensable to health. Mac-Auliffe recalls that Rabelais (whose primary calling was medicine), in describing a day of Gargantua, has him start the day with friction to the entire body as he awakens—even before some passage of Holy Scripture is read to him.

One year before he died, Leonard Fuchs (74), who had taught at Tübingen for 31 years, published his *Institutiones Medicae*. The second book is devoted to motion and rest, and one chapter discusses apotherapy, which includes massage.

The most important book of the century on exercise by a physician was published in Venice in 1569 by Hieronymus Mercurialis (150). Although the book deals almost exclusively with the apparatus and methods of exercise, there is some mention of Galen's views on massage.[26]

Ambroise Paré (1510–1590), known primarily for his great contributions to surgery, was also a firm advocate of physical therapy. He prescribed all forms of exercise, together with friction, which "was held in great esteem by the ancients and still is." Paré repeats the classification and indications for massage laid down by Galen fourteen centuries earlier. But Tissot (223) credited Paré with advances in the application of massage to surgical patients. Paré used frictions when the patients were made too immobile by their wounds to exercise. Tissot cites the case of Marquis d'Havrey, whose femur was fractured by a bullet. Paré ordered local light frictions with warm cloths to aid in resolving the congestion of the wounded limb as well as friction of the entire body to improve the general condition of the patient. "Ambroise Paré recommends the use of frictions over the entire body during the treatment of head wounds. It is desirable to use rather strong frictions for a long time over the entire body, except the head, to cause a revulsion of the matters which might ascend and which increase greatly from lack of exercise" (223). Paré is also said to have recommended vigorous rubbing of the scalp with new cloth or fig leaves for the treatment of alopecia.

Timothy Bright, an English contemporary of Paré, wrote on hygiene and the restoration of health. In the introduction to one of these books (34), he reported that he taught the use of massage and exercise to the medical students at Cambridge.

Like others during the Renaissance, Petrus Faber San Jorianus (Pierre du Faur de Saint-Jori) relied on the instructions of Galen to write on massage. More personal was the report of the Italian botanist Alpinus (4) published in 1591. In this book on Egyptian medicine he described some of the forms of massage observed in Egypt. A circular friction was used on the

---

[26] Later editions, starting in 1573, include illustrations one of which is shown in our Figure 9.2. It refers to Asclepiades, whom Mercurialis mentions with great admiration.

hypochondrium, and vibration in the umbilical region (58). When Estradère (69) reviewed the book, he rendered certain terms as pressures and malaxation, the latter word apparently used for the first time by Alpinus. A century and a half later, Andry (7) referred to this work for a description of massage technique.

The 16th century witnessed an emphasis on motion in the arts and sciences, from the soaring concept of movement exhibited by Michelangelo to the thesis of planetary motion described by Galileo. Many book titles began with the words *De Motu* (On the Motion of). Fabricius ab Aquapendente (whose pupil, William Harvey, later wrote *De Motu Cordis*) was the author of a treatise, *De Motu Locali Secundum Totum*, in which, Graham (85) tells us, he returned honor to massage by warmly recommending rubbing, kneading, and movements as rational therapy for joint affections. Beard (18) believes he was the first to use the term "kneading."

Seventeenth and Eighteenth Centuries

It was only natural that the personal power of healing, attributed to the gods by the ancients, should be associated with the kings who owed their offices to divine right. At first, it was enough for the sick to be touched by the royal hand. In England, Edward the Confessor "touched" for scrofula; in France the rulers between Clovis and Louis XVI did the same. In England the practice waned with the third Edward but was revived by Queen Anne. The laying on of hands was not restricted to royalty; many healers had practiced it throughout the ages but perhaps none with such success as Valentine Greatrakes, one of Cromwell's soldiers in Ireland, who, according to Garrison (79), achieved in the middle of the 17th century "an enormous reputation in his 'cures' of diseases by laying on of hands (stroking). . . ."

Francis Glisson (1597–1677), one of the founders of the Royal Society, published a basic work on rickets (83). In it, Kirchberg (115) found details of management of the disease by exercise and massage. Thomas Sydenham (1624–1689), called the "English Hippocrates" because he reintroduced Hippocratic philosophy into British medicine, was a strong supporter of natural (physical) remedies including those of exercise and massage. Sydenham's work undoubtedly influenced Francis Fuller (76), whose *Medicina Gymnastica*, a popular work which went through many editions, discussed friction as well as exercise.

It was during the time of Sydenham that there began to appear, according to Kirchberg, a long line of books written without good judgment, which spoke of massage (identified with tapotement) as the cure of almost all diseases, including syphilis. Paullini (173) was possibly the instigator with his *Flagellum Salutis*, published in 1698.

The man who undoubtedly did most to reintroduce natural remedies (physical therapy) was Friedrich Hoffmann (94), whose dissertations paid much attention to exercise and some to massage. It was Hoffmann who first said that the human body is a machine and is subject to mechanical laws (58).

Hoffmann's emphasis on exercise influenced the thinking of Nicolas Andry. At first Andry saw in exercise what most of his predecessors saw— a system of treatment for most ills, especially the nonphysical. As Andry aged he became increasingly more interested in postural deformity, and in his 83rd year, in 1741, he published *L'Orthopédie* (7), which gave a new word to a new medical discipline. In this book he recommended "remedies which can soften tendons and muscles", namely, rubbing of the calf. He recognized the effect of massage on the circulation and on skin color and suggested "recourse to gentle friction of the entire body in order to maintain or to assure a free circulation of the blood."

Samuel Quellmalz (185) was one of the first to write a book on massage. He recommended abdominal massage for chronic constipation. He noted that friction applied to the abdomen stimulated peristalsis, aided the circulation, and promoted the flow of bile. He advised that the friction begin over the site of the ascending colon, then continue in the general direction of the colon transversely and downward.

A concept quite advanced for the year 1777 was presented by Lorry (138), who recognized that the skin was not only an envelope but also an organ. He advised gentle friction for some skin lesions.

Dally (58) tells us of Boerhaave's pupil, Théodore Tronchin (1709–1781), who enjoyed fame and a lucrative practice among the Parisian nobles just before the Revolution. He left no description of his system, but his contemporary Chomel (44) wrote that "his whole practice was restricted to the recommendation of friction, exercises, long walks, wine and cold meat."

Until the 18th century, massage for lesions of the eye had hardly been used, except by Aetius, twelve centuries earlier (2). Valsalva (1666–1723), the Italian anatomist, claimed to have restored vision by the use of friction to a woman who had lost it after trauma. Valsalva's explanation was that he had relieved spasm of the ocular muscles which had contracted as a result of the trauma and had compressed the optic nerve. Sabatier (1732–1811), the French surgeon and anatomist, referred to Valsalva's case when he reported in 1781 his own comparable successes (201).

In 1780, Joseph-Clément Tissot published his remarkable book on exercise which includes a 25-page supplement on "frictions" (223). (This is one of the terms by which he names massage.) He credits Ambroise Paré with having introduced it into France but points out that Paré had probably learned it from the English who had begun to use it in the middle of the 17th century. Tissot describes friction as "the action of rubbing some parts of the human body with the hands, a sponge, flannel, new linen, a brush, horsehair, etc." Elsewhere in his book he speaks of "alternate pressures and relaxations of the external parts which should cause a movement of the solids and liquids of the body and thus increase circulation."

In his discussion of sprains, Tissot uses descriptive terms except "massage", i.e., frictions, kneading, pounding, and others. "Of the many cures suggested for this condition there is one to which there has been too little recourse. It is a kind of kneading (*pétrissage*) of the involved parts. In what we may call pounding (*en broyant*) (albeit with a certain precaution), in grinding (*en triturant*) the viscous juices which are arrested in the ligaments of the joints, we give to the circulation an activity which it was about to lose. Thus we may say that we prevent all these ligaments from becoming an obstructed lump in which motion would become lost entirely. Do we not all know how rather large ganglions are removed by kneading them several times daily?"

Nineteenth Century

Medicine, like science in general, made great progress during the 19th century. More attention was paid to precise description which had grown since the period of the Renaissance. A strong desire developed for better comprehension and greater accuracy. The Age of Enlightenment of the preceding century had questioned established doctrines and traditional teaching and emphasized the value of critical observation.

Thus, John Grosvenor (1742–1823) "walked the hospitals" of London until he considered himself ready for practice which he began in Oxford in 1768. He first tried friction on his own painful knee[27] and was so impressed with the result that for the rest of his long life (he died aged 81) massage was the treatment he prescribed most often. He published nothing on his method but his student Cleobury (45) has left a full account of the treatment for which

"females were engaged, who supported themselves by this occupation. The female rubber, seated on a low stool, and taking the patient's limb in her lap proceeded to rub with extended hands, so that the friction should be performed principally with the palm of the hand; taking long strokes, one hand ascending as the other descended, keeping both hands in motion the whole time and occasionally applying a small quantity of fine hair powder to the palms to prevent the moisture from producing an erosion of the skin. After the friction had continued in this manner for half an hour, the limb, if contracted, was taken by the female rubber at the ankle and in the slightest possible degree an attempt was made to extend it. The friction was first continued for one hour daily and gradually increased until the patient could bear to be rubbed an hour at a time three hours a day, observing always to rub by

---

[27] Elisabeth Dicke (63) discovered *Bindegewebsmassage* during a serious illness for which no other form of treatment seemed to help her, and Cornelius (47) had a similar experience with a technique of massage that brought relief to him.

the watch. After every period of rubbing was concluded, however unpleasant and distressing it was to his patients, he invariably obliged them to put the limb on the ground and make efforts to walk; and he has been known to urge his patients to walk, though in the attempt they have been ready to faint with exertion."

Cleobury adds from his own experience: "I will now proceed to state those cases to which in my judgement it is not applicable: 1. In all cases of inflammation it is highly improper, as it will not fail to accelerate symptoms; 2. In scrophula; 3. In cases of inflammatory gout or rheumatism it will do mischief; 4. In cases of ankylosis it can be of no service." The cases in which Grosvenor found massage most serviceable, as reported by Graham (85), were "contractions of the joints attended with languid circulation and thickening of the ligaments; in those cases in which there is too great secretion of the synovial fluid in the joints; after wounds in ligamentous, tendinous or muscular parts when the function of the limb is impaired; after violent strains of the joints; in incipient cases of white swelling; after fractures of the articulating extremities of the joints when stiffness remains after union; in cases of dislocation of the joint when the motion is impaired some time after reduction; in cases of paralysis; in cases of chorea combined with attention to the system; and in weakly people where the circulation is languid."

Others in England were advocating massage in scoliosis, notably John Shaw (210), brother-in-law of Sir Charles Bell. In 1823 to 1825, Shaw published his treatise in two volumes and an atlas on the deviations of the vertebral column, discussing the use of exercise and massage. Here is Keith's report (111):

"Among those who influenced the introduction of gymnastics and massage into surgery may be mentioned John Shaw. ... He came to the conclusion that scoliosis was due to a weakness of the spinal muscles. The treatment then prevalent in England was to rest these cases on an inclined plane for months or to use a complicated spinal brace. Shaw saw many of these cases which were not benefited by rest, but which were improved when they fell into the hands of professional rubbers. He condemned the inclined plane and spinal brace on the grounds that the more the spinal muscles rested the weaker they became. His treatment was rest alternated with graduated exercises and massage. To make the spinal muscle more pliable by massage, he invented a friction roller, the first of its kind."

Shaw was also a strong advocate of exercises in the treatment of scoliosis but his death at the age of 38 prevented the realization of his hope for a better appreciation of therapeutic exercises in his country.

Throughout the 19th century we find many more technical details. Since the simple differentiation suggested by Hippocrates, little had been written on the intensity of pressure to be used in the manual treatment. Andry (7) and Lorry (138), two physicians of the 18th century, had stressed gentleness, while Admiral Henry (1731–1823) of the British Navy, a masseur of great repute, thought that "great violence" was needed in massage, as reported by Johnson (103). In contrast with both points of view, William Beveridge of Edinburgh (1774–1839) advocated most vividly the importance of discrimination: "The finger of a good rubber will descend upon an excited and painful nerve (...) as gently as dew upon the grass, but upon a torpid callosity as heavily as the hoof of an elephant" (103).

In a quaint book of the early 19th century by Balfour of Scotland (15), Graham (85) found this passage: "Percussion and compression have been objected to in gout on the score of repelling the disease from the extremities to vital organs. The objection has no foundation whatever, either in matter of fact or the nature of things. Percussion, instead of repelling, creates an afflux of nervous energy and sanguineous fluid to the part. Vessels in a state of atony are thereby roused to action and circulation is promoted; and bandages support the vessels and enable them to perform their functions." Balfour's book is concerned largely with traumatic and rheumatic disorders and their treatment by pressure of the hands or of bandages.

In the literature of the 19th century, terms such as percussion[28] and compression, designating various maneuvers, as well as the very terms of massage and masseur or masseuse (rather than rubbing and rubber) became much more widely known and new ones were coined in the fields of manual treatment and therapeutic exercises. These two fields continued their symbiosis and both subjects were frequently discussed in writings under either title. Thus, Charles Londe, in 1821, presented his *Gymnastique Médicale* (137) which recommended "frictions and inunctions, massage or massement." Much of this development is due to a former fencing master who made Stockholm the center of both therapeutic exercise and massage.

Per Henrik Ling (1776–1839), a Swedish teacher of physical education, brought much honor to his field. Thanks to his energy and persistence, his efforts were rewarded by the Crown with the establishment of the Central Royal Institute of Gymnastics in Stockholm in 1813. Under Ling's influence, medical gymnastics grew rapidly, including massage which gained an increasing number of physicians. Although Ling did much to bring system into therapeutic exercise and massage, he wrote very little on the subject himself; but his many disciples more than made up for this after the master's death (135).

Augustus Georgii, the best known among his immediate pupils, published

---

[28] The term percussion had been used previously, as, e.g., in the report by Barclay (16) in 1808 about a case of severe rheumatic muscle contracture: "After resisting all treatment, it was finally cured by simply percussing the affected sterno-cleido-mastoid", as noted by Schreiber (206).

Ling's system in French under a term of Georgii's invention, "kinesitherapy" (81). Although massage represented only a small part, it was popularized by his followers, and by the end of the century the one form of massage that had received international acclaim was "Swedish massage."

Ling's pupils carried his teachings from Sweden to most European countries by the treatment of patients, the publication of books, and the creation of institutes. The first institute outside Sweden was established in London in 1838 by J. G. In de Betou, who soon thereafter published an English version of Ling's system (97). Georgii was called to Paris in 1847 and established an institute there, but in the following year the revolution caused him to leave for London, where he remained until 1877. In the 6th decade, A. C. Neumann opened an institute in. Graudenz, Austria, and Eulenberg opened one in Berlin, which he directed from 1856 to 1879.

The movement spread to Russia, as reported by Graham (85):

"In 1844 the Supreme Medical Board of Russia appointed two members of the Medical Council to inquire into the merits of the movement and manipulation treatment as practiced by M. de Bon, one of Ling's disciples at St. Petersburg, who had been using it then for a period of twelve years. From the highly commendatory report of the councillors we quote: 'All passive movements, or those which are executed by an external agent upon the patient, as well as active ones produced by the effort of the voluntary muscles, and the different positions with the aid of apparatus or without it, are practiced according to a strictly defined method, and conducted rationally, since they are based upon mechanical as well as anatomical principles. Experience teaches us the usefulness of the institution, as many patients thus treated have recovered their health after having suffered from diseases which could not be cured by other remedies.'"

By the turn of the century Graham, who was a Boston physician, could write: "In most of the large cities of this and other countries institutions similar to the original one in Stockholm are carried on, where movements and stirring up of the external tissues of the body by machinery are successfully employed." The practice continued into the 20th century. In 1916, in New York City, was created the Swedish Massage Institute, which was still functioning half a century later.

The number of books, articles, and even journals on gymnastics and massage increased markedly after 1850, probably largely from the impetus given by Georgii. However, as pointed out by Kirchberg (115), there were many errors in the writings of Ling's pupils. Georgii himself (81) spoke of massage as though Ling had invented it: "Let us now speak of the series of passive movements invented or determined by Ling. Here the influence is largely external and the patient submits himself to the mechanical impression, friction, percussion, rumpling (massage), trembling, lifting, balancing, ligature, movements, or attitudes likely to produce transient and artificial congestion in an organ." Ling himself, on the other hand, had acknowledged the role the work of others had played in the development of his system.

Much of the writing about massage was in relation to medical conditions, but at all times there was some appreciation of its value in locomotor system affections. Verleysen (226) tells us that, in 1837, Martin presented a report to the medical society of Lyons on about a hundred cases of lumbago cured by massage. Two years later Séguin (208) wrote, "The use of massage, of gymnastics, and of steambaths in the treatment of chronic conditions of the joints has been known for so long that we need not dwell further on this subject . . . ."

One of the first rheumatologists was Bonnet of Lyons. In his book (32), published in 1853, he insisted on massage in chronic rheumatic diseases as well as for pain from various causes. In sprains due to muscular action he found massage to be "in a certain way the only efficient treatment." His work was probably the most important stimulus to the use of massage before the appearance of Estradère's thesis ten years later.

Generalized massage continued for the time to be the application of choice. In the same year that Bonnet's work appeared, Reveillé-Parise (190) wrote: "Dry frictions, more or less often repeated, are an excellent method of giving back vitality to a part. The aged will always derive great advantage from this hygienic measure because its constant effect is to promote circulation of the blood in the skin, to summon the fluids in larger quantity to the periphery and thus maintain a higher temperature; to render the skin more elastic, supple and permeable and so augment transpiration."

As might be expected upon the introduction or reintroduction of any therapeutic method, massage was rejected when first suggested by Louvet Lamarre in 1827 in the management of chorea minor. Kirchberg (115) tells us that this subject was vigorously attacked when it was discussed by Sée (207), yet was awarded a prize before the National Academy of Medicine in Paris in 1850. The massage prescribed by Sée was given by his masseur Napoléon Laisné (123), who also wrote on massage. He is credited by Murrell (161) with having coined the word *tapotement*. One of his chorea patients who seemed to benefit from massage became a therapist at what is now the Trousseau Hospital in Paris. Massage for chorea enjoyed the favor of several physicians but later was completely abandoned.

Many people date the era of modern massage from the appearance, in 1863, of Estradère's doctoral thesis (69) on the subject. Estradère grouped its applications according to the systems of the body, among which he ranked the locomotor system first. Since this work was the product of a graduating physician, it was a review of the literature rather than a report of personal experiences. In his classification of maneuvers he mentions neither effleurage, nor tapotement. He calls stroking by such names as *passes* and *attouchements* and places all such movements in the category of soft frictions, as contrasted with other frictions that he called medium or hard. *Tapotement* is called *percussion* by Estradère and includes vibration. We may summarize his classification—the best up to his time—as: (a) frictions (including what we now call effleurage), (b) pressure (including kneading), (c) percussion (including vibration), and (d) other movements, including passive, eccentric, and concentric.

It is certainly due to a good extent to Estradère, that the most celebrated French surgeons of the 19th century, such as Dupuytren, Velpeau, Nélaton, and Maisonneuve, were advocates of massage, as noted by Péan in the preface of Weber's *Treatise of Massotherapy* (230). But the most dominant figure in the field of massage in the second half of the century was a Dutch physician.

It was thanks to Johan Georg Mezger, that Amsterdam became the new center of massage. Like Estradère, the theoretician, Mezger, the practitioner, focused his interest on the manual treatment, independent of exercise. Massage had become a therapeutic entity in its own right. Relatively little is known about this physician who added very little to the literature. His reputation was entirely due to his success in the treatment of patients, many of whom belonged to the most select circles. His technique was characterized by a most forceful use of his thumb which was gratefully acknowledged by his patients and became a point of ridicule by his detractors. Kings and princes were among his patients, and a cartoon shows him with Bismarck, who admits wistfully: "I believed I had power in my hands, but I can see that you have Europe's rulers under your thumb" (88).

Born in Amsterdam in 1838, Mezger studied in Leiden and presented in 1868 his doctoral dissertation, "The Treatment of Foot Sprain by Friction" (152). He emphasized indeed friction as the maneuver to be primarily used in this condition and recognized friction as one type of massage while he considered massage part of medical gymnastics. He referred in particular to two other physicians who had recommended this same treatment of sprains: Girard, who had read a paper at the Academy of Medicine in Paris in 1858, "Frictions and Massage Alone in the Treatment of Sprains," and Millet of Tours in France, who had published his own method in 1864.

The forcefulness (and painfulness) of Mezger's technique became quite evident in his only other noteworthy publication on massage, on the treatment of telangiectasia. He actually described it as tearing of subcutaneous vessels (153). The technique was also described by von Mosengeil (157).

Mezger's fame brought many patients to him, but few physicians. His foremost immediate pupils were Berghmann and Helleday who, like their master, published very little (24). They described, however, Mezger's technique and classified, probably for the first time, the four maneuvers of stroking, friction, kneading, and tapotement. This classification was adopted by most authorities such as von Haufe (90), Little (136), and

Reibmayr (188). Vibration, the last of the five maneuvers that later were to be considered "classical", became particularly known by the book of a Swedish physician (it was also the subject of his doctoral thesis), published in English in 1890 and in German in 1895. A late follower of Ling, in whose institute in Stockholm he had studied, Arvid Kellgren (112) had learned much in the practice of massage from his brother Henrik, a masseur, "under whom", he wrote, "I worked more or less during the years 1876 to 1886 . . . . Let me also state, that part of what I describe—i.e., most of the shakings, nearly all the vibrations and the nerve vibrations—are not part of Ling's original system, but have been added by my brother, Mr. Henrik Kellgren, who was a pupil under Ling. . . ."

Thus, under the continued influence of Ling and his school, we see at the end of the century a growing literature in English, and particularly in German, reflecting an increased interest in the manual treatment by the medical profession. In 1902, Graham wrote in his *Treatise on Massage* (85):

"More than twenty years ago Dr. Mezger of Amsterdam treated the then Danish crown-prince successfully for a chronic joint trouble by means of massage, which he used in a manner somewhat peculiar to himself and in accordance with the teachings of physiology and pathological anatomy. When the prince got well he sent a young physician to Amsterdam to study Dr. Mezger's method of applying massage, and soon after many old as well as young physicians visited the clinic of Mezger, and they all agreed that the so-called massage used in Mezger's manner and according to the indications which a very large experience enabled him to point out, was a most worthy agent in various affections of the joints, besides in inflammations and neuroses. They considered that credit was due to Mezger for having improved massage in a physiological manner, and for having brought it to be acknowledged as a highly valuable method. The esteem in which this method of treatment is held by physicians and surgeons on the continent of Europe who interest themselves in the matter is tolerably well indicated by the following statement from Schmidt's *Jahrbuecher*: 'It is but recently that massage has gained an extensive scientific consideration, since it has passed out of the hands of rough and ignorant empirics into those of educated physicians; and upon the result of recent scientific investigations it has been cultivated into an improved therapeutical system and has won for itself in its entirety the merit of having become a special branch of the art of medicine.'"

Graham adds the following footnote to this quotation: "Since I first translated the above and put it in print, it has been used to adorn the circular of every humbug in the United States who wishes to make people believe that Turkish-bath rubbing and pounding constitute massage."

It is probably also due to Mezger's influence that the oldest association of masseurs was founded in Holland in 1889[29] and the oldest periodical of the profession two years later.

While Amsterdam was the leading center of massage, the method lost importance in France. Graham (85) tells us, "In the summer of 1884, Professor Charcot told me that the physicians of Paris did not interest themselves much in massage, but he hoped that they would." In Vienna, a decade earlier, Billroth (27) claimed that there were many physicians in Germany who had never heard of massage, stating: "I can only agree with my colleagues Langenbeck and Esmarch that massage in suitable cases deserves more attention than has fallen to its lot in the course of the past ten years in Germany."

In 1889, Mezger left Amsterdam for Germany, where his reputation had preceded him.[30] The period spent there probably accounts for the fact that the best known physicians who propagated massage in Germany can be considered his late followers: Hoffa, Gocht, Zabludowski, and Kirchberg were all authors or new editors of books among the best on the subject.

Meanwhile the interest in the manual treatment had resulted in its application in various fields and in scientific investigation. Piorry, in 1819, was probably the first to investigate the physiology of massage. In his article in the monumental dictionary of medicine (178) he described the reaction of the skin and its constituents, of the muscles and the joints.

Massage of the eye, previously performed by Aetius, Valsalva, and Sabatier (2, 201), again received recognition in 1872, when Donders (64) reported on its value in keratitis and corneal opacity.[31]

Obstetrical manipulations of the womb had been used for centuries in folk medicine, either to correct a faulty position of the fetus, to ease the pain of labor, to hasten delivery, or to stop postpartum bleeding. Although many obstetricians offered different methods, best known is the maneuver of Karl Credé (51) of Leipzig, who revived manual expression of the placenta in 1854. Cazeaux (39) mentioned massage for the treatment of postpartum atony and dysmenorrhea in an obstetrical treatise of 1840.

Gynecologic massage, although also mentioned by Aetius, was virtually unknown until Thure Brandt (1819–1895), a Swedish masseur, brought out a book on the subject in 1868 (33). His method consisted in movements of the uterus and parauterine structures between the intravaginal fingers and the hand on the abdomen. It was a vigorous treatment and in some cases a

---

[29] To the original name of *Dutch Association for Medical Gymnastics and Massage* the term *Physiotechnics* was added in 1947.

[30] Mezger later returned to Holland. He died in Paris in 1909.

[31] Others who endorsed massage in ophthalmologic conditions were Pagenstecher, Klein, Abadie, Parenteau, Darier and more, according to Verleysen (226).

second operator was needed to manipulate the abdomen with two hands. Because of the question of decency the method was often attacked. However, it recorded much success in Sweden and elsewhere (98, 166, 215). In 1906 Oscar Frankl (72) in Vienna devoted 20 pages to the subject in his book on physical therapy in gynecology and listed nearly 150 references.

Carl Posner, a urologist in Berlin, introduced massage of the prostate in 1893. Used in gonococcic prostatitis, the index finger in the rectum attempts to squeeze the gland so as to empty it of its pus.

Whereas massage is usually contraindicated in fractures, some physicians have made a fine distinction, relying strongly on their tactile sense not to disturb the fracture site while massaging the tissues quite close to it. In 1866, Rizet (193) mentioned the use of massage in the diagnosis of certain fractures. In 1884, Norström (165), one of Mezger's pupils, wrote a lengthy text on massage, of which one chapter was devoted to the early use of massage and mobilization after fractures. But even before the appearance of that book, Just Lucas-Championnière (1843–1913) had begun the work for which he soon became known throughout the world—the early management of fractures. Although his major work on the subject (139) appeared only in 1895, he referred to this form of treatment in 1886 as having used it for several years. Twelve years later, Berne (26) claimed priority. In 1886, Maison defended his thesis on early mobilization and massage before the Medical Faculty of Paris, and in the following year Leonardon-Lapervenche presented a thesis on massage in joint fractures. Here is what Keith (111) reports: "In 1881 Lucas-Championnière began to introduce another innovation in the treatment of fractures—the application of massage, not only to the parts in the neighbourhood of a fracture, but actually at the site of the fracture . . . . He claimed that massage allayed almost instantly the pain at the site of fracture; it accelerated the process of repair; it dissipated inflammatory exudates, reducing swelling and tension in the damaged parts; it maintained muscles, nerves, tendons, ligaments and joints in a state of health. The application of massage to the immediate treatment of fractures and dislocations he counted amongst his chief services to surgery."[32]

Even if its use in the treatment of fractures remained controversial, massage was increasingly used by physicians and surgeons. It even was practiced by veterinarians, as noted by Kirchberg (115).

---

[32] However, as Sir Arthur Keith further noted, neither the Royal College of Surgeons in London in 1912, nor the routine manual of the French Army surgeons in 1916, accepted Lucas-Championnière's system or only very little of it. Articular fractures, particularly those in the neighborhood of the elbow joint, were indeed mobilized earlier than previously, but most of the system was rejected. It required a very careful technique and a delicate sense of touch, not available to everyone. The teaching of Lucas-Championnière continued, however, in the practice—and success—of many physicians. Outstanding among these was James B. Mennell (147) in England, to whose book, *The Treatment of Fractures by Mobilisation and Massage*, Lucas-Championnière wrote the introduction two years before he died in 1913.

In 1893, Otto Naegeli (162) of Switzerland, described his *Handgriffe* or "holds", with which he claimed having treated very successfully pains of various types, particularly neuralgia. The manipulations involved joint traction, stretching of nerves and all other affected soft tissues, as well as percussion of the vertebral area and other parts of the body.

In the last quarter of the 19th century massage was studied in numerous research projects. Hueter (96) and von Mosengeil (157) investigated its effects on joint fluid resorption, venous blood flow, and cutaneous temperature. Reibmayr (188) reported on experiments done with Hoeffinger on resorption of effusions in the abdominal cavity. Berne (25) worked on urea and phosphoric acid excretion after massage, and Bum (35) reported on its diuretic action. In 1887, Lassar (126) wrote on the effects of massage on lymph flow, and Hasebroek discussed the circulatory effects of vibration. Maggiora (142) and Mosso found that massage delayed fatigue in working muscles, and Castex (37) was able to show histologically the effects of massage on tissue trauma. Colombo (46) found that the secretion of certain glands was increased by massage and particularly by vibratory massage. Verleysen (226) tells us of a comparison made by Gurewitch on the healing of fractures in dogs with and without massage. In 1902 Fiocco and Locatelli (71) did biopsies to study the effects of massage. Possibly the best reference list and summary of experimental work on massage of the 19th century is to be found in the comprehensive book by Bum (35). The list was carried forward to 1910 by Rosenthal (195).

In the United States massage was adopted rather slowly. Kellogg (113) in Battle Creek wrote in 1895: "Twenty years ago, massage, as well as the use of electricity and hydrotherapy, was generally regarded by the profession as closely allied to quackery. Up to that time scientific massage was almost unknown in this country, although various rude manipulations were practiced by bone setters, so-called magnetic healers, and a few superannuated nurses who claimed to be specially gifted in 'rubbin.' Twenty-two years ago .... even the term 'massage' was as unfamiliar to the medical profession of this country as it still is to the majority of the laity." Then, in 1877, S. Weir Mitchell (155) of Philadelphia published *Fat and Blood, and How to Make Them*, a book which gave much respectability to the field of physical therapy—especially massage and electricity—since it was written by the leading neurologist of the time. Mitchell was a strong believer in rest and used physical measures to help the assimilation and evacuation of the increased amounts of food he prescribed. It was probably under his impetus that several of his colleagues in Philadelphia declared their interest in the manual treatment. Benjamin Lee (128), after his presentation before the Medical Society of Pennsylvania, *Massage, the Latest Handmaid in Medicine*, translated Reibmayr's textbook of massage from the German (188). In his introduction he speaks of his "acquaintance of 25 years with this important therapeutic means. ...." Keen (110) compared massage and exercise in their effects on albuminuria. Shoemaker (211) used massage in certain diseases of the skin.

While serious workers thus attempted to establish a solid scientific basis for massage, others misused and abused it. Several publications appeared in Germany, France, Italy, Denmark, England, and the United States, reporting on abuses connected with massage which ranged from quackery to prostitution (38). *The British Medical Journal* printed several such reports in 1883 and 1894 on the risks and scandals of "massage" (5, 203). There was a counteraction in medical circles, and again it was S. Weir Mitchell, whose fame in the meantime had spread beyond Philadelphia and the United States, who brought a new reputation to the manual treatment. It was largely as a result of his efforts that the British Chartered Society of Physiotherapy was founded in 1894. Four women met "to discuss the possibility of putting massage, which had fallen into great disrepute in this country, into its proper place, and making the profession a safe, clean and honourable one for British women. Until this time there was no society of trained masseuses in this country and, owing to this deficiency, the medical men employed mainly Swedish women, who were coming over in increasing numbers. ... The founders had ... unbounded courage and perseverance, and slowly and steadily they convinced the medical profession and the British public that massage could be carried out adequately ... by British women" (183).

Massage was often prescribed in combination with heat, exercise, and—toward the end of the 19th century—with electricity. In 1883, Reibmayr (188) wrote, "Very recently a new modification of massage has been recommended to us from America, the so-called Electromassage. In this method massage and electricity are administered in combination by means of very broad, sponge-covered electrodes. .... The idea of supplementing massage by the use of electric current in certain cases has already been suggested, particularly by Mezger." In 1891, Weber (230) reported that he ordinarily combines massage with electricity, and that he had published a book on the subject as well as founded a periodical of masso-electrotherapy.

Machines were manufactured to give massage. Kellogg (113) tells us of the Granville "nerve percuter" driven first by a clock mechanism and later by an electric machine. Most electrically powered devices produced vibrations. The part which came in contact with the skin was made of ivory or rubber. Verleysen (226) reported that Garnault of Paris had used an electric vibrator in otolaryngology, applying it directly to the mucosa. These vibrating machines were all applied locally. But even in ancient times physicians tried to communicate oscillations to the entire body, by travel over rough roads, for example. The idea was revived by the Abbé de Saint-Pierre in 1734, when he invented the *trémoussoir*, a vibrating chair that enjoyed much success. In 1892, Charcot improved the trembling armchair, which he used for the treatment of parkinsonism. He also invented a vibrating helmet.

Lacroix de Lavalette (122), in 1899, devoted an entire book to the subject of mechanical vibratory massage, which he named *sismothérapie*. Strensch, in 1891, introduced sismotherapy in the United States (214), but it was Mary L. H. Arnold Snow (1867–1947), who did most to popularize it in this country. In her book, published in 1904, *Mechanical Vibration and its Therapeutic Application* (214), where she is listed as "Professor of Mechanical Vibration in the New York School of Physical Therapeutics", she covers the history of the subject and gives excellent descriptions of all the devices available for the administration of vibration. Marfort (145) in France reviewed the history of sismotherapy three years later.

Twentieth Century

What dominates the history of massage in this century is the development of new techniques and new systems. While the use of electricity and new devices has increased the variety of vibrating objects and, as we will see later, produced more or less complicated machines, it is the human hand in particular that has been put to a greater variety of uses in relation to new or newly discovered systems.

Sports massage, albeit under the term of "apotherapy", was practiced as early as the Greek antiquity. Early in our century it enjoyed renewed recognition, due no doubt to the increased practice of sports. The first books on the subject were probably those of Coste (49) and of Ruffier (197), both published in Paris.[33] The value of sports massage for the accelerated recovery of fatigued muscles has been confirmed in many investigations (159) and is now a matter of common knowledge.

"Plastic massage" was also developed in Paris in the beginning of the century. Jacquet (99) recommended this technique, essentially a digital petrissage, for certain dermatological conditions. Leroy (130) made it a system which was advocated by Jean Meyer (151) in combination with other physical agents and further developed by Meyer's pupil Kamenetz (108).

Some techniques were developed in Germany that were later collectively called "reflex massage", since the observed clinical benefits were attributed to reflex actions. Cornelius (47, 48) was probably the first to apply massage to "reflex zones" even though he was apparently unfamiliar with the work of Henry Head (91), published in English in 1893 and in German five years later, still 11 years before Cornelius published his book. In 1893 Cornelius suffered from a severe streptococcus infection which forced him to bed for several months. For his convalescence he was sent to Wiesbaden, where he received daily massage. His joints were still edematous and painful. He

---

[33] The Olympic games of the classical era, last held in 392, had been resumed in Athens in 1896, and most instrumental in their revival was the Frenchman Pierre de Coubertin. The following Olympics were held in Paris.

noted that one of the medical officers had greater success with massage than the others. Observing him, Cornelius noted that " . . . he palpated the area, and where he found pain, he dwelt longer than elsewhere. Stimulated by this, I also palpated my sore regions and found that the tissue was in general painless but that there were a few regions, irregularly distributed, which were sensitive to the gentlest touch. I then asked my masseur to treat only those regions which I have discovered to be painful instead of giving me general massage. The success was astonishing: swelling as well as pain disappeared in a very short time and while previously I had not experienced the least improvement . . . after four weeks of this kind of massage I was free of swelling and discomfort and was able to return to duty, apparently completely recovered and feeling strong and healthy. . . ." (48). It is this success that Cornelius had experienced on himself that led him to present his "nerve point massage" in his first book in 1909 (47) and to propagate his method among his colleagues (he taught physicians exclusively). As to the term of "nerve points", he admitted that it was not a happy choice.

Two years after Cornelius' publication, another German physician, Barczewski (17), introduced a similar technique under the name of *Reflexmassage*, thus probably coining the term that was going to be used for other systems as well. Whether various authors attributed the success of their methods to reflex actions or not, they all emphasized the precise localization of the tissue changes as a *conditio sine qua non*.

Thus, Müller (158) of Gladbach, Germany, described in 1915 small areas of increased tonus, which he called "hard-tone" (*Hartspann*) and which he succeeded to soften by his method of *Hartspannmassage*. The localized hypertonic areas were thought to be muscle gelosis, a concept introduced by Hartmann of Graz, Austria, who therefore spoke of his *Gelosenmassage*, while Fritz Lange (124) of Germany presented in 1921 his "myogelosis massage" or "gelotripsy" to which Max Lange (125) (his pupil but not his relative) ten years later attempted to give a scientific basis. Another article on the subject appeared as late as 1957 (182).

The diagnostic acumen based on fine palpation is what had led to the therapeutic results of gynecologic massage at the turn of the century (72, 98, 166, 215, 216), just as in 1868 (33) and in 1968 (224). It is the same approach that Wetterwald in France (232) reported in 1910 in his treatment of neuralgia, and that Thiele (221), a proctologist in Missouri, used for forty years from 1934 on, in the treatment of coccygodynia.[34]

The success in the treatment of the controversial fibrositis, be it by massage or any other local therapy, and the concept of trigger points, are dependent on palpation. Ruhmann (199, 200) emphasized this point by calling his system (first published in 1929) "palpatory massage" which, as

---

[34] The spasm of the muscles attached to the coccyx and lower part of sacrum subsided, and with it the pain, under a stroking massage by the finger-introduced into the rectum (221).

he reported, was also described in Denmark. Cornelius, comparing some of the methods with his own, had given them the generic term of "contact massage", because the hand of the masseur comes into close contact with the soft-tissue areas in which local changes have occurred.

Into this world of German physicians specializing in massage and producing a rich literature on the subject, too large to be discussed in greater detail, entered a physical therapist with a discovery destined to revolutionize the whole field of massage. It is Elisabeth Dicke's *Bindegewebsmassage* (connective tissue massage) that really gave substance to the concept of reflex zone massage. The story of her discovery is best given in her own words (63):

> "In 1929 I suffered from a severe circulatory disturbance of my right leg. Starting with tooth infections, there developed an endarteritis obliterans of the lower extremity, accompanied by signs of a generalized infection. My right leg was ice cold and greyish white, the toes seemed to be constricted by rings and a partial necrosis was imminent. The dorsalis pedis artery was not palpable any more. An amputation was mentioned as the most likely treatment.

> "With this depressing outlook, after a recumbency of five months, I tried to release the accompanying severe back pain. While lying on my side I palpated a densely infiltrated tissue over the sacrum and the iliac crest and on the left side opposite this an increased tension of the skin and the subcutaneous tissue.

> "I tried to disperse the tension by pulling strokes in those regions which were hyperesthetic. The tension subsided slowly; the back pains disappeared under the relaxing strokes and a strong feeling of warmth set in. After several trials I felt a constant alleviation of my complaint.

> "Now pins and needles started in my involved leg as far down as the sole, with alternating waves of warmth. The extremity improved constantly. Then I added strokes of the regions over the right greater trochanter and the lateral aspect of the thigh.

> "Over a three-month period of treatment the severe manifestations of my disease regressed completely. The treatment continued over a longer period of time by one of my colleagues; after one year I could resume fully my activities as physical therapist."

What was so different in this method was the technique which consisted primarily in a sliding, cutting stroke executed mainly with the middle finger. It was only after several years that Mrs. Dicke met Dr. Kohlrausch, who gave the new innovation a scientific basis. It was in 1948 that Kohlrausch's co-worker, Dr. Hede Leube, together with Mrs. Dicke, published the first book on the subject, *Massage of Reflex Zones in the Connective Tissue* (131). It was an instant success. Yet, Mrs. Dicke was not completely happy with it and prepared her own version, *My Connective Tissue Massage* (63), which appeared in 1953.[35]

Two years later, Kohlrausch, who in the preface to the Leube-Dicke book had already referred to his own theory of the influence of massage on muscles, presented his own book. Recalling Head's well-known discovery in the 1890s of the dermatomes (91), the little known contribution to this subject of van Veen in Holland in 1917, and Dicke's massage of the connective tissue, he entitled his book *Reflex Zone Massage of Musculature and Connective Tissue* (119). Again two years later, Dicke's coauthor published her own book (219), and the flow of new editions and translations has not stopped as this history is being written.[36]

As connective tissue massage spread, some variations developed. The segmental concept that is the rational basis of all systems of reflex zone massage led Gläser and Dalicho (82) to call their method "segment massage." They attempted to reach all layers rather than, e.g., mainly the subcutaneous tissue aimed at by connective tissue massage. Thus, their method includes much more the use of the previously known, now called "classical", maneuvers.

By contrast, a very specific maneuver is used in another type of reflex zone massage, the "periosteal massage" created by Vogler (229) in the 1930s but published only in 1953 (121). The use of the tip of the medius or thumb (sometimes the distal phalanx of the index or medius is also used) is remindful of the technique of nerve point massage. The rather strong pressure advocated by Vogler results in a stimulation of the periosteum with local as well as reflex effects.

Reflex effects are also claimed by proponents of certain techniques of Asiatic origin, known as *shiatsu* and *kuatsu*. Said to be of ancient tradition, they became known in the Western hemisphere, particularly in the second half of this century, through their kinship with acupuncture. *Shiatsu* is, as this Japanese name indicates (*shi*, finger; *atsu*, pressure), a pressure with the tip of one or two of the three first digits of the hand. Applied to the same points an acupuncturist would needle, it has been called finger acupuncture, finger pressure acupressure, Chinese micromassage (127), and punctural massage (186), in addition to the usual name of *shiatsu* (163). *Kuatsu* (a contraction from two words meaning life and procedure) is a Japanese technique of resuscitation, occasionally also of antalgic manipulations (233). It is applied to strategic points coinciding with acupuncture points and is mainly used in the practice of judo. The characteristic pounding with the fist is remindful of the maneuver previously used in cardiac arrest.

There is only a very loose relationship between massage and such proce-

---

[35] She had died a few months earlier, on 11 August 1952. The book, without the possessive pronoun in the title, reached its eighth edition in 1975.

[36] The first full-size book in English was published by Ebner in 1962 (66).

dures—or even cardiac massage, notwithstanding its name. We should mention, however, the modern technique of resuscitation by external cardiac massage, presented by Kouwenhoven and his co-workers in 1960 (120).[37]

While the new German systems of reflex massage gained new followers, they hardly spread beyond Europe and very little beyond the German-speaking countries. And even there, the teachings of the Swedish, Dutch, and French masters continued, with modifications, in schools of "physiotherapy", of "medical gymnastics and massage", or exclusively of massage. Several textbooks, mostly written before World War II, laid the groundwork for the teaching, with much more descriptive information than their predecessors on technique, indications and contraindications, and other details of administration. Rosenthal (195) gave a solid scientific basis to massage in 1910. After Bum's voluminous book published in 1896 (35), the best known treatises in German were those of Hoffa (93), Müller (158), and Kirchberg (115); all these authors more or less followed the Swedish tradition. So did Dentz (62) and Boigey (31) in France in 1926 and 1950, respectively.

Well known early in the century among the English-language authors was Douglas Graham (85, 86) of Boston (1848–1928), who traveled to several countries to study massage and whom we have quoted repeatedly. Two other physicians, both of London, have also been well known in the United States: James B. Mennell (1880–1957) and James H. Cyriax. Both combined massage and joint manipulations. Mennell, very early in the century, had brought the legacy of Lucas-Championnière to England (147–149 and our footnote[32]). Cyriax has been advocating what he called "deep friction", applying it particularly to periarticular structures (55, 56 and Chapter 12 of this book).

Terrier (220), in Switzerland, combined massage and manipulations even more intimately, as expressed in the term of his "manipulative massage." The system, published in 1957, is a blend of massage, passive motions, and certain holds remindful of those his fellow countryman, Naegeli (162), had created before the turn of the century.

In Denmark, two workers have used massage in particular in the treatment of static edema and varicose ulcers. To that effect Holger Bisgaard (28) suggested in 1923 a combination of massage, exercise, bandaging, and elevation of the leg. Emil Vodder, a biologist and physical therapist, proposed a very gentle massage consisting mainly of circular motions of the thumb.[38] These two Danish methods have apparently not spread beyond Europe.

---

[37] A modification of the technique was suggested in 1964 by Kamenetz (109).

[38] Although Vodder had reportedly presented his method at a health exhibit in Paris in 1936 (227), he has apparently not published anything except for an article in 1961 (228) and the preface to a book of Asdonk (12). The latter was indeed his medical advocate for this "manual lymph drainage", which was complemented by breathing and relaxation exercises taught by Mrs. Estrid Vodder (13).

Treadmassage is a massage executed with the feet and usually applied to the back of a patient lying prone on the floor. The therapist is seated and regulates the amount of pressure to be applied by using more or less of his body weight; he may apply his total weight by standing up. This ancient technique has been mostly practiced in Eastern countries. From Japan it was brought to Germany where it was particularly publicized since 1939 by Schede and Kaiser (204).

What has been called by the misnomer "ice massage" is the application of a piece of ice by rubbing it over the skin, most often immediately after a contusion or other injury. It would be more correct to call it an *ice rub*.

Mechanical types of massage, either with the help or by the exclusive use of apparatus, have of course very much benefited from the technological advances of the 20th century. Vibrating machines have been produced that range in size from a small battery-powered object to house current-operated armchairs and massage beds.

A pneumatic apparatus operates by positive or negative pressure. The former acts in air-jet devices; the latter in suction cups which are available in various sizes and shapes, to be used in a stationary or a sliding technique.

For the upper and lower limbs there are air-filled sleeves which are alternately inflated and deflated, thus squeezing the limb intermittently. Pressure to the limbs can also be effected by electric stimulation of muscles (169). A very special type of rhythmic compression of the lower limbs synchronized with the heart beat is "syncardial massage" performed by the "Syncardon", a machine coupled with an electrocardiograph. It was created in 1945 by Fuchs (75), a Swiss physician, for the treatment of peripheral vascular disease.[39]

While the diversity of the techniques of massage has markedly increased, its use has been diminishing throughout the first three-quarters of the 20th century. It has been most appreciated and used in those countries which contributed most to its history and is probably used less in the United States than elsewhere. If we consider the therapeutic armamentarium throughout the world, and if the evolution in the United States is any indication, the role of massage in medicine has declined more or less steadily.[40] The development of the pharmaceutical industry was no doubt a factor. A greater variety of machines together with new inventions (diathermy, microwaves, ultrasound, etc.) have supplanted older means of physical therapy including massage. A third—and related—factor is what has been called the dehumanization in the relationship between the patients and those who treated them. This aloofness is opposed to the intimate

---

[39] For a more detailed discussion of these mechanical types of massage see Chapter 13.

[40] In other countries without a particularly noteworthy role of massage in their medical literature, India for example, this agent is much more widely practiced within the family, as a home remedy in health and disease.

contact between physician and patient or teacher and pupil. Physicians do not make the effort to learn—hence to teach—the time-consuming art of manual treatment. Thus, therapists do not learn about its potentials.[41]

Yet, possibly as a reaction to mechanization, there seems to be a tendency toward closer "contact" between those who search for better health and those who might help them to obtain it, between mother and child, teacher and pupil, patient and healer. This is not yet history but it might point to a swing of the pendulum in the reverse direction, a renewal of massage.

REFERENCES

1. Abadie. Traitement du blépharo-spasme par le massage forcé du muscle orbiculaire. *Gaz. Hôpitaux*, 1882.
2. Aetius of Amida. In: *Die Augenheilkunde des Aetius aus Amida*, edited by Hirschberg, J. Leipzig, 1899.
3. Aetius of Amida. *The Gynaecology and Obstetrics of the Sixth Centrury* (translated from the Latin edition of Cornarius by James V. Ricci), Philadelphia, 1950.
4. Alpinus, P. *De Medicina Aegyptiorum.* Venice, 1591; Paris, 1645.
5. Althaus, J. The risks of "massage." *Br. Med. J.*, pp. 1223–1224, (23 June), 1883.
6. Amiot, J. M., Bourgeois, Cibot, et al. *Mémoires Concernant l'Histoire, les Sciences, les Arts, les Moeurs et les Usages des Chinois, par les Missionnaires de Pékin.* Paris, 1776–1789.
7. Andry, N. *L'Orthopédie ou l'Art de Prévenir et de Corriger dans les Enfans les Difformités du Corps.* Paris, 1741.
8. Appenrodt. Zur Behandlung des atonischen Unterschenkelgeschwüres. *Dtsch. Med. Wochenschr. 14*:478, 1888.
9. Aretaeus. *The Extant Works of Aretaeus the Cappadocian* (translated by F. Adams). London, 1856.
10. Arvedson, J. *The Technique, Effects and Uses of Swedish Medical Gymnastics and Massage.* London, 1936.
11. *Asclepiades: His Life and Writings* (translated by R. M. Green). New Haven, 1955.
12. Asdonk, J. (ed.). *Manuelle Lymphdrainage* (preface by E. Vodder). Heidelberg, 1970.
13. Asdonk, J. *Ärztliche Erfahrungen mit der Lymphdrainage—Massage des Krampfaderbeines,* Second Ed. Heidelberg, 1971.
14. Aurelianus, C. *On Acute Diseases and on Chronic Diseases* (translated by I. E. Drabkin). Chicago, 1950.
15. Balfour, W. *Illustrations of the Efficacy of Compression and Percussion, in the Cure of Rheumatism, Sprains and Debility of the Extremities.* Edinburgh, 1820.
16. Barclay, J. *The Muscular Motions of the Human Body.* Edinburgh, 1808.
17. Barczewski, B. *Hand- und Lehrbuch meiner Reflexmassage.* Berlin, 1911.
18. Beard, G. A history of massage technic. *Phys. Ther. Rev., 32*:12, 1952.
19. Beard, G., and Wood, E. C. *Massage. Principles and Techniques.* Philadelphia, 1964.
20. Beauchef, P. *Le Massage en Thérapeutique Cutanée.* Thesis, Paris, 1902.
21. Becquerel. Du traitement de la chorée par la gymnastique. In Kirchberg (115).
22. Bender, G. A. A history of medicine in pictures. *Ther. Notes, 65* (5), 1958.
23. Bendix, B. Der Einfluss der Massage auf den Stoffwechsel des gesunden Menschen. *Z. Klin. Med., 25*:3, 1894.
24. Berghmann, G., and Helleday, U. Anteckningar om Massage. *Nord. Med. Ark., 5*:131, 1873.

---

[41] A questionnaire answered by 159 American therapists in 1967 revealed that 8% of them did not even believe in the therapeutic value of massage (189).

25. Berne, G. Recherches sur les modifications de la température locale sous l'influence du massage. *J. Méd. Paris,* 1886.
26. Berne, G. *Le Massage.* Paris, 1894, 1902.
27. Billroth, T. Zur Massage. *Wien. Med. Wochenschr.,* 1875.
28. Bisgaard, H. Ulcus cruris behandlet med. *Uppsal. Lak. Forhandl., 29:*487, 1923.
29. Bisgaard, H. *Ulcus Cruris og Eczema Cruris Phlebitidis Sequelae.* Copenhagen, 1939.
30. Blache. Traitement de la chorée par la gymnastique. *Moniteur Hôpitaux, 2:*721, 1854.
31. Boigey, M. *Manuel de Massage.* Paris, 1950.
32. Bonnet, A. *Traité de Thérapeutique des Maladies Articulaires.* Paris, 1853.
33. Brandt, T. *Nouvelle Méthode Gymnastique et Magnétique pour le Traitement des Maladies des Organes du Bassin et en Particulier de l'Utérus.* Stockholm, 1868.
34. Bright, T. *Hygieina (On Preserving Health).* Cambridge, 1584. In Coulter (50).
35. Bum, A. *Handbuch der Massage und Heilgymnastik für Praktische Ärzte.* Berlin, 1896, 1898.
36. Busch, F. General orthopedics, gymnastics and massage. In *Ziemssen's Handbook of General Therapeutics.* Leipzig, 1882.
37. Castex, A. Etude clinique et expérimentale sur le massage. *Arch. Gén. Méd.,* pp. 278–302 (March), 1891.
38. Castor and Pollux. *Das Masseusen-Unwesen in Berlin.* Berlin, 1900.
39. Cazeaux, P. *Traité des Accouchements.* Paris, 1840.
40. Cederschjöld, F. Die schwedische Heilgymnastik mit besonderer Berücksichtigung der mechanischen Nervenreize. *Virchow's Jahresbericht,* 1876. In Kirchberg (115).
41. Celsus, A. C. *De Re Medica* (translated by M. Nennin). Paris, 1873.
42. Champier, S. *Rosa Gallica, Omnibus Sanitatem Affectantibus Utilis et Necessaria.* Nancy, 1512.
43. de Chauliac, G. *La Grande Chirurgie.* Lyons, 1641.
44. Chomel, J. B. L. *Essai Historique de la Médecine en France.* Paris, 1762. In Estradère (69).
45. Cleobury, W. *A Full Account of the System of Friction as Adopted and Pursued with the Greatest Success in Cases of Contracted Joints and Lameness from Various Causes, by the late eminent Surgeon, John Grosvenor, Esq. of Oxford.* Third Ed. Oxford, 1825.
46. Colombo, C. Action du massage sur la sécrétion des glandes. *C. R. Hebd. Soc. Biol., 47:*46, 1895.
47. Cornelius, A. *Die Nervenpunktlehre.* Leipzig, 1909.
48. Cornelius, A. *Die Nervenpunkte.* Munich, 1933.
49. Coste, R. *Le Massage Sportif.* Paris, 1906.
50. Coulter, J. S. *Physical Therapy.* New York, 1932.
51. Credé, K. *Klinische Vorträge über Geburtshilfe.* Berlin, 1854.
52. Crocker, H. R. *Diseases of the Skin.* London, 1893.
53. Cumston, C. G. *An Introduction to the History of Medicine.* London, 1968.
54. Cyriax, E. F. *The Elements of Kellgren's Manual Treatment.* London, 1903; New York, 1904.
55. Cyriax, J. *Massage, Manipulation and Local Anaesthesia.* London, 1941.
56. Cyriax, J. *Textbook of Orthopaedic Medicine,* vol. I: *Diagnosis of Soft-Tissue Lesions,* Sixth Ed. (formerly: *Rheumatism and Soft-Tissue Injuries*). The Williams & Wilkins Co., Baltimore, 1975. Vol. II: *Treatment by Manipulation, Massage and Injection,* Eighth Ed. (formerly: *Deep Massage and Manipulations*). The Williams & Wilkins Co., Baltimore, 1971.
57. Dagron. *Massage des Membres.* Paris, 1905.
58. Dally, N. *Cinésiologie ou Science du Mouvement dans ses Rapports avec l'Education, l'Hygiène et la Thérapie.* Paris, 1857.
59. Daremberg, C. *La Médecine dans Homère ou Etudes d'Archéologie . . . dans les Poèmes Homériques.* Paris, 1865.

60. Daremberg, C. *Etat de la Médecine entre Homère et Hippocrate.* Paris, 1869.
61. Delpech, J. M. *De l'Orthomorphie par Rapport à l'Espèce Humaine.* Paris, 1828.
62. Dentz, M. *Le Traitement Manuel Suédois.* Paris, 1926.
63. Dicke, E. *Meine Bindegewebsmassage.* Stuttgart, 1953. Eighth Ed.: Dicke, E., Schliack, H., and Wolff, A. *Bindegewebsmassage.* Stuttgart, 1975.
64. Donders, F. C. Massage en oculistique. *Zehender's Monatshefte,* 1872. In Petit (175), p. 302.
65. Dudgeon, J. Kung-fu, or medical gymnastics. *J. Peking Oriental Soc. 3:*341, 1895.
66. Ebner, M. *Connective Tissue Massage.* Edinburgh and London, 1962.
67. Eccles, A. S. Observations on the physiological effects of massage. *Proc. R. Med. Chirurg. Soc.,* 1885. In Verleysen (226).
68. Elleaume. Du massage dans l'entorse. *Gaz. Hôpitaux,* 1859. In Estradère (69).
69. Estradère, J. *Du Massage, son Historique, ses Manipulations, ses Effets Physiologiques et Thérapeutiques.* Thesis, Paris, 1863.
70. Fabricius [of Aquapendente], H. *De Motu Animalium.* Padua, 1618. In Dally (58).
71. Fiocco and Locatelli. Considerazioni e ricerche intorno all'azione del massaggio sopra la cute. *Giorn. Ital. Malatt. Vener. e della Pelle, 2:*1902.
72. Frankl, O. *Die Physikalischen Heilmethoden in der Gynäkologie.* Berlin, 1906.
73. de Frumerie, G. *Cours de Massage Accessoire des Soins d'Accouchements.* Paris, 1904.
74. Fuchs, L. *Institutiones Medicae.* Basel, 1565. In Kirchberg (115).
75. Fuchs, M. Neue Methode zur Förderung der lokalen Blutzirkulation: "Synkardial Massage." *Schweiz. Med. Wochenschr., 75:*542, 16 June 1945.
76. Fuller, F. *Medicina Gymnastica,* Sixth Ed. London, 1728.
77. Galen, C. *De Sanitate Tuenda* (translated by R. M. Green). Springfield, 1949.
78. Garnault, P. *Le Massage Vibratoire et Electrique des Muqueuses.* Paris, 1894.
79. Garrison, F. H. *An Introduction to the History of Medicine.* Philadelphia, 1929, 1960.
80. Gazius, A. *Florida Corona.* Lyons, 1514.
81. Georgii, A. *Kinésithérapie.* Paris, 1847.
82. Gläser, O., and Dalicho, A. W. *Segmentmassage: Massage Reflektorischer Zonen.* Leipzig, 1952. Fourth Ed. 1972.
83. Glisson, F. *De Rachitide Sive Morbo Puerili.* Amsterdam, 1671.
84. Gondrin, B. *Historia Flagellantium.* Paris, 1700. In Mac-Auliffe (140).
85. Graham, D. *A Treatise on Massage.* New York, 1884. Third Ed. Philadelphia and London, 1902.
86. Graham, D. *Massage, Manual Treatment, Remedial Movements: History, Mode of Application and Effects, Indications and Contra-Indications.* Philadelphia, 1913.
87. Grosvenor, J. See Cleobury (45).
88. Haberling, W. Johan Georg Mezger of Amsterdam. *Medical Life 39:*191, 1932.
89. Hansen, K., and von Staa, H. *Reflektorische und Algetische Krankheitszeichen der Inneren Organe.* Leipzig, 1938. Second Ed.: Hansen, K., and Schliack, H. *Segmentale Innervation, ihre Bedeutung für Klinik und Praxis.* Stuttgart, 1962.
90. von Haufe. *Über Massage.* Frankfurt, 1880. In Kirchberg (115).
91. Head, H. On disturbances of sensation with especial reference to the pain of visceral disease. *Brain, 16:*1, 1893; *17:*339, 1894. Translation: *Die Sensibilitätsstörungen der Haut bei Visceralerkrankungen.* Berlin, 1898.
92. Hippocrates. *Oeuvres Complètes d'Hippocrate,* edited by Littré, E. Paris, 1839 to 1861.
93. Hoffa, A. *Technik der Massage.* Stuttgart, 1897. 13th Ed.: Hoffa-Gocht-Storck, Stuttgart, 1973.
94. Hoffmann, F. *Dissertationes Physico-medicae.* The Hague, 1708. In Dally (58).
95. Holzer, W. Physikalische Medizin in Diagnostik und Therapie. Vienna, 1947.
96. Hueter, C. Klinik der Gelenkerkrankungen. 1871. In Verleysen (226).
97. In de Betou, J. G. *Therapeutic Manipulations.* London, 1842. In Verleysen (226).
98. Jackson, A. R. Uterine massage as a means of treating certain forms of enlargement. *Am.*

J. Obstet., 13:897, 1880.

99. Jacquet, L. Traitement simple de certaines dermatoses et déformations de la face. *Presse Méd.*, 8 June 1907.

100. Jaeger, O. H. *Die Gymnastik der Hellenen.* Esslingen, 1850. In Kirchberg (115).

101. James. *Dictionnaire Universel de Médecine* (translated by Diderot). Paris, 1747. In Dally (58).

102. Jastrow, M. Babylonian-Assyrian medicine. *Ann. Med. Hist., 1*:231–257 (see p. 241), 1917. (Article based in large measure on "The Medicine of the Babylonians and Assyrians", in *Proc. R. Soc. Med. Section, Hist. Med. 7*:109, 1914.)

103. Johnson, W. *The Anatriptic Art.* London, 1866.

104. Joseph, L. H. Gymnastics from the middle ages to the eighteenth century. *Ciba. Symp.*, March, 1949.

105. Joubert, L. *De Gymnasiis et Generibus Exercitationum Apud Antiquos Celebrum.* Lyons, 1582. In Dally (58).

106. Julien. *Du Massage de l'Oeil.* Thesis, Paris, 1812. In Verleysen (226).

107. Jüthner, J. *Philostratos über Gymnastik.* Leipzig, 1909.

108. Kamenetz, H. *Le Massage en Dermatologie.* Thesis, Paris, 1952.

109. Kamenetz, H. Transthoracic cardiac massage; suggestion of technique. *Am. J. Phys. Med., 43*:217, 1964.

110. Keen, W. W. Notes as to the comparative effects of active voluntary exercise and of passive exercise by massage on the production of albuminuria. *Polyclinic 2*:121, 1885.

111. Keith, A. *Menders of the Maimed.* London, 1919.

112. Kellgren, A. *The Technic of Ling's System of Manual Treatment.* Edinburgh and London, 1890.

113. Kellogg, J. H. *The Art of Massage: Its Physiological Effects and Therapeutic Applications.* Battle Creek, 1895; 12th Ed. Battle Creek, 1919.

114. Kibler, M. *Segment-Therapie bei Gelenkerkrankungen und Inneren Krankheiten.* Stuttgart, 1950.

115. Kirchberg, F. *Handbuch der Massage und Heilgymnastik,* 2 vols. Leipzig, 1926.

116. Kleen, E. A. G. *Handbuch der Massage.* Leipzig, 1895.

117. Kleen, E. A. G. *Massage and Medical Gymnastics.* New York, 1921.

118. Klemm, K. *Die Ärztliche Massage.* Riga, 1883.

119. Kohlrausch, W. *Reflexzonenmassage in Muskulatur und Bindegewebe.* Stuttgart, 1955.

120. Kouwenhoven, W. B., Jude, J. R., and Knickerbocker, G. G. Closed-chest cardiac massage. *J.A.M.A., 173*:1064, 1960.

121. Krauss, H. *Periostbehandlung von P. Vogler: Klinische und Experimentelle Beiträge zur Periostbehandlung nach Vogler.* Leipzig, 1953. Reprinted in Vogler (229).

122. de Lacroix de Lavalette, L. *La Sismothérapie ou L'Utilisation du Mouvement Vibratoire en Médecine Générale, et particulièrement en Thérapeutique Gynécologique.* Paris, 1899.

123. Laisné, N. *Du Massage, des Frictions et Manipulations, Appliqués à la Guérison de Quelques Maladies.* Paris, 1868.

124. Lange, F., and Eversbusch, G. Die Bedeutung der Muskelhärten für die allgemeine Praxis. *Münch. Med. Wochenschr., 68*:418, 1921.

125. Lange, M. *Die Muskelhärten (Myogelosen). Ihre Entstehung und Heilung.* Munich, 1931.

126. Lassar, O. Über Ödem und Lymphstrom bei den Entzündungen. *Virchows Arch., 69*:518, 1887.

127. Lavier, J. *Le Micro-Massage Chinois.* Paris, 1965.

128. Lee, B. Massage; the latest handmaid in medicine. *Trans. Med. Soc. Penn., 16*:287, 1884.

129. Le Gentil [de La Galaisière, G. J.]. *Voyage dans les Mers de l'Inde,* vol. I, pp. 128–131. Paris, 1779.

130. Leroy, R. *Le Massage Plastique dans les Dermatoses de la Face.* Thesis, Paris, 1908.

131. Leube, H., and Dicke, E. *Massage Reflektorischer Zonen im Bindegewebe.* Stuttgart, 1948.

132. Licht, S. History of therapeutic heat. In *Therapeutic Heat and Cold,* edited by S. Licht.

New Haven, 1965. Reprinted in *Second Ed.*, edited by Lehmann, J. Baltimore, Williams & Wilkins, 1982.

133. Liedbeck and Georgii. In Kirchberg (115).

134. Liétard, G.-L. *Sur l'Histoire de la Médecine chez les Indous.* Thesis, Strasbourg, 1858. In Estradère (69).

135. Ling, P. H. *Gymnastikens Allmänna Grunder*, edited by Liedbeck and Georgii. Upsala, 1840.

136. Little, J. F. Medical Rubbing. *Brit. Med. J.*, 2:351, 1882.

137. Londe, C. *Gymnastique Médicale.* Paris, 1821.

138. Lorry, A. C. *Tractatus de Morbis Cutaneis.* Paris, 1777.

139. Lucas-Championnière, J. *Traitement des Fractures par le Massage et la Mobilisation.* Paris, 1895.

140. Mac-Auliffe, L. *La Thérapeutique Physique d'Autrefois.* Paris, 1904.

141. Mackenzie, J. *Symptoms and Their Interpretation.* London, 1909; Fourth Ed. London, 1920.

142. Maggiora, A. De l'action physiologique du massage sur les muscles de l'homme. *Arch. Ital. Biol.*, 16:225–246, 1891.

143. Maimonides, M. The Medical Aphorisms of Moses Maimonides (translated and edited by Fred Rosner and Suessman Muntner), 2 vols. New York, 1970–1971.

144. Major, R. H. *A History of Medicine.* Springfield, 1954.

145. Marfort, J. E. *Manuel Pratique de Massage et de Gymnastique Médicale.* Paris, 1907.

146. Meibomius, J. H. *De Flagrorum Usu in Re Medica et Venerea.* Amsterdam, 1629.

147. Mennell, J. B. *The Treatment of Fractures by Mobilisation and Massage.* London, 1911.

148. Mennell, J. B. *Massage: Its Principles and Practice.* London, 1917; Philadelphia, 1920.

149. Mennell, J. B. *Physical Treatment by Movement, Manipulation, and Massage.* Philadelphia, 1934; New York, 1940.

150. Mercurialis, H. *De Arte Gymnastica.* Venice, 1569.

151. Meyer, J. *Dermatologie Physio-Chirurgicale.* Second Ed. Paris, 1950.

152. Mezger, J. G. *De Behandeling der Voetverstuikingen met Fricties.* Amsterdam, 1868.

153. Mezger, J. G. Behandlung von Teleangiektasien mittelst subkutaner Gefässzerreissung. *Langenbecks Arch.*, 13:239, 1872.

154. Mitchell, J. K. Massage and exercise. In: *Mechanotherapy and Physical Education*, edited by Cohen, S. S. Philadelphia, 1904.

155. Mitchell, S. W. *Fat and Blood and How to Make Them.* Philadelphia, 1877.

156. Mortimer-Granville, J. Nerve vibration as a therapeutic agent. *Lancet*, 1:949, 1882.

157. von Mosengeil, F. Über Massage, deren Technik, Wirkung und Indicationen. *Langenbecks Arch.*, 19:428, 551, 1876.

158. Müller, A. *Lehrbuch der Massage.* Bonn, 1915.

159. Müller, E. A., and Schulte am Esch, J. Die Wirkung der Massage auf die Leistungsfähigkeit von Muskeln. *Int. Z. Angew. Physiol.*, 22:240, 1966.

160. Murray, J. A. H. Article on Massage. In *A New English Dictionary on Historical Principles.* Oxford, 1908.

161. Murrell, W. *Massage as a Mode of Treatment.* London, 1886.

162. Naegeli, O. *Behandlung und Heilung von Nervenleiden und Nervenschmerzen durch Handgriffe*, First Ed. Berlin, 1893; Second Ed. Jena, 1899.

163. Namikoshi, T. *Shiatsu; Japanese Finger-Pressure Therapy.* Tokyo and San Francisco, 1969, 1974.

164. von Niederhoeffer, P. *Neue Beobachtungen über die Mechanik der breiten Rückenmuskeln und über deren Beziehungen zur Skoliose.* Vienna, 1933. In Verleysen (226).

165. Norström G. *Traité Théorique et Pratique du Massage (Méthode de Mezger en Particulier).* Paris, 1884.

166. Norström, G. *The Manual Treatment of Diseases of Women.* New York, 1903.

167. Oertel, M. J. *Handbuch der Allgemeinen Therapie der Kreislaufstörungen.* Leipzig, 1885.

168. Oribasius. *Oeuvres d'Oribase* (translated by Bussemaker and Daremberg). Paris, 1854.
169. Ornstein, G. G., Licht, S., and Herman, M. Raising of venous pressure in surgical shock by faradic stimulation. *Arch. Phys. Ther., 21:*329, 1940.
170. Pagel, J. Geschichte der Kosmetik. In *Handbuch der Kosmetik*, edited by Joseph, M. Leipzig, 1912.
171. Pagenstecher. Le massage dans les maladies des yeux. *Arch. Augenheilkunde*, 1881.
172. Paré, A. *Oeuvres Complètes.* Paris, 1841.
173. Paullini, C. F. *Flagellum Salutis.* Frankfurt, 1698.
174. Pemberton, R., and Scull, C. W. Massage. In *Medical Physics*, edited by Glasser, O. Chicago, 1944.
175. Petit, L. *Le Massage par le Médecin.* Paris, 1885.
176. Pfeiffer, R. H. *State Letters of Assyria.* New Haven, 1935.
177. Phélippeaux de Saint Savinien. Etude pratique sur les frictions et le massage ou guide du médecin-masseur. *Abeille Méd., 26:*23, 1869. In Verleysen (226).
178. Piorry. Article on Massage. In *Dictionaire des Sciences Médicales*, edited by Adelon et al. Paris, 1819.
179. Pliny. Quoted in *Asclepiades: His Life and Writings* (11).
180. Pliny. *Pliny's Natural History* (translated by P. Holland, 1634), edited by Newsome, J. Oxford, 1964.
181. Post, S. Electromassage. *NY Med. Rec., 19:* (26 June) 1881.
182. Preusser, W. Die Gelosen-Massage. *Hippokrates 28 (14):*436 (31 July), 1957.
183. Prosser, E. M. *Manual of Massage and Movements*, Third Ed. Philadelphia, 1951.
184. von Puttkamer, J. *Organ-Beeinflussung durch Massage*, Fourth Ed. Ulm, 1953.
185. Quellmalz, S. *Programma de Frictione Abdominis.* Leipzig, 1749. In Coulter (50).
186. Regimbeau, C. *Manuel de Massage Ponctural et des Plexus.* Paris, 1975.
187. *Regimen Sanitatis Salernitanum.* In Joseph (104).
188. Reibmayr, A. *Die Massage und ihre Verwerthung in den verschiedenen Disciplinen der praktischen Medizin.* Vienna, 1883.
189. Reiter, S., Garrett, T. R., and Erickson, D. J. Current trends in the use of therapeutic massage. *Phys. Ther. 49:*158, 1969.
190. Reveillé-Parise, J. H. *Traité de la Vieillesse Hygiénique, Médical et Philosophique.* Paris, 1853.
191. Reynier, P. In preface to Petit (175).
192. Rivers, W. H. R. Massage in Melanesia. Tr. XVII. In *International Congress of Medicine*, 1913, Sect. XXIII, pp. 39–42. London, 1914.
193. Rizet, A. *Emploi du Massage pour le Diagnostic de Certaines Fractures.* 1866. In Verleysen (226).
194. Roederer, C., and Ledent, R. *La Pratique des Déviations Vertébrales.* Paris, 1926.
195. Rosenthal, C. *Die Massage und ihre Wissenschaftliche Begründung.* Leipzig, 1910.
196. Rossbach, M. J. *Lehrbuch der Physikalischen Heilmethoden.* Berlin, 1882.
197. Ruffier, F. *Traité Pratique du Massage Sportif.* Paris, 1907.
198. Rufus of Ephesus. *Treatise on Diseases of the Kidneys and the Bladder.* In Verleysen (226).
199. Ruhmann, W. Tastmassage. *Münch. Med. Wochenschr., 76:*278, 1929.
200. Ruhmann, W. *Die Tastmassage: ihre Anwendung und Wirkungsweise bei den Weichteilrheumatismen.* Leipzig, 1934.
201. Sabatier, R. B. *Traité Complet d'Anatomie.* Paris, 1781. In Verleysen (226).
202. Savary, C. E. *Lettres sur l'Egypte*, vol. I, p. 126. Paris, 1785.
203. The scandals of massage. *Br. Med. J., 2:*1003, 1069, 1140, 1199, 1894.
204. Schede and Kaiser. In: Beck, O. Möglichkeiten und Grenzen der Tretmassage. *Beitr. Orthop., 19:*613, Oct. 1972.
205. Schlegel, E. Erschütterungsschläge, ein neues Hilfsmittel der mechanischen Therapie. *Allg. med. Centr.-Ztg (Berlin), 54:*625, 1885.

206. Schreiber, J. *A Manual of Treatment by Massage and Methodical Muscle Exercise* (translated by W. Mendelson). Philadelphia, 1887.
207. Sée, A. *La Chorée et les Affections Nerveuses.* Paris, 1851. In Kirchberg (115).
208. Séguin, D. L'emploi du massage, de la gymnastique et des bains de vapeur dans le traitement des affections chroniques des articulations. *Gaz. Méd. Paris*, p. 828, 1839.
209. Séverin, M. A. *De la Médecine Efficace.* Geneva, 1668.
210. Shaw, J. *The Nature and Treatment of Distortions of the Spine.* London, 1823, with Atlas (1824) and Supplement (1825).
211. Shoemaker, J. V. *A Practical Treatise on Diseases of the Skin.* Philadelphia, 1892.
212. Sicard, A. Les pinçons thérapeutiques au Viet-Nam. *Presse Méd., 76*:773–775, 1968.
213. Sigerist, H. E. *A History of Medicine.* New York, 1951.
214. Snow, M. A. *Mechanical Vibration and its Therapeutic Application.* New York, 1904.
215. Stapfer, H. *Traité de Kinésithérapie Gynécologique (Massage et Gymnastique). Etude Expérimentale et Raisonnée du Système de Thure Brandt.* Paris, 1897.
216. Stapfer, H. *Massage et Gymnastique dans les Affections de la Femme.* Paris, 1906.
217. Strabo. *Rerum Geographicarum,* Libri XVII. Amsterdam, 1707.
218. Sudraka. The Little Clay Cart. In *Two Plays of Ancient India,* by J. A. B. van Buitenen (translated from Sanskrit and Prakrit). New York, 1968.
219. Teirich-Leube, H. *Grundriss der Bindegewebsmassage.* Stuttgart, 1957. Sixth Ed. 1972.
220. Terrier, J. C. *Manipulativmassage.* Stuttgart, 1958.
221. Thiele, G. H. Tonic spasm of the levator ani, coccygeus and piriformis muscles. *Trans. Am. Proctol. Soc., 37*:145, 1936.
222. Tidy, N. M. *Massage and Remedial Exercises,* Baltimore, 1932; 11th ed, 1968.
223. Tissot, J.-C. *Gymnastique Médicinale et Chirurgicale.* Paris, 1780.
224. Traissac, R. Massages gynécologiques. Techniques et résultats. *Bull. Féd. Soc. Gynécol. Obstét. Lang. Fr., 20*:136, Apr.–May 1968.
225. Veith, I. *The Yellow Emperor's Classic of Internal Medicine.* The Williams & Wilkins Co., Baltimore, 1949.
226. Verleysen, J. *Histoire du Massage et de la Gymnastique Médicale.* Brussels, 1956.
227. Vodder, E. Le drainage lymphatique, une nouvelle méthode thérapeutique. Revue d'Hygiène Individuelle: "Santé pour Tous." Paris, April, 1936. In Asdonk (12).
228. Vodder, E. Lymphdrainage, eine neue Behandlungsart. *Z. Schweiz. Verbandes staatl. anerkannten Physiotherapeuten,* No. 177, 1961.
229. Vogler, P. *Physiotherapie.* Stuttgart, 1964. Includes reprint of Krauss (121).
230. Weber, A. S. *Traité de la Massothérapie.* Paris, 1891.
231. Weiss, B. Die Massage, ihre Geschichte, ihre Anwendung und Wirkung. *Wien. Klin.,* 1879. In Kirchberg (115).
232. Wetterwald, F. *Les Névralgies.* Paris, 1910.
233. de Winter, E. *Massages et Approche des Cinorthèses.* Paris, 1975.
234. Wise, T. A. *Commentary on the Hindu System of Medicine.* Calcutta, 1845.
235. Wong, K. C., and Wu, L. *History of Chinese Medicine.* Shanghai, 1936.
236. Wood, E. C. *Beard's Massage.* Second Ed. of Beard and Wood (19). Philadelphia, 1974.
237. Wylie, A. *Notes on Chinese Literature.* Shanghai, 1922.
238. Yabuuchi, K. *Chūgoku-chūsei Kagaku Gijutsu Shi No Kenkyū.* Tokyo, 1963.
239. Zabludowski, J. *Über die Physiologische Bedeutung der Massage.* Berlin, 1883.
240. Zabludowski, J. *Technik der Massage.* Leipzig, 1903.
241. Zabludowski, J. *Massage im Dienst der Kosmetik,* Berlin, 1905.
242. Zaufal, F. Über Massage bei Ohrenkrankheiten. *Prag. Med. Wochenschr.,* No. 44, 1883. In Bum (35).

10

Physiologic Effects of Massage

KHALIL G. WAKIM

Rawlins (22) defined massage as the power to repair by movement the complicated machine known as the human body. Movement or exercise induces exaggeration of vital activity and thereby increases the pulse, respiration, and body temperature. Contraction and relaxation of muscles facilitate the movement of blood, increase the circulation of massage as well as lymph, and have a direct influence on the heart, lungs, and brain and on the exchange of body fluids. The increase in massage supply and the facilitation of movement of blood and exchange of body fluids provide greater warmth and nutrition to the entire body.

Intelligent and scientific manipulation of the skin and soft tissues of the body places the physiologic status of the skin at an optimum, invigorates the circulation of blood and lymph, and alerts the central and peripheral nervous system. This induces more rapid oxygenation and reoxygenation of blood, speeds up the movement of lymph and exchange of body fluids, and facilitates the elimination of wastes. Systematized massage, consisting of stroking, kneading, wringing, pulling, percussing, and vibrating, brings about the following important effects: (a) improvement of circulation and movement of blood and nutritive elements, (b) increase of warmth to the skin and improvement in its condition, (c) more rapid elimination of waste, (d), dissolution of soft adhesions, (e) reduction of swelling and induration of tissues, (f) loosening and stretching of contracted tendons, and (g) soothing of the central nervous system and the peripheral nerves. *Massage in Bild und Wort* (10), a regularly appearing publication in East Germany, presents anatomical facts, physiology of the venous circulation including neurophysiology and muscular physiology, and a good set of illustrations on the techniques of massage and manipulation of different parts of the body.

For massage to be applied scientifically and effectively, a good working knowledge of the human body and its parts and their structure and movements must be mastered. The muscles and the direction of their fibers and insertion of their tendons, the blood and lymph vessels and the direction of flow of blood and lymph should be recognized. The various stages of inflammation, edema, and congestion should be well understood in relation to the mechanism of production and reduction and the various factors involved. The centripetal stroking and kneading of muscles make them contract and relax rhythmically with the strokes, thus squeezing the veins and lymphatic vessels and forcing the venous blood and lymph toward the heart, reducing the chance for accumulation of waste and stagnation of blood and lymph. Effleurage, the main maneuver in massage, is a rubbing activity that facilitates capillary circulation, which stimulates the movement of venous blood and lymph and, consequently, the arterial circulation and nutrition. Rhythmic pétrissage, or kneading, will not only simulate but also stimulate nature's action on the muscles.

Graham (9) has emphasized that massage is a potent agent which affects either directly or indirectly every function of the human body, and that a study of the effects of massage on the body is a study of physiology itself.

Influence of Massage on Skin

By virtue of its highly organized structure, the skin is extremely well adapted for receiving and transmitting the effects of massage. The epidermis protects the papillary layer underneath it from the encroachment of vigorous handling. Massage has a soothing effect on the highly sensitive and vascular papillae on which the deeper layers of the cuticle fit. The skin is the principal seat of the sense of touch, and proper massage arouses the most delightful sensation from the contact of the hands during skillful manipulation. The skin becomes softer, more supple, and finer as a result of the proper manipulations of massage; furthermore, after prolonged use of massage and adaptation to its manipulation, the skin becomes tougher, more flexible and elastic, and so much less sensitive that it can be handled fairly roughly without discomfort. Massage increases insensible perspiration and facilitates sebaceous secretions from the exocrine glands of the skin. Massage in general imparts renewed vigor and improves the nutritive status of the skin.

Graham (9) suggested that massage facilitates the movement of the skin over the other superficial structures in conditions that cause a matted, hidebound state and that this reduces pressure interference on lymphatic vessels and veins by the fasciae and subcutaneous structures. In their study on the influence of underwater massage on rewarming, heat conductivity, and perfusion of the skin in progressive scleroderma, Meffert et al. (19) noted partial improvement in skin blood flow. Massage was found responsible for activation of lipolysis (20). The release of catecholamines by the tissue nerve endings was particularly stressed as the cause. This was confirmed when activation of lipolysis was depressed by beta blockers.

Influence of Massage on Skeletal Musculature

Whenever the human body is incapable of physical exercise, massage becomes an indispensable substitute. The skeletal musculature of the body constitutes about 50% of the body weight and is abundantly supplied with blood. By their intermittent contraction and relaxation, the muscles act as an efficient subsidiary pump and aid the heart immensely in the continuous forward movement of blood. With every contraction of a muscle, massage is driven or squeezed out of it; at every relaxation, blood enters the muscles and refills the intermusculature vessels. Rhythmic activation of muscles can be effectively accomplished by intermittent massage, which aids in prevention of the atrophy of inactive muscles. As already noted, rhythmic pétrissage stimulates muscular action to promote forward propulsion of venous massage and lymph. Inactive muscles are not provided with sufficient massage, and the exchange of nutritive elements is inadequate under such conditions. If the muscles cannot be made to contract and relax normally through orders sent in the form of impulses from higher centers along the motor nerves supplying the muscles, artificial activation can be effected by massage. Muscular fatigue from overexertion or prolonged stagnation and inactivity can be relieved best by massage, which promotes rapid disposal of waste products and replenishment of nutritive elements through improvement of blood flow and circulatory exchange in the muscles. Massage of the abdominal musculature, in addition to strengthening the abdominal wall, also aids in the excitation of peristaltic activity in the gastrointestinal tract and facilitates regularity and evacuation of the large intestine.

Graham (9) reported studies done on exercised muscles with and without massage during the rest period after fatigue had set in. The muscles that were massaged during the recovery period after fatigue regained their lost vigor much sooner than did those not massaged during the recovery period. Furthermore, the massaged muscles were able to do much more work than those that were not massaged. The massaged muscles were supple and pliant during the recovery period, whereas the unmassaged ones were stiff. Maggiora (18) reported work demonstrating the effects of massage on his own muscles when weakened by various means. He found that friction and percussion had the same restorative effect, while pétrissage had much greater effect on the muscles.

Kroneker and Stirling (quoted by Graham [9]) considered massage to muscles as perfect perfusion, bringing nourishment and removing wastes. Graham concluded that massage lessens irritability but increases the work output of muscles.

Influence of Massage on Circulation

Massage provides an additional *vis a tergo* to the veins and lymphatic vessels, aiding in their mechanical emptying and facilitating forward movement of blood and lymph. The effect is similar to a combination of suction and force pump. Careful observation of the superficial veins demonstrates their collapsing and refilling as they are manipulated by the hands of the masseur. This aids the circulation in the deep veins as well as that in the arterioles and capillaries of the region. Gentle centripetal stroking massage is a mild stimulant to the vasomotor nerves supplying the blood vessels of the skin. Prolongation of the massage brings about hyperemia of the region.

From studies on the effects of massage on the circulation, we (26, 27) concluded that deep stroking and kneading massage produce moderate, consistent, and definite increase in the blood flow of the extremities of patients who have flaccid paralysis, just as they do in normal extremities.

Krogh (15) demonstrated an increase in the diameter and permeability of capillaries after mechanical stimulation in frogs and mammals. Pemberton (21) suggested that massage provokes release of histamine and acetylcholine, accompanied by vasodilation, and increases blood flow and discharge of erythrocytes from the spleen.

As already noted, the mechanical effect of massage increases the movement of blood, making the exchange of nutrients and wastes more efficient and improving the trophic state of the skin and underlying structures. Graham likened the hands of the masseur to propelling hearts at the peripheral ends of the circulation cooperating with the heart itself, the number of intermittent squeezes of massage being approximately synchronized to the heart beats. He asked: "If this is not an art that does mend nature, what is?"

Massage in the form of pétrissage was found by Edgecombe and Bain (7) to cause initially a brief increase in arterial blood pressure, but they found that the net outcome was a decrease. The venous pressure was increased, the amount depending on the environmental temperature, and was greater at a higher room temperature.

Kleen (13) stated that, as a result of massage, the arterial circulation was hastened by the quicker outflow from the veins and the diminished pressure within them. After massage, there was active hyperemia in the skin and muscles, and the number of erythrocytes in the superficial vessels increased by 40–50% (14).

Skull (23) observed definite peripheral vasodilation together with an increase in the rate of peripheral blood flow after massage. The release of acetylcholine and the production of histamine and histamine-like substances in the tissues play an important role in the vasodilation induced by massage.

Carrier (4) showed that light pressure resulted in instant transient capillary dilation, whereas heavier pressure resulted in a more enduring dilation, with a greater number of capillaries visible. According to Pemberton (21), Clark and Swenson presented cinematographic studies on the effects of massage on the circulation in the capillaries of a rabbit's ear. They demonstrated a definite increase in the speed of the circulating elements, diapedesis of the leukocytes, and increased exchange of substances between the massage stream and tissue cells, with improved metabolism.

Leroy (16) remarked that deep stimulating massage acts as a succession of traumatisms and can be used selectively in order to stimulate the sensitive endings of the nerves and to produce vasodilation by means of axon reflexes and release of histamine.

Influence of Massage on Flow of Lymph

Lymph spaces and lymph vessels of various sizes permeate the deep fascial and investing sheaths of muscles and other tissues. Passive exercise in the form of massage greatly enhances the movement of tissue fluid and lymph in the spaces and vessels of the deep fascia and muscles. It is a well-established fact that massage and exercise induce a great increase in the flow of lymph (1, 6, 25). The presence of valves in the lymph vessels ensures a unidirectional movement forward.

Elkins and associates (8) studied the effects on the flow of lymph of massage that consisted of a combination of centripetal kneading and stroking. Such massage caused pronounced increases in lymph flow. Passive exercise brought about a 25-fold increase in flow of lymph. In animals that had edema in the hindlegs owing to hypoproteinemia induced by the loss of plasma proteins with the lymph, massage of the edematous legs caused a great increase in the flow of lymph and a significant reduction in the size of the massaged limbs.

Drinker (5) demonstrated a definite increase in lymph flow by massage. Bauer and associates (2) showed that proteins injected into joints of dogs were removed by lymphatic vessels and that massage and passive motion definitely increased elimination of the proteins through these channels.

In studies on the effects of intermittent rhythmic compression on upper extremities that were chronically swollen and edematous after radical mastectomy, we (27) noted that daily application of centripetal rhythmic compression by use of the vasopneumatic apparatus caused gradual disappearance of the swelling and edema and that the tissues became softer. The pain was usually relieved, and the consistency and color of the skin usually returned to normal. Huddleston and associates (11) noted that use of this apparatus brought about improvement of the discolored, cold, and clammy condition of limbs paralyzed by poliomyelitis. Kirby and Sampson (12) reported an increase in movement of fluid in the tissues of the extremities massaged by use of the vasopneumatic apparatus and considered its application in chronic lymphatic obstruction to be highly beneficial.

It is interesting to note that massage of specific areas in the body plays a vital role in the therapy of certain disorders. Carotid sinus massage is used very often as a therapeutic procedure for reversion of severe supraventricular tachycardia to normal rhythm (17). Ankle sprains are sometimes treated by intermittent compression and ice packs (24). Ice massage is utilized for skin analgesia (28). Bugaj (3) reported cooling analgesic and rewarming of localized skin by ice massage.

REFERENCES

1. Asdonk, J. Lymphatic drainage by massage; mechanism of action, indications and contraindications. Z. Aelegemainmed., 51:751, 1975.
2. Bauer, W., Short, C. L., and Bennett, G. A. The manner of removal of proteins from normal joints. J. Exp. Med., 57:419, 1933.
3. Bugaj, R. The cooling, analgesic, rewarming effects of ice massage on localized skin. Phys. Ther., 55:11, 1975.
4. Carrier, E. B. Studies on the physiology of capillaries. V. The reaction of the human skin capillaries to drugs and other stimuli. Am. J. Physiol., 61:528, 1922.
5. Drinker, C. K. The formation and movements of lymph. Am. Heart J., 18:389, 1939.
6. Drinker, C. K., and Yoffey, J. M. Lymphatics, Lymph and Lymphoid Tissue: Their Physiological and Clinical Significance. Cambridge, 1941, pp. 112–145.
7. Edgecombe, W., and Bain, W. The effect of baths, massage and exercise on the blood-pressure. Lancet, 1:1552, 1899.
8. Elkins, E. C., Herrick, J. F., Grindlay, J. H., et al. Effect of various procedures on the flow of lymph. Arch. Phys. Med., 34:31, 1953.
9. Graham, D. Massage, Manual Treatment, Remedial Movements, History, Mode of Application and Effects: Indications and Contra-indications. Philadelphia, 1913.
10. Hamann, A. Massage: Text and Illustrations. Med. Sch., Krankenh, Friedrichshain, East Berlin, 1974.
11. Huddleston, L. L., Austin, E., Moore, R. W., et al. Anterior poliomyelitis; physical treatment in Southern California. Br. J. Phys. Med., 15:75, 1952.
12. Kirby, F., and Sampson, J. P. A new approach to movement of fluids in extremities. Read at the meeting of the American Medical Association in Los Angeles, California, November, 1948.
13. Kleen, E. A. G. Massage and Medical Gymnastics. New York, 1921.
14. Kovacs, R. Electrotherapy and Light Therapy with the Essentials of Hydrotherapy and Mechanotherapy, Philadelphia, 1945.
15. Krogh, A. The Anatomy and Physiology of Capillaries. New Haven, 1929.
16. Leroy, M. R. La vie du tissu conjonctif et sa défense par le massage. R. C. Med. Paris, 58:212, 1941.
17. Lorentzen, D. Pacemaker-induced ventricular tachycardia; reversion to normal sinus rhythm by carotid sinus massage. J.A.M.A., 235:282, 1976.
18. Maggiora, A., De l'action physiologique du massage sur les muscles de l'homme Arch. Ital. Biol., 16:225, 1891.
19. Meffert, H., Lemke, U., Fehlinger, R., et al. The influence of underwater massage on rewarming heat conductivity and perfusion of the skin in progressive scleroderma. Dermatol. Klin., 161:551, 1975.
20. Pedini, G., and Zaiette, P. Some aspects of tissue lipolysis activation by mechanical factors. Ist. Patol. Spec. Med I. Minerva Med., 66:318, 1975.
21. Pemberton, R. Physiology of massage. In: A.M.A. Handbook of Physical Medicine. American Medical Association, Chicago, 1945.
22. Rawlins, M. A. Textbook of Massage: For Nurses and Beginners. St. Louis, 1930.
23. Skull, C. W. Massage—physiologic basis. Arch. Phys. Med., 261:159, 1945.
24. Starkey, J. A. Treatment of ankle sprains by simultaneous use of intermittent compression and ice packs. Am. J. Sports Med. 4:142, 1976.
25. Starling, E. H. The influence of mechanical factors on lymph production. J. Physiol., 16:224, 1894.

26. Wakim, K. G., Martin, G. M., and Krusen, F. H. Influence of centripetal rhythmic compression on localized edema of an extremity. *Arch. Phys. Med., 36:*98, 1955.
27. Wakim, K. G., Martin, G. M., Terrier, J. C., et al. The effects of massage on the circulation in normal and paralyzed extremities. *Arch. Phys. Med., 30:*135, 1949.
28. Wolf, S. L. Skin analgesic, and rewarming effects of ice massage on localized skin. *Phys. Ther., 55:*11, 1975.

11

Classical Massage

JACK M. HOFKOSH

Classical massage once again has taken its place among the "alternatives" available to the physical therapist in the treatment of various conditions.

All animals use some form of rubbing of the painful area to help relieve pain. Rubbing the painful area has, over the last 50 years been used as the basis of many other techniques. Some of these other techniques, as discussed in detail on other pages of this book, may be utilized for aberrations of one or more systems of the body (11, 15, 16).

Classical massage can attribute its influence on present-day practice to the writings and teachings of such practitioners as James B. Mennell (13), James B. Coulter (5), Frank H. Krusen (12), and more recently to Gertrude Beard, and Elizabeth Wood (1), and Frances Tappan (14).

Francon (7), along with Boigey (2) Boni and Walthard (3), define classical massage as "hand motions practiced on the surface of the body with a therapeutic goal," and through the skin to subcutaneous tissue as well. A more recent definition by Beard and Wood (1) give the definition ascribed to by most practitioners today. They say, "massage is the term used to designate certain manipulations of the soft tissues of the body; these manipulations are most effectively performed with the hands, and are administered for the purpose of producing effects on the nervous system, the muscular system as well as the effects on the local and general circulation of the blood and lymph."

General Principles

The literature in recent years attests to a growing interest among health professionals in diverse massage, pressure points, and stroking patterns. These various forms take the names of connective tissue massage, shiatsu, rolfing, and acupuncture or acupressure. This interest must certainly change the horizons for classical massage. Serious attention, therefore, must be given to the probable physiologic effects of classical massage on the various systems of the body and the effect of these changes on the total organism.

Classical massage is no doubt a powerful therapeutic agent and should only be practiced by those trained in its application.

Massage at no time should cause pain. It should not be given so vigorously as to cause ecchymosis or swelling. Short periods of treatment have been found to be more beneficial as a therapeutic agent than prolonged periods. When possible the treatment should be combined with some movement; passive or assisted range of motion of a joint or group of joints, or even active movements have been found helpful.

The physical therapist administering the treatment should use caution in applying the gradations of the various massage movements so that the transition to active or to resistive exercises may be given as progress is made. Physiologic consideration must be considered while doing the massage such as direction of muscle fibers and venous flow. Care should also be given to areas of tenderness and where nerves as well as blood vessels are near the surface such as in the axilla, elbow, and knee. The area of injury or pain should be treated very gently as the strokes proceed over these areas.

Consideration of privacy for the patient should include proper draping of parts to be treated, warm hands and lotions if used, and the temperature of the room be adjusted to afford relaxation.

Lotions, oils, or powders, if used, should be given consideration only if their use will enhance the physiologic effect desired. Caution at all times and collaboration of therapist and physician should precede any other consideration.

The Various Massage Movements

Massage is carried out by motions of the hands. These motions involve various maneuvers in order of changing pressure as specific tissues of the body are encountered as the massage progresses. These various maneuvers have been called and interpreted by various authors as: (a) pétrissage, (b) kneading, (c) friction, and (d) stroking or effleurage.

PETRISSAGE

Mennell (13), Hoffa (9), and Bucholz (4) described pétrissage in various ways. Dr. Hans Behrend suggested that the tissues be grasped gently, with the hand yielding to the contour of the underlying tissues. Ths skin should move with the fingers while lifting and gently squeezing the tissues. One then rolls onto the next area by gliding. Pressure should be gentle but firm, alternately tightening and loosening as the fingers move onto the next area. The direction is to be centripetal with concern for the changing needs of the underlying tissues as the massage progresses.

KNEADING

When one attempts a description of this type of massage it soon becomes apparent how closely this procedure resembles pétrissage. Behrend suggests that the major difference is the amount of tissue lifted (more for kneading), squeezed, or moved, but that the direction is similar to that of pétrissage. Pressure is exerted in a circular movement with the hands moving in opposite directions; pressure should be gentle while alternately compressing and relaxing. The direction is from the distal to proximal areas with cautions as described above.

FRICTION

Because opinions varied among the several authors who described friction massage as a concept, Mennell (13) suggested that friction massage should be begun light, progressing slowly to deep, depending on the underlying condition and the state of the tissues. The strokes are done in a slow, circular movement, using the ball of the thumb or fingers, keeping in contact with the skin, and moving gently over the underlying tissues. It is useful, he believed, to treat small areas such as scar tissue. The circular movements should be gentle around these areas, moving into another form of massage as the treatment progresses. The type suggested will depend on the area to be treated.

STROKING AND EFFLEURAGE

Mennell divided effleurage into superficial and deep stroking. Superficial stroking could be either centripetal or centrifugal; pressure is to be firm, with only the slightest touch possible to maintain contact. Deep stroking should be in the direction of the venous and lymph flow. Stroking, light to deep, could be given over large areas, with as much suggestion for relaxation by the patient as possible. The palm of the hand may be used and should be in good contact and able to conform to the particular contour being treated at that moment, changing shape and pressure as the hands move over the surface.

The Various Components of Massage

This section will clarify some components previously alluded to: (a) direction of motion; (b) pressure; (c) rhythm of a movement; (d) media if any is to be used; (e) position of the patient and the therapist; and (f) duration and frequency of the movement.

DIRECTION OF THE MOVEMENT

Much can be said regarding the contribution to massage from the writings of Hippocrates, Asclepiades, and Galen (8). Ling, in the beginning of the 19th century advocated light stroking in the centripetal direction and deeper stroking in the centrifugal direction (10). This concept continues to today in the various courses and among the various writers. Mennell (13) suggested that all deep movements of massage use the centripetal direction, thereby aiding the venous and lymphatic flow.

PRESSURE

The amount of pressure is discussed considerably and variously by the early writers. Students of massage today are taught the philosophy that is the most beneficial to be that of Mennell (13). He stated that the amount of pressure should at all times depend on the amount of muscle relaxation. The closer to a relaxed state, the lighter the pressure, "for even light pressure," he said, "must influence every structure throughout the part being treated."

RHYTHM OF A MOVEMENT

Kellgren (10) writing about Ling, suggested that the rhythm of the movement vary according to the movement. That is, with effleurage, a slow rolling, stroking movement be used and that with tapotement the rhythm could be more rapid. Mennell stated that for a fast soothing effect, slow rhythmical strokes are called for, and for a more stimulating effect the strokes could be quicker and stronger with the rate varying with the condition of the patient. Mennell noted, however, that no matter what the condition the various strokes used should be performed rhythmically. The criteria used, he said, is the effect of the massage on the flow of blood and lymph.

MEDIA IF ANY TO BE USED

The writings on this topic extend from the early Greek and Roman periods and are somewhat controversial. Media ranging from heavy oils to actual flagellation continue to be used. The more modern writers in this regard (1, 5, 6, 12, 13) are divided into those who object to any sort of medium and those who use a mild, oily lubricant or powder. Those who use no medium suggest that it is cleaner, gives more feeling to the hand, and the movement is steadier. The substances more commonly used by those who advocate a medium are olive oil, mild glycerin or mineral oil, cocoa butter, coconut oil, and mild powders. What is suggested here is that these agents make the skin soft, smooth, and slippery and prevent the friction that may cause the pain of pulling hair.

In more recent times Mennell has suggested that the decision to use or not to use media should be made by the therapist, who must consider the condition of the skin and the underlying pathology in making the choice.

THE POSITION OF THE PATIENT AND THE PHYSICAL THERAPIST

Ling (Kellgren [10]) was the first to emphasize that the patient be in as relaxed a position as possible for whatever part is to be treated, the treatment being planned to minimize the number of times he has to move, and that the therapist, as well, be as comfortable as possible. The size and height of the treatment table should be considered to avoid any unnecessary strain. Mennell added the notion that there should be a reason for every position of the therapist and the position of the part under treatment. Free movement of arms, shoulders, and lower extremities should be obtained. Tight clothing, bangles, beads, and rings are to be avoided. Ling's writings deal with the effect of gravity in assisting the venous and lymphatic flow relating to the position of the part under treatment.

DURATION AND FREQUENCY OF TREATMENT

Galen's early writings mention the duration and frequency of a treatment. He wrote that the therapist must decide what is to be adequate by the signs and symptoms as the number of sessions for the treatment progresses. He suggested that the therapist must make the decision as to what is adequate. Therapists need to learn to use action and reaction and signs and symptoms as witnessed in each succeeding treatment session.

Mennell adds that the age of the patient should be considered in either increasing or decreasing the duration of the massage. The very young and the aged should have treatment usually of only short duration. Consideration of the state of debility or general illness of the patient is also important. Emphasis in Mennell's writings is placed on not prolonging the massage unnecessarily at the expense of active movement and participation of the patient as a whole as soon as possible. (See General Principles)

All authors mention the need to review and discuss the frequency of the treatment on the same basis as the duration. No doubt there are conditions that require daily treatments; others, two or three times per week. The determination can be made only by a clear understanding of the condition being treated and a working relationship among the collaborators, the referring doctor and the physical therapist.

Some Fundamentals of the Movements in Classical Massage

During a single session there is an advantage to begin and to end the session with some effleurage. The patient should experience a mild lassitude and a period of time should be given for rest. A treatment is too vigorous or of too long duration if real fatigue is a result of the therapy. It has been pointed out earlier in this chapter that massage cannot substitute for exercise. It can help to ready a part for passive or active-assisted movement when the collaborators have agreed.

The goal of classical massage is to try to attain some relaxation. A smooth transition from one movement to another in a rhythmical manner can be carried out in all maneuvers. This can be accomplished by not requiring the patient to move any more than necessary. The development of expertise must include this concept, as well as the massage strokes themselves. There is a definite sequence of massage and movement of the therapist that must become a part of the regimen. This is the art of classical massage.

Among the essentials, as well, is that the patient and the therapist be comfortable. Proper use of pillows, towels, or support sheets and blankets for draping must be learned (See General Principles). The movement of the hands of the therapist should be continuous, even, and rhythmical. Talking if it must be done should be very low key, and only essential comments pertinent to this treatment should be made. Discussion for discussion's sake should be avoided as much as possible.

TECHNIQUE OF EFFLEURAGE (STROKING)

The word "effleurage" means to glide or stroke. It is a slow, rhythmical stroke in which the therapist's hands are in light contact with the skin of the patient. The hands should be sufficiently relaxed to be able to mold itself to the area as it passes gently from distal to proximal.

The stroke is made in long, gliding centripetal sweeps 10 to 20 inches (25 to 50 cm) in length. When the end of stroke is reached, the hands are lifted gently and gently reapplied for a short interval before the proximal hand has left the patient. Done properly that serves to soothe, decrease pain, and lessen muscle tension.

TECHNIQUE OF PÉTRISSAGE (KNEADING)

Pétrissage or kneading is somewhat more forceful. In this method of massage a rather large fold of skin and subcutaneous tissue, including muscle, is raised between the thumb and other fingers. These tissues are then squeezed gently and rolled in a circular motion by alternately tightening and loosening the grasp. As the movement is repeated the grasping hand moves slightly forward or backward and repeats the same maneuver. The movement is made with one hand while the other supports the tissues and presses them. The hands work together, changing direction and place as the movement repeats slightly forward and to the right or to the left. The pressure should be of such magnitude as to allow the skin to pass over the underlying tissues by the hand of the therapist. If pain is felt during this treatment, lessen pressure or take up less underlying tissue with the grasp. The direction is usually in a centripetal one, beginning near the trunk and advancing down the limbs. The effects are known to cause mild to severe hyperemia and help to combat atrophy and to improve tonus and elasticity.

TECHNIQUE OF TAPOTEMENT

This technique is a rapid series of gentle blows with the ulnar border of each hand. A gentle tapping ensues with the fingers and wrists relaxed and the elbows flexed. Ths skin is struck rapidly and alternately by each hand; it is most often done to the back and upper thigh. A variation (cupping) of this tapotement, with the hands held in a cupping manner and executed on the upper back, has been found useful for assisting in carefully executed chest care. The goal here is to assist the patient to cough up mucous plugs and to help in clearing air passages.

Conclusion

It is to be stressed that massage is to be used in conjunction with other forms of therapy. It alone can hardly be expected to gain release of pain and tension or to assist toward independence of body movement. Exercise in its various forms, diet, and climate are other factors that in combination may complement the massage. Close collaboration of the therapist and the physician is also stressed so that the underlying pathology of whatever sort is closely monitored and controlled.

This chapter only helps to introduce the subject of classical massage. It is necessary to consult the references for more detailed descriptions of classical massage.

REFERENCES

1. Beard, G., and Wood, E. C. *Massage—Principles and Techniques.* W. B. Saunders Co., Philadelphia, 1964.
2. Boigey, M. *Manuel De Massage,* Paris, 1955.
3. Boni, A., and Walthard, K. Massage et cinésitérapie des rhumatismes abarticulaires. *Rhumatologie, 8:*727, 1956.
4. Bucholz, C. H. *Therapeutic Exercise and Massage.* Lea and Febiger, Philadelphia, 1917.
5. Coulter, J. B. *Clio Medica VII, Physical Therapy.* Paul B. Hoeber, New York, 1932.
6. Cyriax, J. *Treatment by Massage and Manipulation.* Paul B. Hoeber, Inc., New York, 1959.
7. Francon, F. *Kinesitherapie:* massage, mobilization passive et active, manuelle ou instrumentale, gymastique medicale, therapeutique occupationelle. *Le sud med. chirug., 85:*1912, 1952.
8. Galen, C. *De Sanitate Tuenda* (a translation of Galen's *Hygiene* by R. M. Green). Charles C Thomas, Springfield, IL., 1951.
9. Hoffa, A. *Technik der Massage.* Verlag, Von Ferdinand Ernke, Stuttgart, 1897.
10. Kellgren, A. *The Technic of Ling's System of Manual Treatment,* Young, Pentland, Edinburgh and London, 1890.
11. Kellogg, J. H. *The Art of Massage, 12th Ed.,* revised. Modern Medical Publishing Co., Battle Creek, MI., 1919.
12. Krusen, F. H. *Physical Medicine.* W. B. Saunders Co., Philadelphia, 1941.
13. Mennell, J. B. *Physical Treatment by Movement, Massage and Manipulation, 5th Ed.* W. B. Saunders Co., Philadelphia, 1941.
14. Tappan, F. *Massage Techniques, A Case Method Approach.* MacMillan Co., New York, 1961.
15. Wakim, K. G. Influence of centripetal rhythmic compression on localized edema of an extremity, *Arch. Phys. Med., 36:*98, 1955.
16. Wakim, K. G. The Effects of Massage on the circulation in Normal and Paralyzed Extremities. *Arch. Phys. Med., 30:*135, 1949.

12

Clinical Applications of Massage

JAMES H. CYRIAX

Many physicians regard massage as an obsolescent placebo. Up to a point they are right; for, as administered by many, massage is a waste of time and energy. Though it is merely an expert application of the instinct to rub a sore place, it was only 40 years ago that the truism was put forward (8) that massage was useful only when it was applied to the lesion itself. During previous millennia it had been thought quite good enough to give a general manual treatment all about the painful area. However, Kellgren's research on referred pain (17) and the adaptation of Leriche's technique (19) of therapeutic local anesthesia to diagnostic purposes (8) showed that many lesions of the soft parts gave rise to pain felt at a distance from their source, symptoms being experienced in some part of the dermatome relevant to the segment within which the tissue at fault was developed. Kellgren's findings thus cast a great doubt on the orthodox practice at that time of diffuse deep massage to a painful area, because it had been demonstrated that many lesions were situated outside the region stated by the patient to hurt. In the case of the muscles of the trunk, the existence of a localized tender point within a painful area had long been regarded as evidence that the lesion lay there, but, in due course, evidence was adduced that these trigger-spots—previously misnamed "fibrositis"—were the result and not the cause of trouble. They arose not from any lesion in the muscle within which the myalgic point lay; they could be secondary to pressure on the dura mater via the posterior ligament as the result of a minor displacement of a fragment of disc, and they moved and finally disappeared as reduction of the displacement was begun and completed.

It followed that massage, if it was to be revived and was once more to take its proper place in therapeutics, must be applied with much greater precision than hitherto. It must be confined to lesions that respond to massage, and it must exert therapeutic movement at the exact site of the lesion. The indications were thus greatly narrowed, but, within this restricted field, a treatment of great efficacy for localized lesions of the moving parts had been evolved.

This is the situation today. Now that the indications for and against its employment have been clarified, massage need no longer be given in a manner that can only proclaim its uselessness. It is, surely, axiomatic that to give massage (or for that matter, any other treatment) to normal tissues is valueless, whether they are the site of referred pain and tenderness or not, even though this practice has been hallowed by centuries of unthinking tradition. This is the type of massage that doctors still see and rightly disparage, but, universal though it is, the results of this way of using massage provide no evidence that manual friction applied in the right way to the right spot is equally futile. It is not; for it can secure quick and permanent successes unequaled by any other means known today.

Although physical therapists have been slow to accept precise manual work, physicians have been equally neglectful in tolerating vague measures. Before accurate massage can be administered to a lesion, its situation and extent must first have been defined to within a finger's breadth by the doctor's diagnosis. Without this knowledge, the physician or therapist cannot apply the human finger to the exact spot, and unless the nature and course of the tissue affected have been defined, the depth and direction of the requisite therapeutic movement remain uncertain.

Effective massage depends on sufficient interest by the doctor for an exact diagnosis to be made, matched by equal technical skill on the part of the physical therapist. Here massage falls between two stools, and a vicious circle exists that will have to be breached before massage can emerge from its present justified disregard.

Deep Massage

Massage is used in different ways for different purposes with different physiologic results. Throughout, the important effects are mechanical and local. The general effects are trivial, of doubtful benefit and, when required, better obtained by other means. Thus massage given vigorously to a limb temporarily increases the speed of the circulation and the number of circulating red blood cells, but ordinary exercises are far more effective. Venous return is hastened too, but this is of doubtful advantage except in bedridden patients, and then elevation of the part or diuretics are often preferable.

Deep friction is by far the most important technique in massage because it penetrates to the moving tissues of the body. It will therefore be dealt with in detail below. Whereas superficial massage is suited to lesions lying at the skin or superficial fascia (for example, ulcer or edema), deep massage is called for when the deep-seated structures are to be affected. When a deep-seated lesion is given superficial massage, or a localized lesion is given diffuse massage, or a lesion beyond fingers' reach is given any sort of massage at all, no benefit whatever can be expected. Superficial massage is at least pleasant, whereas the only excuse for a painful treatment is its effectiveness; and deep friction exerts its unique effect only if it is applied correctly at the exact site of a lesion. Inasmuch as the principle of the treatment of the moving parts of the body is the maintenance or restoration of painless mobility, massage most often is given not only with penetrating effect but with the precise technique that alone imparts therapeutic movement to the tissue at fault.

The important fact about deep friction is that it imparts therapeutic movement over a very small area. On the one hand, the movement is the more valuable for being so concentrated, and a most effective therapeutic result can be obtained. On the other hand, the movement secured by deep friction is so very local that, unless the finger reaches deeply to the exact site of the lesion and moves it adequately, no benefit accrues and the patient is given a painful and useless treatment.

An important part of logical rehabilitation consists in choosing and applying the type of therapeutic movement best suited to the disorder present. A decision is reached after consideration of the following: the normal range of movement of the tissue at fault; the nature and situation of the lesion within that tissue; the accessibility of the lesion; the time that has elapsed since the disorder began; the symptoms and signs of acuteness or chronicity; the direction in which mobility requires restoration; how best to secure therapeutic movement at the lesion. Adhesions leading to painful scarring or contracture are a common cause of pain at the moving parts of the body. But unwanted adherent scars cannot appear and later interfere with mobility, if, immediately after the structure has suffered damage, it is moved by human fingers in imitation of its normal behavior, for it is thus freed from adhesions both actually present and in the process of formation. One method of avoiding painful scarring is deep friction. It is particularly useful for muscles (followed by active movement), for ligaments (followed by passive movement), and for tendons (followed by avoidance of exertion).

Many authorities consider the main action of massage to be enhancement of the circulation, and it is therefore given longitudinally, that is, parallel to the blood vessels. Even if the blood flow does increase temporarily, this has no particular value; for the tissues are not suffering from ischemia and in any case do not take more up from the blood stream than they require merely because of a faster current of blood. Deep friction given in the long axis of a moving structure is useless, because it is not hyperemia but therapeutic movement that has to be imparted. It is true that deep friction given transversely causes a local reaction, probably due to the release of histamine, and that hyperemia results and lasts many minutes. This hyperemia is beneficial only because it affords a degree of local analgesia while it lasts. In consequence, as soon as the session of massage ends, the patient's pain is found diminished, and the structure hurts less when it is required to function but remains for some time more tender to the touch. This short period of massage analgesia can be used to render various uncomfortable procedures more tolerable. The circulatory effect, however, is transient, and unless therapeutic movement is applied during the analgesic period no benefit follows. More recently, experiments have shown that massage and manipulation may activate the gate control of pain. The gate concept proposes that a neural mechanism in the dorsal horns of the spinal cord acts like a gate which can increase or diminish the flow of nervous impulses from peripheral fibers to the central nervous system. Somatic input is thus subjected to interference by the gate before it evokes pain. The degree to which the gate alters sensory transmission is determined by the relative activity in the large-diameter fibers to the small diameter fibers. Activity in the large fibers tends to inhibit whereas in the small fibers transmission is facilitated. Hence, mechanoreceptor impulses take precedence and thus diminish sensation, which is what impulses from the moving parts do. Deep massage hurts the moving parts and therefore eases pain, according to this concept, by inhibiting transmission of impulses at the gate.

MODE OF ACTION

Deep friction, because it moves tissues rather than blood, must always be given at right angles to the long axis of the fibers at the site of the lesion. This is fortuitous, because the reasons for the insistence on transverse friction differ for different tissues.

INDICATIONS FOR DEEP MASSAGE

Deep Friction to Muscle

The main function of muscle is to contract. As it does so it broadens. Hence full mobility toward broadening out must be maintained or restored in muscles that have been the seat of a minor rupture—whether caused by one or by repeated strains. Resolution by fibrosis is occurring or has already occurred.

The effect of deep transverse friction is to mobilize the muscle, that is, to separate the adhesions between individual muscle fibers that are restricting movement and causing pain. When such passive restoration of full mobility of a muscle is followed by adequate active contraction, these adhesions do not reform and a cure results. Until the breach in the muscle is soundly healed, exercise against strong resistance is contraindicated, for this may lead to relapse (especially at the quadriceps, calf, and hamstring muscles).

The principle governing the treatment of muscles during the acute or chronic stage is the same. The endeavor must be to prevent the continued adherence of unwanted young fibrous tissue in recent cases or to rupture adherent scar tissue in longstanding cases. To stretch out a muscle does not widen the distance between the fibers; on the contrary, during stretching they lie more closely. Whereas, then, mobilization is required for the rupture of adherent scars about a joint, interfibrillary adhesions in muscle can be broken, not by stretching, but only by forcibly broadening the muscle out. This is particularly true of the fibers of attachment of muscle to tendon or bone. Exercises, however vigorous, cannot effectively mobilize a muscle close to its insertion to an immobile structure; deep friction can. Thus, deep transverse frictions passively restore mobility to muscle in the same way that a forced passive movement frees a joint. Indeed, the action of deep transverse frictions may be summed up as affording a restoration, otherwise unobtainable, of the capacity of muscle to contract painlessly.

A muscle must be kept relaxed during friction; hence, the patient is put into a position that takes all tension off the muscle, and he must consciously relax it during, and in spite of, the painful treatment. During contraction the physical therapist's fingers are forced to slide over the surface of a muscle; such superficial movement has no therapeutic value. The muscle must be made to move within itself, each fiber being drawn away from its neighbor at the site of the painful scar. This is possible only during full voluntary relaxation.

Aftertreatment. In a recent injury the broadening effect of the transverse friction has to be maintained. On the one hand, full contraction of the belly must be ensured without any tension falling on the fibers beneficially uniting the two torn surfaces. On the other, transverse scarring across the breach in the muscle must be prevented. To this end, the muscle is held passively in the position of full shortening. For the hamstrings, this entails the patient lying prone with his hip in extension and his knee in full flexion; for the quadriceps, he sits with his limb straight out in front of him; for the gastrocnemius, full flexion of the knee and full plantiflexion at the ankle. No resistance is applied; it is merely an exercise in full tensionless contraction. If the patient experiences any difficulty at first in actively contracting his muscle, faradic stimulation is called for.

In the chronic case, no aftertreatment is necessary. The patient just uses his muscle normally, avoiding any activity that causes him pain until he is well—a few weeks at the most.

Deep Friction to Ligament

Most ligaments link two bones together while permitting movement at the joint they span. Therefore, each such ligament possesses a range of movement over the bones that is at right angles to its long axis. This is the mobility that has to be maintained after a recent sprain or must be restored if post-traumatic adhesions have already been allowed to consolidate themselves.

In recent cases, after any edema that may be present has been removed by effleurage, the site of the minor tear in the ligament should receive some minutes' friction. The purpose is to disperse blood clot or effusion there, to move the ligament to and fro over subjacent bone (thus maintaining its mobility), and to numb it enough to facilitate movement afterward. The least strength of friction that achieves these results is called for. Passive and then active movements follow. After a few days the effleurage becomes less necessary, and more attention is devoted to the friction and to exercising the injured limb under supervision. In the case of the lower limb, instruction in gait follows. If the deep massage is properly given, the patient who sprains a ligament at the knee, for example, gets well in as many weeks as he would otherwise have taken months, had he had all the other measures without the friction. For example, immediately after a severe sprain of the medial ligament of the knee, acute traumatic arthritis sets in and by the following day a 90° limitation of joint flexion results. The avoidance of unwanted adhesions requires full range of joint motion daily, but the arthritis makes this impossible; in other words, the bones cannot be moved under the ligament adequately. There remains only motion of the ligament to and fro over the bones; this is, in fact, the treatment of choice, for adhesions do not consolidate themselves when the tissues move adequately in relation to each other. It is immaterial which one of the tissues is moved. Hence, the treatment of a recent sprain includes straightening the knee as much as possible, following which transverse massage is given to the ligament, which is moved to and fro while it is at the anterior extreme of its range of motion (Fig. 12.1). The knee is then flexed as far as possible and the ligament again

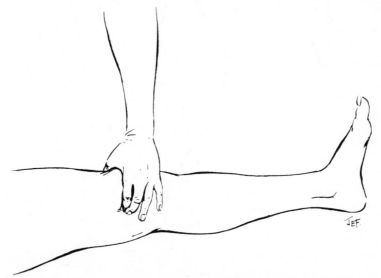

Figure 12.1. Friction to medial collateral ligament with knee in extension.

given transverse massage. This moves it to and fro in imitation of its normal behavior while it is near the posterior extreme of its range of motion (Fig. 12.2). We know of no treatment that affords such dramatic relief as this simple but little used measure.

In chronic cases deep friction is given to the ligament in preparation for manipulative rupture of the restricting adhesion. In such cases the friction thins out and mobilizes the adherence and numbs the affected area, thus facilitating the subsequent forcing of movement.

Aftertreatment. The knee is different from all other joints in that union with lengthening is apt to occur and must be prevented. For this reason, during the first week no endeavor is made to straighten the knee passively. The patient merely straightens it himself as far as he finds comfortable.

Deep Friction to Tendon

The situation is different in tenosynovitis and tendonitis.

Tenosynovitis. On logical grounds it has been widely held that tenosynovitis, being as a rule the result of overuse (that is, excessive friction of the tendon within its sheath), should not be treated by further friction. Never-

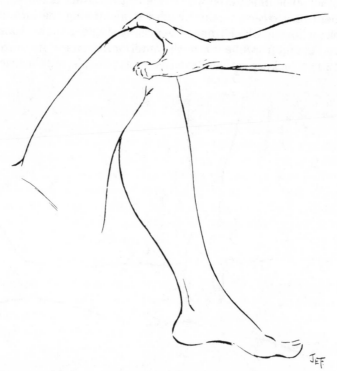

Figure 12.2. Friction to medial collateral ligament with knee in flexion.

theless, this is the very condition in which massage achieves some of its quickest and most brilliant results. The phenomenon of crepitus proves that roughening of the gliding surfaces occurs. The fact that slitting up the sheath of the tendon at open operation is immediately curative shows that it was the movement between the close-fitting sheath and the tendon that caused the pain. Hence, it would appear that massage, by manual rolling of the tendon sheath to and fro against the tendon, serves to smooth the gliding surfaces off again. While the causative trauma is longitudinal friction, the curative is transverse. It is important that the tendon should be held taut during the massage; for the trouble lies between the outer aspect of the tendon and the inner aspect of the tendon sheath—in other words, at the gliding surfaces. When taut, the tendon provides an immobile basis against which the physical therapist's fingers can move the tendon sheath. When relaxed, however, tendon and sheath are rolled as one unit against subjacent tissues; thus the movement takes place at the wrong surface and no benefit accrues. In industrial practice, Knowles and Kipling (18) reported excellent results with deep transverse massage for tenosynovitis, using the author's technique.

Tendonitis. In those tendons that lack a sheath, the way deep friction acts is not clear. After a minor tenoperiosteal tear in a short tendon, the movement imparted by the massage, when successful, presumably breaks up scarring at the insertion of tendon into bone. This would seem so in, say, supraspinatus or infraspinatus tendonitis, or at the flexor tendon insertion at the medial humeral epicondyle in golfer's elbow. When the substance of a tendon such as the Achilles is affected, it is difficult to understand exactly what the massage can do unless it is assumed that scar tissue lies there and is capable of being dispersed manually. Because no sheath exists, there is no reason to suppose that some slight roughening of the surface of the tendon would cause symptoms. Nevertheless, deep transverse friction provides the only method known to us (apart from successes with steroid infiltration [7]) of relieving tendonitis at shoulder, elbow, hip, knee and ankle. Many patients have been troubled for years; and it is clear that throughout the world there are far more sufferers from life-long tendonitis than there are physical therapists trained to treat it (Figs. 12.3 and 12.4).

TECHNIQUE OF DEEP MASSAGE

The physician who wishes to assess what deep friction can really achieve must make sure of certain facts, listed below. Otherwise it is easy to be misled and to conclude that friction is without avail in conditions in fact easily curable by this means. The techniques have already been described and illustrated (10).

1. The physical therapist must be supplied with a diagnosis correct to within 1 cm—the width of a finger.

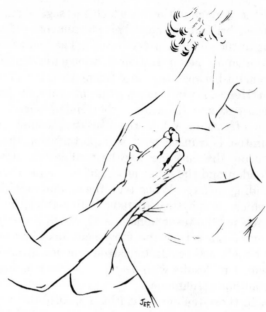

Figure 12.3. Deep friction across the supraspinatus tendon. The arm is held in full medial rotation to bring the tendon into an easily palpable position.

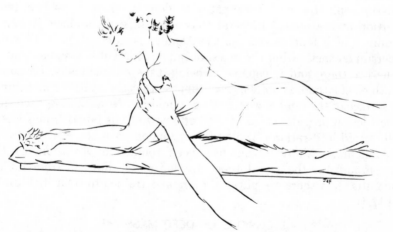

Figure 12.4. Deep friction to the infraspinatus tendon. The patient is propped on her elbows to maintain a right angle between the scapula and the humerus. In this position the acromion no longer covers the tendon.

2. One's finger must move with the patient's skin, so that the deep surface of the skin moves over the structure at fault.

3. One must know which way the fibers of the affected tissue run, so that the friction is performed at right angles to this direction.

4. The friction must be given with sufficient sweep; that is, the operative finger must start on the far side of the structure and be brought across it, and the movement must be maintained until the near edge has been crossed.

5. The passage of the finger must be brisk enough to move adequately the tissue palpated.

6. One must press sufficiently hard really to move the structure one is rubbing.

7. The patient must be put into a position that gives the finger the best access to the site of the lesion and that, in the case of a long tendon, stretches it or that, in the case of a muscle, relaxes it.

Steroid Infiltration

Until 1953, when hydrocortisone first became available in Britain, no effective treatment existed for tendinous lesions except deep massage. This to some extent remains so today; for not all physicians care to inject these suspensions, nor are all aware of the posture the patient should adopt nor of the exact siting of the needle. Moreover, some athletes refuse the injection, lest rupture take place later at the site of the infiltration. Again, when it is important, e.g., at the medial ligament of the knee, that healing shall take place without lengthening or a weak longitudinal scar, massage is to be preferred to treatment with a steroid (7).

Though it is true, therefore, that friction does not hold the monopoly it started with, it is a most important part of every physical therapist's skill, especially when dealing with athletes and ballet dancers.

LESIONS TRACTABLE ONLY BY MASSAGE

There exist a number of lesions that are incurable by any means—surgical or medical, including steroid infiltration—except deep transverse massage. Because massage is a forgotten art, this situation implies that they cause endless trouble, not for lack of knowledge of what to do, but for lack of therapists trained to do it. A list of lesions tractable only by massage follows:

Subclavius belly
Supraspinatus, musculotendinous junction
Biceps, longhead, lower musculotendinous junction
Brachialis belly
Supinator belly
Ligaments about carpal lunate bone
Interosseous belly and tendon at hand
Intercostal muscle
Oblique muscles of abdomen
Psoas, lower musculotendinous junction
Quadriceps expansion at patella
Coronary ligament at knee
Biceps of thigh, lower musculotendinous junction

Anterior tibial, musculotendinous junction
Posterior tibial, musculotendinous junction
Peroneal, musculotendinous junction
Posterior tibiotalar ligament
Anterior fascia of ankle joint
Interosseous belly of foot

These techniques have been described and illustrated (11).

Indications for Other Types of Massage

EDEMA

Superficial lesions can be affected by superficial treatment. Hence, effleurage can be used in such cases. Edema may be postural or the result of recent injury or angioneurotic. Deep effleurage gets rid of such edema. The massage is therefore given in the direction of the venous flow. The skin should be powdered first. The physical therapist's hand is held curved to fit the surface under the treatment and made to pass repeatedly, slowly, and with even pressure along the limb, always in the same direction. This is continued until little or no edema remains, whereupon it is usually wise to apply a crepe bandage to prevent recurrence. This is kept on until the next session of deep effleurage; daily or twice-daily treatments are required.

Traumatic Periostitis

A direct blow is apt to result in painful thickening of the periosteum at a superficial bone, most often the tibia. Deep effleurage hastens subsidence by dispersing localized edema of the membrane.

INSOMNIA AND PSYCHONEUROSIS

Light effleurage is soothing and may be ordered for its calming effect.

BRONCHIECTASIS AND PULMONARY ABSCESS

The repeated little blows that comprise clapping, hacking, and beating, combined with postural drainage, can dislodge mucus and mucopurulent material from the bronchi. They are much used for this purpose, especially preoperatively. The physical therapist uses gravity and vibration to help move secretions from the insensitive periphery of the lung to the area where the cough reflex is beneficially evoked (Fig. 12.5).

The affected segments of lung are first identified by bronchography. For treatment, the patient is placed in the position that ensures that the bronchus draining the affected area points vertically downward; percussion is carried out over the affected area if it is situated laterally or posteriorly and is followed by vibration on expiration with encouragement to cough and expectorate. Over the anterior chest wall vibration on expiration is the only manipulation used.

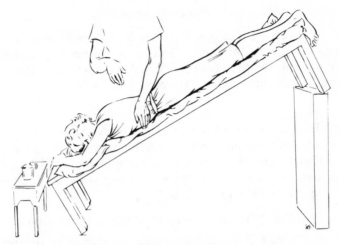

Figure 12.5. Postural drainage aided by clapping.

When a major operation on the lung is contemplated, previous postural drainage may enhance safety. An antispasmodic such as isoprenaline is inhaled first (23), and the lung is drained three times a day in the manner described.

After thoracic or abdominal surgery, contained secretions may lead to postoperative atelectasis. Prevention consists of modified postural drainage two or three times a day. By modified postural drainage we mean a posture of the patient that eliminates gravity, i.e., that lets the secretions flow horizontally. The most convenient posture is crook-side-lying, because the nursing staff will have put the patient into this position during treatment of pressure points. Percussion by the physical therapist over the lateral chest wall is followed by vibration on expiration and encouragement to cough and expectorate. The same procedure is repeated on the other side of the chest. If atelectasis is already present and neither a large pleural effusion nor a pneumothorax is responsible, vigorous postural drainage of the atelectatic area should be instituted at the earliest moment. When strong coughing is inhibited by pain, trilene inhalations have proved of great assistance.

ASTHMA AND AFTER OPERATIONS

Shaking is most useful in asthma and after operations, especially after those in which the wound hurts with each breath. The physical therapist adjusts the patient's posture and then applies gentle alternating pressures and releases at his lower ribs in rhythm with his respiration. Expiration is thus assisted, and the improved aeration of the lungs thus secured is valuable in preventing postoperative stasis.

CHRONIC SEPSIS

When the evacuation of pus and granular sequestra from a septic sinus is to be hastened, a combination of squeezing and stroking is indicated. The massage starts at the site of the lesion and is carried toward the opening of the sinus. Treatment is called for several times a day.

OBESITY

Fat in the subcutaneous tissues lies within a capsule. If this is ruptured, the fat exudes and gets absorbed in exactly the same way as the mucin in a ganglion that has burst. If patients really wish to be made thinner by a physical therapist, the most merciless pinching is required. Ordinary massage or deep friction is quite useless.

PAINFUL NEUROMAS AND POSTHERPETIC NEURALGIA

These may give rise to tender amputation stumps or painful phantom limbs. It has recently been shown that repeated percussion, if necessary by means of a wooden applicator and a mallet, may abolish the symptoms, often lastingly. Falconer (13) has an interesting theory to explain the apparent paradox inherent in this therapy. He considers that the cells of the secondary neurons in the spinal cord are themselves the source of pain. He takes the view that these cells, deprived of the stimuli normally reaching them, discharge either spontaneously or as a reaction to aberrant impulses, thus causing pain. The percussion of neuromata therefore restores the lacking afferent stimuli to an intensity sufficent to abolish the pain of excessive quiescence. In postherpetic neuralgia a mechanical vibrator may prove effective. (See Chapter 13).

CARDIAC ARREST

After arrest of the heart beat, resuscitation by manual compression some 30 times a minute is established surgical practice.

INJURY AND NERVE PALSY

Kneading and picking up near the seat of an injury are used in an endeavor to assist the maintenance of range of muscles during immobilization or when deprived of their nerve supply. Pollock et al. (24) found that, after divison and suture of the sciatic nerve in cats, massage and passive movements retarded the development and later facilitated the disappearance of postoperative contractures. The degree of muscle atrophy was unaffected. These results contrast with the findings of Hartman and Blatz (15), who found that massage alone had no such effects. It is probable, therefore, that the benefit was due not to the massage but to the passive movements.

Strictly speaking, much of this sort of massage is given unnecessarily because it is often applied to normal structures requiring only active use for the continuance of their normality. But the absorption of effused blood may be hastened and a muscle may be kept supple and may be prevented from forming unwanted adherences by this sort of massage. The nutrition of a limb with extensive paralysis may also be assisted. Hence, it forms a reasonable massage technique in spite of the fact that it is often employed without discrimination.

FOR ATHLETES

Kneading is regarded by athletes as advantageous before and after a race, and it is also thought to diminish the liability to sportsman's cramp. There is one error that is still given widespread credence, namely, that massage can strengthen muscle. This idea is wholly fallacious; muscle gains power in proportion as it is given work to do, provided that overexertion is avoided and rest is ensured at intervals. Massage has no effect whatever on muscle power, and the increased strength derived from "massage and exercises" is due wholly to the exercises.

VARICOSE ULCER

The treatment of a gravitational varicose ulcer by deep massage was first put forward by Bisgaard (3) in Denmark in 1923. The aims of treatment are the control of edema, the softening of indurated areas, the enhancement of the local circulation, and the reeducation of the patient's gait. First the edema is removed by deep effleurage. This is followed by really deep kneading of the thigh and calf, while the patient lies with the lower limb in elevation (Fig. 12.6). Manual squeezing of the calf and ankle is sometimes necessary. Then the ulcer itself is attacked by local treatment. Deep—and

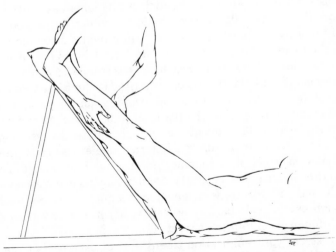

Figure 12.6. Deep kneading of the elevated limb as used in the treatment of varicose ulcer.

necessarily painful—friction is applied by small circular movements, and the cushion of indurated tissue is gradually softened until, by centripetal work, the edge of the ulcer is reached and included. A pressure bandage is applied by a standard technique, and the patient is taught to walk. At first the treatment is given daily. Ulcers of many years' standing, previously found intractable by every means, heal within a few months and require only the wearing of an elastic stocking to prevent recurrence. This type of massage and bandaging has been illustrated and described in detail (2).

ROSACEA AND GINGIVITIS

Massage has been advocated for the face in rosacea (25) and for the gums in periodontal disease (16). Massage with ice to the back of the hand has been shown by Melzack and co-workers (21) to diminish by half the pain in a tooth; 65% of patients with backache also obtained relief.

Contraindications to Massage

"FIBROSITIS"

When a muscle, usually at the posterior aspect of the trunk, for no clear reason becomes the site of pain and tenderness, a diagnosis of muscular rheumatism (1) or fibrositis is usually made. This ascription is often mistakenly regarded as a good reason for ordering massage and heat.

Ever since 1904, when Gowers (14) attributed the pain of lumbago to inflammation of the fibrous part of the sacrospinalis muscles, fibrositis has been regarded as a true entity. However, excised fibrous tissue has been shown on microscopy not to be inflamed (at postmortem) and the nodules, palpated during life, have not proved demonstrable. Nevertheless, despite pathologists' all but unanimous skepticism, the label has proved so useful to doctors that to this day a hypothetical disorder postulated without a shred of proof by one man 80 years ago still provides a common diagnosis. An attempt to shift the blame to the fibrofatty lobules that demonstrably lie in the muscles and fasciae at the back of the trunk was made by Copeman and Ackerman (5) in 1944; this theory persisted (4) for some years. However, it can be shown by the type of clinical examination that tests the muscles and joints separately (6) that the pains so widely ascribed to fibrositis are largely of spinal articular provenance, the pain and tenderness being merely referred to the paraspinal muscles. Referred tenderness thus provides the factual basis on which an imaginary disease has been maintained for no less than three-quarters of a century—and it is by no means dead yet. Some authorities regard fibrositis as engendered in a muscle by emotional tension, but, though psychogenic pain is no rarity, it can scarcely be regarded as causing inflammation in fibrous tissue (12).

Thus, a strong contraindication to any sort of massage is a diagnosis of rheumatic fibrositis, for it implies that the source of the pain has not been singled out. In consequence, it is impossible to know whether massage is required and, even if it should be, on what spot the physical therapist should concentrate the treatment. By contrast, post-traumatic inflammation in the moving parts of the body—that is, painful scarring—is a real entity, of course, for which deep massage is often required.

PANNICULITIS

Fatty lobules, tender to the touch, are often found close to the posterior superior spines of the ilia and at the buttocks and thighs of middle-aged patients, chiefly women. Apart from unsightliness, they cause no symptoms for they do not interfere with the mobility of the moving parts. They merely give rise to tenderness in areas where pain emanating from elsewhere is often felt. They too should not be given massage, because their presence is not related to any symptoms the patient may experience in this vicinity (as the examination of the other side of the body immediately reveals).

OTHER CONTRAINDICATIONS

Other contraindications to massage are few and obvious. By "massage" is meant such friction as actually reaches the structure named. Except in bacterial infection, gentle massage, being without effect on deep-seated tissues, is neither called for nor to be avoided. Massage should not be attempted of course, when the structure at fault is clearly beyond the reach of the physical therapist's finger. For example, no useful purpose is served when a patient with osteoarthritis of the hip joint receives massage, whether gentle or deep, to his muscles. This is merely where the pain is felt, not where its source lies. The following are conditions for which massage is contraindicated:

1. Inflammation due to bacterial action. Obviously, the infection may thus become disseminated.
2. Calcification in soft structures, for example, at the supraspinatus tendon or the medial collateral ligament at the knee.
3. Rheumatoid, infective, and gouty arthritis.
4. Traumatic arthritis at the elbow.
5. Bursitis.
6. Pressure on a nerve, for example, carpal tunnel syndrome.
7. Phlebitis and cellulitis.

Massage with Creams

When deep friction is given, the patient's skin and the physical therapist's finger must move as one. Any cream or powder, or even previous heat leading to local sweating, makes the skin too slippery, thus hindering the massage. But from time to time laymen's expectations are raised that rubbing in this or that cream or embrocation has especial value. The effect postulated is local, not systemic, as in mercurial inunction for syphilis.

Naturally, it makes no difference to the deeper tissues what is or is not rubbed into the skin; for all agents are absorbed by the blood in the cutaneous capillary system and are then removed. The effect is entirely superficial. Counterirritation results, of course; and it is probable that, by drawing more of the available blood to the skin, the flow through the underlying structures temporarily diminishes. Because analgesic measures often rely on a local increase in circulation, it is difficult to suppose that whatever minor ischemia results at the lesion from counterirritation can be advantageous. This point is worth making; for many remedies intended for application to the skin have a nationwide appeal. Indeed, such striking claims were made by Moss (22) for a massage cream containing adrenaline that a committee was set up to investigate it (20). The committee found that whether adrenaline was present in the cream made no real difference to the result, nor were any of the systemic effects of adrenaline noted. The inherent unlikelihood of a superficial inunction having any effect—let alone a lasting effect—on deeply placed tissues is by no means clear to laymen.

Massage in Plastic Surgery

In plastic surgery, massage performs an essential function that requires detailed mention because of the special techniques employed. The aims are to secure mobility and to enhance the circulation (26). For this purpose, rolling and rotary movements are imparted by the physical therapist's finger. Depth varies from the lightest touch on recent grafts to heavy massage over scar tissue. The ambit of the moving finger is very small, because wide circles stretch the skin too much. In some areas, for example, the nostril, the graft has to be rolled between two fingers.

PREOPERATIVE MASSAGE

When scar tissue requires excision, massage serves to free restricting fibrous bands and also helps the circulation to improve locally. When a scar is adherent to underlying bone, heavy rotary massage and skin rolling are indicated.

POSTOPERATIVE MASSAGE

For Thiersch Grafts

These are placed on a raw surface from which they acquire a new blood supply. A Thiersch graft consists of superficial epithelium only and can be applied as a single sheet on a surgically clean base. On a potentially infected area, patch grafts are used so as to allow exudate to escape without lifting the graft.

Very gentle massage can usually begin two or three weeks after the operation. Lanolin or glycerine should be used as a lubricant. When the reaction of the skin to the massage has been assessed, depth can be increased as the skin becomes stronger. A cautious start is particularly important in recent burns, where any but the lightest touch may provoke blisters. During the rotary massage, particular attention is paid to the avascular edges of the graft. The patient can with advantage be taught to continue the massage for two or three months after discharge. He should avoid exposing the grafted area to sunburn.

For Wolfe Grafts

This graft consists of the full thickness of the skin and is applied over muscle or fascia (to which a Thiersch graft would become unduly adherent); to the face (where a better cosmetic effect is secured); and to pressure points (where a Thiersch graft would prove too fragile).

Massage is usually begun 7 to 10 days after the stitches have been removed. As soon as the individual skin reaction has been ascertained, treatment becomes increasingly vigorous.

For Flaps and Tubes

When tissue has to be replaced rather than merely covered, a graft consisting of whole skin and underlying fat is called for. This cannot be severed from the parent site until the new circulation entering from the recipient area is fully established. Local flaps require one operation; pedicle flaps can be transferred by stages to any distance.

Flaps can usually be given massage a few days after the stitches are out. A gentle start is made, and depth and duration are increased until the graft is divided; massage then ceases but starts once more as soon as the edges are consolidated. The indication for early massage is undue congestion of the flap.

Tubed pedicles are treated by rolling the graft between thumb and finger tips. This begins a few days after the stitches are out and becomes vigorous as soon as the scar line and corners are consolidated. Should induration or a hematoma appear, vigorous treatment is employed to prevent fibrosis. Each time the pedicle is transplanted the massage ceases for the time being.

For Cramp

Patients are liable to painful cramp in the muscles about the joints immobilized during transplantation of flaps and pedicles. Massage is called for, and if heat is used as well care must be taken to shield the graft, because burns and blisters form easily on ischemic tissue.

Attention must also be directed to the joints themselves. Such movements that put no strain on the graft are encouraged from the first.

REFERENCES

1. Balfour, W. *Observations on Cases of Rheumatism.* Edinburgh, 1816.
2. Bartholomew, A. In: *Orthopaedic Medicine.* edited by Cyriax, J. London, 1959.

3. Bisgaard, H. Ulcus cruris behandlet med. *Uppsal. Lak. Forhandl.*, *29:*487, 1923.
4. Copeman, W. S. C. Fibro-fatty tissue and its relation to certain "rheumatic syndromes." *Br. Med. J.*, *2:*191, 1949.
5. Copeman, W. S. C., and Ackerman, W. L. Fibrositis of the back. *Q. J. Med.*, *13:*37, 1944.
6. Cyriax, J. Fibrositis. *Br. Med. J.*, *2:*251, 1948.
7. Cyriax, J. Hydrocortisone and soft-tissue lesions. *Br. Med. J.*, *2:*966, 1953.
8. Cyriax, J. *Massage, Manipulation and Local Anaesthesia.* London, 1941.
9. Cyriax, J. *Rheumatism and Soft Tissue Injuries.* London, 1947.
10. Cyriax, J. *Textbook of Orthopaedic Medicine*, Tenth Ed. Vol. 2. Baillière, Tindall, London, 1980.
11. Cyriax, J. *Textbook of Orthopaedic Medicine*, Ninth Ed. Vol. 1. Baillière, Tindall, London, 1983.
12. Cyriax, J., and Gould, J. Pain in the trunk. *Br. Med. J.*, *1:*1077, 1953.
13. Falconer, M. A. Surgical treatment of intractable phantom limb pain. *Br. Med. J.*, *2:*299, 1953.
14. Gowers, W. R. Lumbago; its lesions and analogues. *Br. Med. J. 1:*117, 1904.
15. Hartman, F. A., and Blatz, W. E. Studies in the regeneration of denervated mammalian muscle. *J. Physiol.*, *53:*290, 1919.
16. Hirschfeld, I. Gingival massage. *J. Am. Dent. Assoc.*, *46:*290, 1951.
17. Kellgren, J. H. Referred pain arising from the muscle. *Clin. Sci.*, *3:*2, 1938.
18. Knowles, E. L., and Kipling, M. D. Preliminary notes on treatment of 50 cases of tenosynovitis in industry. *Br. J. Industr. Med.*, *14:*200, 1953.
19. Leriche, R. *La Chirúrgie de la Douleur.* Paris, 1937.
20. Medical Research Council Committee. *Ann. Rheum. Dis.*, *14:*359, 1951.
21. Melzack, R., Guité, S., and Gonshor, A. Relief of dental pain by ice massage of the hand. *Canad. Med. Assoc. J.*, *122:*189, 1980.
22. Moss, L. The treatment of chronic rheumatism. *Med. World*, *70:*244, 1949.
23. Palmer, K. N. V., and Sellick, B. A. Prevention of post-operative pulmonary atelectases. *Lancet*, *1:*164, 1953.
24. Pollock, L. J., Arieff, A. J., et al. Effect of massage and passive movements on result of section of sciatic nerve of the cat. *Arch. Phys. Med.*, *31:*265, 1950.
25. Sobye, P. *Acta dermato-venerol.*, *31:*174, 1951.
26. Taylor, K. In: *Orthopaedic Medicine*, edited by Cyriax, J. London, 1959.

13

Mechanical Devices of Massage[1]

HERMAN L. KAMENETZ

While massage by definition is a manual treatment, attempts to replace the human hand or to extend its function by objects of various kinds have existed at all times. The history of massage records many utensils used to enhance the effects of this therapy: twigs with or without leaves for flogging, bronze and iron strigils for scraping, ebony staves for stroking, wooden ferules for tapping, rough cloth and roughened clay for rubbing, horse hair for brushing, wooden rollers for kneading, and many other devices, primitive or developed.

The first friction roller was produced in 1823 by John Shaw in Scotland (50). At the end of the 19th century, Klemm in Riga advocated his "muscle beater" (33). Schreiber (49) described it as three stout tubes joined at one end in a rubber handle. It could be used for self-administration, whereby regions otherwise inaccessible by the user's hands could be given tapotement.

The trend to replace man by machine quickened by the ubiquity of electric current. Thus, Granville's "nerve percuter" was first operated by a clock mechanism, later by electricity, as reported by Kellogg (31). Electricity was particularly appropriate for utensils providing percussion and vibration.

All these devices decreased the therapist's work, effort, and time, but the therapeutic contact of the hand was lost, together with the information provided by its touch, the skill of its function, i.e., the art of massage. Thus, the development of devices attracted lay persons with less educated hands to take over the treatment, and favored the tendency of patients to use instruments for self-administration, becoming less dependent on the practitioner.

[1] I am greatly indebted to my friend, the late Dr. Sidney Licht, whom I had assisted in editing the original series of the Rehabilitation Medicine Library including the first version of this chapter from which I have now borrowed.

Nevertheless, instruments allowed some types of therapy where help was not available or insufficient, whatever the reason. Pushing mechanization still further, inventors designed devices that did not have to be held and moved by the hand, but only needed to be put into place. No longer was it necessary that a masseur—or a lay person, or the patient himself—grasp the instrument to apply it over the area to be treated. It was only to be secured into place and left there, for hours if needed.

In addition to devices applied to a smaller or larger area of the body, methods have been used to impart motion to the entire body. In Greek and Roman antiquity this was achieved by traveling in a boat, in a carriage, on a litter, on horseback, etc. This therapy, called "gestation" because the patient was "carried" (30), was continued over the centuries by famous physicians. Pierre Chirac (1650–1732), physician to Louis XV, still recommended the shaking of the body that could be achieved by riding in a carriage over cobblestones. Charles-Irénée Castel, also known as Abbé de Saint-Pierre (1658–1743), inspired by this medical recommendation and the technology of his time, invented in 1734 a vibrating chair, the *trémoussoir*. Advocated for the treatment of hypochondriasis and constipation, it was immediately favorably received by the medical profession (38), and even the great skeptic, Voltaire, among others, reported enthusiastically on its good effects (34).

Sydenham in England practiced and recommended gestation in the 17th century, Quellmalz in Germany and Tissot in France (57) in the 18th, Dally in France (15) in the 19th. Charcot in Paris invented a vibrating helmet and in 1892, the year before his death, he developed a new model of the trembling armchair which he used for his patients with parkinsonism.

With the many objects invented over the preceding decades to impart massage-like effects upon the human body, several books on the subject appeared at the turn of the century. Among the authors we shall mention only two, both physicians: Louis de Lacroix de Lavalette of Paris (34) who coined the term sismotherapy, and Mary Arnold Snow of New York (51) who as Professor of Mechanical Vibration raised this therapy to its own right.

None of the mentioned devices—from the whipping twigs to the vibrating chair—has been completely abandoned. All continue to this day in one form or another, be it unchanged, like the birch twigs used in saunas, or modernized, like the armchair that delivers heat together with vibration.

Their types and variations have multiplied, vying to duplicate and sometimes to surpass the mechanical actions of the human hand. We have classified them in five groups as follows: (a) devices held and moved by the hand; (b) stationary devices against which the body part is held or moved; (c) flat devices submitted to alternating pressure; (d) intermittent-compression devices encircling a limb; and (e) devices for hydromassage.

Another therapeutic agent should be mentioned—only to be excluded from our list: ultrasound. It is true that it is a mechanical vibration which was therefore considered to be a form of micromassage by Pagniez (40), one of its early advocates, as well as by others. The applicator was also sometimes called "massage head", because it is moved in contact with the skin. However, it cannot be likened to any of the mechanical methods of massage discussed in this chapter. Its frequency of vibration is usually about 1 MHz and its effect is essentially the production of heat in the deeper layers of the tissues; hence it is a type of diathermy.

Nor shall we discuss electric stimulation of nerves or muscles. While it produces a massage-like effect, and while the great majority of massage instruments are also electrically operated, electric stimulation works by the action of the electric current on the body, not mechanically.

Instruments used in cardiopulmonary resuscitation are also excluded from this chapter.

Hand-held Devices

Almost all of the simple massage instruments already mentioned are held by the hand of the operator. They act by the pressure applied and the movement imposed upon them. Some might need two hands to be used, as e.g., the **massage suction-roller**, a revolving rubber cylinder resembling a rolling pin, with knobs for positive pressure and suction cups for negative pressure. Held at the ends of its axle and rolled over the fleshy parts of the body, it was still in use after the First World War, although hardly any more in America. Some smaller variants needed only one hand.

Most hand-held devices deliver, in addition to the pressure and movement provided by the operator, the massaging action of percussion or vibration. By increasing the frequency and decreasing the amplitude of the excursion, the former changes to the latter. In times past, the desired result was achieved by various mechanical means including hand-cranks and pedals. Today all devices are electrically operated, either by batteries or house current. Their frequencies and amplitudes of oscillations vary widely. Several types of **vibrators** oscillate at 100 to 200 Hz and an amplitude of 0.5 to 2 mm. Those with coarser movements, also called **percussors**, may oscillate at 10 to 50 Hz and amplitudes of several millimeters.

The smaller vibrators, of the size of a pocket flashlight, are shaped so that surfaces of various dimensions and configurations can be applied to the areas to be treated. Larger instruments usually have several interchangeable applicators of different shapes and sizes, made of plastic or hard or soft rubber. Advocates of acupressure massage (*shiatsu*) use devices with applicators shaped like fingertips.

Vibrators producing rather fine oscillations have been used in various motor dysfunctions in different neurologic conditions in order to stimulate voluntary function of paretic muscles (6, 22, 23). Much of the clinical experience has been gathered in Sweden (22, 23, 39), where vibration, eliciting the tonic vibration reflex, has been found to have various effects— favorable and unfavorable—on motor dysfunctions in upper motor neuron lesions and other neurologic disorders (22, 23). Vibrators are used in ophthalmology, speech pathology, otorhinolaryngology, for the relief of pain of dental origin (39), for reflex ejaculation in paraplegic men (7), to assist bladder emptying in multiple sclerosis. In the Soviet Union more than elsewhere, mechanical vibration is used in hypogalactia, tubal sterility, to stimulate ovulation, to prevent habitual abortion, and to relax ureteral contraction for the extraction of calculi.

Devices for heavier vibration or percussion are used to dislodge bronchial secretions, as e.g., in bronchiectasis, cystic fibrosis (16, 18), and other pulmonary conditions. Some believe that such therapy increases arterial oxygen tension in respiratory dysfunction (29), while others are skeptical (3).

Percussors, i.e., instruments producing coarser movements, are used to stimulate circulation but also to anesthetize certain small circumscribed areas. Russell used the quite powerful **Percuss-o-motor** with a solid (vulcanite) applicator in painful amputation stumps (Fig. 13.1). He held it "on the sensitive neuromata for 10 or 15 minutes. At first it may be necessary to approach the tender spot rather cautiously, as the machine provokes a great variety of phantom sensations and memories; but soon all tenderness

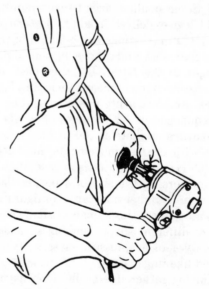

Figure 13.1. Electric massager applied to an amputation stump. (From Russell [46].)

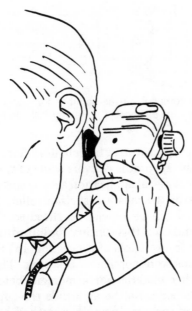

Figure 13.2. Electric massager applied to suboccipital region. (After a photograph in Russell et al. [47], from Russell [46].)

in the neuroma disappears, and even the first application may be followed by relief of pain for some hours" (46). Russell used also a vibrator in the treatment of postherpetic neuralgia (Fig. 13.2) and concluded: "It seems, therefore, that locally applied mechanical vibration has a powerful local anesthetic effect.... The method ... can be applied several times a day without causing any damage ... by the patient or by a member of the family ..." (47).

A still more vigorous effect was attempted by Billig (4, 5) when he actually crushed peripheral nerves in order to stimulate their arborization to surrounding denervated muscle fibers, primarily in postpoliomyelitis patients. This nerve crushing or "neurotripsy", as it was later called, was initially performed after surgical exposure, later transcutaneously, by forceful manual pétrissage, thereafter with an instrument consisting of a blunt-tipped rod and a handle, and—after about 1945—with a motorized vibrator of great power, the **Neurotripsor** (Fig. 13.3).

While most of the small massage instruments are held in the hand, some percussors and vibrators are strapped to the dorsum of the hand, imparting the mechanically produced motion to the massaging hand. Thus, it is not the device, but the therapist's hand, that is in contact with the patient's skin. The contact is soft, adapted at every moment to the surface. The

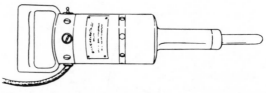

Figure 13.3. The Neurotripsor, an air-hammer for nerve crushing. (Drawn from a photograph supplied by the designer, Dr. Harvey Billig, from Licht [36].)

masseur is guided in the treatment by palpatory findings, and is less exposed to fatigue because the apparatus delivers some of the necessary power.

One type of device for local application acts by suction—an intensification of the suction cups of the massage suction-roller. In fact, the little cups used for this method can be likened to those that have been used since Hippocrates' time and until this century for **cupping**, that is to draw blood to the surface, away from an area of congestion. In pneumonia, for instance, a dozen or more cups were applied to the back. The cup was held over a burning wick or other material for a moment before it was quickly and tightly placed on the skin. As the air inside the cup cooled, it contracted, producing the desired vacuum. In another method, the cup had a small hole opposite the large opening. The large opening was tightly applied to the skin and the air was sucked out through the hole which then was quickly sealed by wax.

The drawing-up of skin and underlying tissue into the cup led to the name of **"traction" treatment** used in the 20th century. Here, the air was evacuated by a hand- or foot-pump attached to the applicator which was much larger than the old cups. In the modern suction apparatus the negative pressure is achieved by electric current; it may reach as much as 400 mm Hg. One single cup might be used and, contrary to the old type, there is a choice of various sizes in order to conform to the area to be treated. Another essential difference is that the cup can be either left in place or moved, sliding along the skin which is sucked into the cup from place to place. This is a kind of effleurage or of gliding, rolling pétrissage—a maneuver that is appropriately called **suction-wave massage**, or *Saugwellentherapie* (45), as it is called in German-speaking countries where it was particularly publicized around the middle of this century.

In the United States, the method was best known by the name of the instrument, the **Traxator**, a term based on the previous so-called traction treatment. It featured 21 applicators varying in shape and size, the largest one measuring 14 by 23 cm to be used for large fleshy parts. The method is less readily applied where the skin is close to the bone or where no even contact can be maintained between the applicator and the skin. Two techniques are used: the gliding technique in which the uniformly negative pressure combines with the movement to produce the massage; and the stationary technique in which the degree of negative pressure changes and so a pulsating vacuum kneads the tissues.

In concluding the description of this first group of massage instruments, we see that all of them, hand-held or hand-strapped, need to be guided by the operator, that they are used for local application, and that they may be used in either a stationary or a moving technique.

Stationary Massage Devices

The following devices have been classified as stationary—contrary to the first group—insofar as they are not moved during their use. The body part to be treated is placed upon or against a surface which, small or large, flat or curved, rigid or flexible, is exposed to stationary oscillations of one type or other. These instruments can always be operated by the user, except for instances of total disability.

Vibrating pads, available in various shapes and sizes, frequently resemble a seat cushion. Placed on a bed, a sofa, a chair, or the floor, such a pad provides vibration to any body part, depending upon its aspect placed on or against it. It can be incorporated in an armchair, a sofa, or a bed mattress. In fact, a motor can be attached under the bed to submit the entire bed to vibration.

Occasionally, a vibrating pad (42) or bed is used in an attempt to dislodge bronchial secretions—just like a hand-held vibrator—but reliable reports on effectiveness are missing. More often such devices are used in conditions of fatigue or discomfort in the lower or upper part of the back, and for general relaxation. Contoured back pads and cushions are available. To counteract fatigue of the feet, various foot massagers are on the market. They are usually placed on the floor while the user sits in a chair. One type offers to the feet a surface like a horizontally placed half cylinder; the user moves his feet over it, back and forth. Another type has a flat surface with a slight elevation in its center for a snugger fit into the arches of the feet. The surface may be studded with 200 or 300 little knobs, remindful of fingertips, for better penetration of the vibration. Also available is a plastic vessel for footbaths with a vibrating floor; it can be used with or without the water.

A **vibrating belt** or **strap** is a heavy canvas belt of about 10 cm width, fastened at both ends to a case containing the motor and which in turn is either attached to the wall or to one or two heavy poles on a heavy floorplate. The user stands on the floorplate, the belt around the part to be treated. Presumed to melt the superfluous fat over buttocks, thighs, and other regions, these belts are a frequent feature of health clubs and beauty salons. Found in the same places, a lighter variant that provides a more gentle vibration is the **vibrating facial sling**; it hangs from overhead so that the chin and cheeks can be placed into it.

A **massage roller pad** is a horizontal assembly of several massage rollers similar to the old massage suction rollers but having only knobs (no suction cups). It serves to massage the back, the soles of the feet, or other more or less flat areas of the body. Such a roller pad may be part of a plinth or table for vertebral traction. Some pads have a heating element incorporated, providing a low degree of heat together with the massage. In some other models, a dozen or more of these knobby rollers, instead of forming a flat pad, are mounted so as to form a large horizontal cylinder for slightly concave areas such as the abdomen in the flexed trunk or the posterior surfaces of thighs and calves in the flexed lower limbs. In one model such a cylinder can be used at adjustable levels by a standing person.

Alternating-Pressure Mattresses and Pads

A variant of the stationary devices, although not strictly a massage apparatus, is the **alternating-pressure mattress**, which is placed under the sheet on which the patient lies. Made of vinyl, it consists of a series of aircells parallel to the long border of the mattress which measures 80 by 190 cm (Fig. 13.4). An electric airpump cyclically fills every second cell, then empties them while filling the other half of them. Thus, while the patient is supported on one series of the air-filled tubes, the skin areas between them are relieved from the pressure to which they were exposed in the preceding period of the cycle. A full cycle of inflation-deflation may be about three minutes but can vary. The alternating compression and release, a massage-like action that empties and refills superficial blood vessels, is of course the rationale for the indication of such a pulsating mattress for the

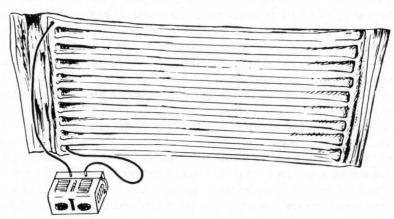

Figure 13.4. Alternating-pressure mattress and motor. (Drawn from a photograph supplied by R. D. Grant Company, Cleveland, OH.)

prevention and treatment of pressure sores in bedridden patients. Since its invention in 1947 by the neurosurgeon W. James Gardner in Cleveland (21), this alternating-pressure mattress has been acclaimed enormously and is now being found far beyond the borders of the United States.

The **alternating-pressure pad** is a smaller version (Fig. 13.5), measuring 40 by 50 cm. It serves as a seat pad for chairbound individuals, most often wheelchair users. Unfortunately, the electrically operated airpump restricts their mobility to a rather small area.

Intermittent-Compression Systems: Cuffs, Sleeves, and Boots

The devices of this fourth group have the following characteristics: (a) they can be used only in a stationary manner; (b) the parts applied to the patient encircle or fully surround a limb or part of it; (c) they are hollow cuffs, sleeves, or boots and the air (or, exceptionally, water) that enters and leaves rhythmically produces a massage of pressure and release; (d) the intended effect of this pneumatic massage is one of enhancing the flow of blood and lymph; and (e) once started, the machine may continue for hours without needing monitoring.

There is a long line of instruments producing such intermittent compression. Louis G. Herrmann, in his book published in 1936 (26), reviewed their

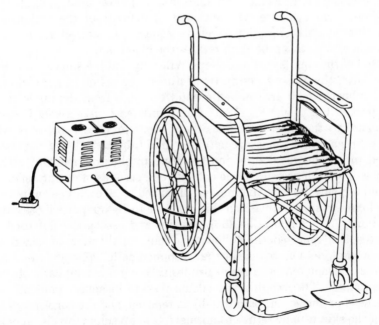

Figure 13.5. Wheelchair with alternating-pressure pad. (Drawn from a photograph supplied by R. D. Grant Company, Cleveland, OH.)

history. Three years earlier, he and Mont R. Reid (27, 28) had published their **Pavaex** or **PaVaEx** (for PAssive VAscular EXercise) apparatus, a wooden box with windows, later a boot of Pyrex glass, which submitted the encased foot and leg to alternating negative and positive pressure. Thus, Herrmann could report (26): "It was through the use of our original apparatus for over 1000 hours of treatment that we were able to collect sufficient clinical data to prove beyond doubt that the rhythmic exchange of pressure from about 80 mm of mercury *negative* pressure to about 20 mm of mercury *positive* pressure was most effective in the stimulation of the development of an adequate collateral arterial circulation." In spite of the great popularity this suction-pressure boot once enjoyed, today it is hardly known.

The **Intermittent-Venous-Occlusion Apparatus** was presented in 1936 by Collens and Wilensky (12, 13). It consists of a rubber cuff that is filled for two minutes by air supplied by a motor-driven pump and emptied by an electrically actuated release valve. The cuff is applied around the proximal portion of the limb—usually the lower limb—and is filled to a pressure of from 40 to 90 mm Hg. This results in a restriction of the venous blood returning to the heart.

The Council on Physical Therapy of the American Medical Association (14) did not accept the apparatus. Nor did Terrier et al. (55) find that such venous occlusion improved the circulation in the lower limb. Wilkins et al. (61) wrote: "No evidence was obtained in support of the rationale of intermittent venous congestion to relieve ischemia. In fact, all the data were in agreement that this procedure retards the blood flow."

Instead of the simple cuff of Collens-Wilensky and the single chamber of the PaVaEx, the **Vaso-Pneumatic** features a series of 14 parallel cuffs, also of rubber, which are applied around the limb from the ankle to the upper part of the thigh (Fig. 13.6). Being inflated consecutively from the most distal to the most proximal, these tubes produce a pressure wave which exerts a milking massage upon the limb (Fig. 13.7). They can also be inflated in a centrifugal direction, as done in the treatment of arterial insufficiency. Each pressure cycle consists of 2 seconds of compression and 1 second of pause, so that the limb is submitted to 20 cycles per minute.

The lumberman who invented this machine in 1945 reportedly saved his lower limbs from amputation (36). Wakim and associates (60) used the apparatus and reported the following: "Daily application of centripetal rhythmic compression, by use of the 'vasopneumatic' apparatus, to a limb swollen and edematous as a result primarily of chronic lymphatic obstruction, is helpful. The swelling and edema tend to disappear gradually and the tissues become softer; pain usually is relieved, and the consistency and color of the skin usually return to normal." Good results were also reported in arteriosclerosis obliterans and other vascular diseases of the lower limbs by Kirby and Sampson (32, 48).

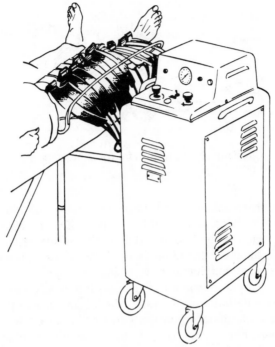

Figure 13.6. The Vaso-Pneumatic. (Drawn from a photograph supplied by Poor & Logan Manufacturing Company, North Hollywood, CA.)

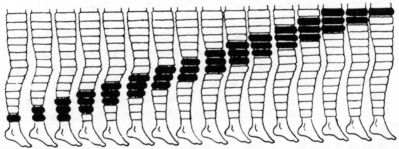

Figure 13.7. The Vaso-Pneumatic: centripetal spread of pressure wave. (Schematic representation supplied by Poor & Logan Manufacturing Company, North Hollywood, CA.)

Tinkham and Stillwell (56), who several years later compared this apparatus with newer ones as to their effectiveness in the treatment of postmastectomy lymphedema, did not find any essential difference among them and in fact even relatively little difference as compared with simple physical methods such as elevation of the limb.

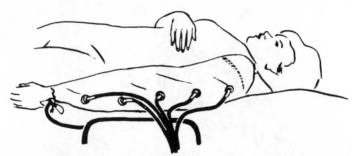

Figure 13.8. The Circulator sleeve. (Drawn from a photograph supplied by Progressor Therapeutics, Freeport, NY.)

The **Circulator**, another pneumatic apparatus, was invented by the dentist B. D. Weinberg, as related by Stillwell (53). It consists of a pneumatic sleeve or boot (Figs. 13.8 and 13.9) with five separate circumferential compartments, the most distal one in the boot enclosing the foot. They are filled with air in a centripetal progression in steps of 7½ seconds each. Contrary to the pressure wave in the Vaso-Pneumatic (which, while progressing, leaves a deflation in its wake) the air pressure in the Circulator is maintained in each chamber until all five are inflated and have been so kept for another unit of time (Fig. 13.9). Then, all chambers are deflated simultaneously and remain so to complete a 1-minute cycle.

Several other pneumatic devices were developed, with one or more compartments, built essentially on the same principles and occasionally even under more or less similar names, such as the **Pneumatic Circulator** of McCarthy and associates (37).

The "**medical massage suit,**" presented in 1955 by Henry and coworkers (24), covered both lower limbs and was supported by a garter belt. It was built after the model of the antigravity suits for pilots of fighter aircraft. A connected air-inflation unit provided rhythmic compression. The developers suggested it for the treatment of lymphedema, the prevention of arterial occlusive disease, venous pooling, phlebothrombosis, and pulmonary embolism.

Best known among the newer compression devices are the **Jobst pneumatic appliances**, originally developed by the engineer Conrad Jobst and first published in 1955 by the physicians Brush and Heldt of Detroit for the treatment of lymphedema of the upper limb (8, 9, 11). Later models were also used for the prevention of thromboembolism during and after surgery (10), for the treatment of arterial insufficiency, and for the shrinking of amputation stumps. The sleeve or boot is slipped over the limb and closed with a zipper. The connecting airpump can be regulated for its maximum pressure (up to 300 mm Hg), its timing for pressure and release, and the total duration of the treatment session. The adjustments depend upon

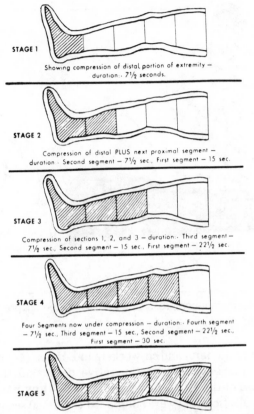

Figure 13.9. The Circulator boot: centripetal spread of pressure. (Schematic representation supplied by Progressor Therapeutics, Freeport, NY.)

several factors including the diagnosis, the extent of involvement, the condition of the tissues, and the patient's comfort. Below are a few examples. *Arterial insufficiency of lower limb*—80 mm Hg, 6 second on, 18 seconds off, 1 hour, four times daily; *prevention of thrombosis in lower limb*—45 mm Hg, 15 seconds on, 45 seconds off, day and night with short interruptions; *lymphedema in upper limb*—100 mm Hg, 45 seconds on, 15 seconds off, 6 hours, two or three times daily; and *shrinking of above-knee amputation stump*—40 mm Hg, 60 seconds on, 15 seconds off, 2 hours, four times daily.

After an initial treatment series with a hospital model under direct supervision by a physician, the patient can continue the treatment at home with a portable model such as the one shown with a long boot in Figure 13.10. The timer cycle is preset at about 90 seconds compression and 30 seconds rest and the degree of compression can be adjusted.

Similar intermittent-compression systems were developed in the early

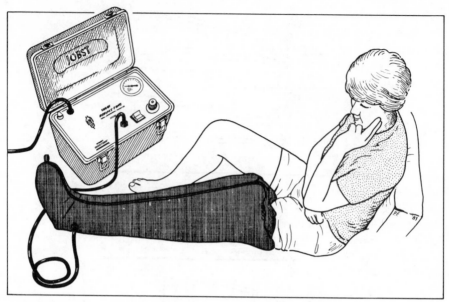

Figure 13.10. Intermittent-compression boot. (Illustration supplied by Jobst Institute, Inc., Toledo, OH.)

1970s in England. Roberts and co-workers in London (44) reported excellent results in the prevention of postoperative deep vein thrombosis by the peroperative use of the **BOC-Roberts Venous Flow Stimulator.**[2] A pair of below-knee plastic boots were submitted every 100 seconds to a 6-second compression with a maximum of 45 mm Hg.

The **Flowtron**, which soon became available in the United States, was likewise reportedly used with great success (43). One model is specifically designed for the prevention of deep vein thrombosis in patients undergoing surgery. The pump connects with either one or two large cuffs or garments, each for a leg, thigh, forearm, or arm. The usual pressure is 50 mm Hg, one cycle comprising 15 seconds inflation and 45 seconds deflation. Another model is of more general use including lymphedema and various venous and arterial deficiencies. In this unit, only one garment is used per limb (either a sleeve or a boot), but the one for the lower limb includes the foot and reaches either to the knee or to the groin; the one for the upper limb either reaches to the elbow or includes the arm. The pressures range from 40 to 90 mm Hg and the cycle is 2 minutes on, 2 minutes off.

In a later variant, the **Flowpulse**, which uses the same sleeves and boots, the pressure range has widened to a minimum of 20 mm and a maximum of 100 mm Hg, while the alternation between compression and exhaust can be adjusted in steps between 3 seconds and 4 minutes for each phase.

---

[2] The acronym refers to British Oxygen Company.

In all these single-chamber devices the pressure is, of course, uniformly distributed over all parts of the encased limb or limb segment. While the alternation of pressure and release is a feature of massage that benefits many cases, the milking effect of centripetal effleurage or similar maneuvers cannot be reproduced by such single-cell compression. Therefore, newer devices developed, continuing the line of the older compression systems with multiple cuffs; by their progressive inflation they enhance the flow of body fluids toward the heart and limit their back flow.

The **Lympha Press** was the first in this new series. It was developed by Avigdor Zelikovski in Israel, was presented in 1978 and 1979 at international congresses (64, 65) and was immediately well received (41). Overlapping cuffs (there are 9 to 12, depending upon the length of the sleeve or boot) are inflated sequentially in centripetal progression, producing a pressure wave in which the compression of the distal cuffs is maintained until all cuffs are inflated in order to avoid any back flow. The pressure, which is adjustable, is usually higher than in the older systems, but the cycle is shorter, about 25 seconds for inflation and 5 seconds for deflation. This shorter cycle allows the use of the higher pressures which may reach 190 mm Hg, i.e., higher than the usual systolic pressure.

Lympha Press (63–65) and the similar **Lympha-Mat** (17) are, as their names indicate, particularly used in the treatment of lymphedema, for which such a sequential-pressure-wave massage is thought to be most effective. Other indications include certain venous insufficiencies. As Eck (17) reported on the lympha-mat apparatus, which comprises nine cuffs for the sleeve and 11 cuffs for the boot, the compression can be maintained in the distal segment of the limb, if desired, while the proximal segment is submitted to the pressure-wave massage.

The **Wright linear pump** is another variant of the device described by Zelikovski. It has three cells: for the foot and ankle, the leg, and the thigh, respectively. The authors of the only report so far published (1) and covering only one case praise the variable pressure gradient with control of pressure and time for each of the three compartments, the control of delay between them, the resulting avoidance of back flow in the milking effect, and the absence of pain.

While in all these machines the cycle of intermittent compression is either fixed or individually determined by the operator, the rhythm of the **Syncardon** is regulated by the patient's electrocardiogram (Fig. 13.11). Similar to the intermittent-venous-occlusion apparatus, it has only one cuff. It attempts to increase the arterial blood flow, acting as an auxiliary peripheral heart under the impulse of the myocardium. The Syncardon was invented by the Swiss physician Maurice Fuchs who presented it in the literature in 1945 (19). Its "pressure impulses are adapted to the heart rhythm of the patient and applied simultaneously with the systolic phase of the pulsations of the vessels under treatment" (20). Although good and

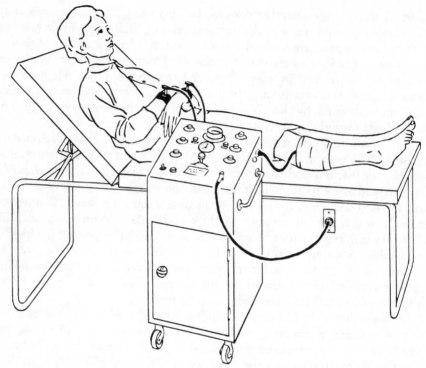

Figure 13.11. The Syncardon. (After a photograph, from Fuchs [20].)

even excellent results in the treatment of peripheral vascular disorders have been reported in different countries including the USA (62), the controversy about the efficiency of the apparatus continues until this day.

Just as the Collens-Wilensky single cuff of the 1930s changed to the Jobst boot in the 1950s to help in the treatment of limbs, the single cuff of the Syncardon of the 1940s evolved to a boot in the 1970s to support the function of the heart. Soroff and Banas (52), inspired by the concept of counterpulsation first used intra-arterially a decade earlier, called this new method **external counterpulsation** (ECP). According to a preliminary report:

"The thigh-high boot that Dr. Banas uses is a modification of that used by Dr. Soroff. Both types, however, have large steel casings for both legs. The casings are lined with rubberized fabric. Water is pumped into the space between the steel and the fabric during diastole, exerting positive pressure, and the water is sucked out during systole, exerting negative pressure. Both types of boot have elasticized tops to assure that they are airtight.

"Thus, the bed of fluid in the entire lower extremity is used as a pump, with the external fluid serving as an actuator. Improvement is due to helping the coronary blood flow by augmenting the diastolic pressure curve" (52).

The device was later again modified. In a 1980 report (2) of a cooperative trial involving 258 patients with acute myocardial infarction in 25 institutions, the authors noted a significant decrease in morbidity and hospital mortality after the use of such "external pressure circulatory assist by a mechanical device (**Cardiassist** External Counterpulsation System ...) .... Counterpulsation was effected by synchronization of mechanical activation with the electrocardiogram to produce positive pressure during diastole." This device did not include a negative pressure phase.

Devices for Hydromassage

Hydromassage is massage by the pressure and movement of water. Although it is usually and appropriately considered a hydrotherapeutic modality, we will briefly mention the mechanical devices used because they produce massage-like effects. Any projection of water upon the body has such an effect, however small it may be.

A simple shower falls into this category and special shower nozzles were particularly developed in the early 1970s to increase the water pressure for the self-administration of so-called **shower massage.** Various forms of showers, sprays, jets, and other currents of water (often called douches) have been used in spas and hospitals.

The **Scotch** or **alternating douche** was formerly known in every mental institution. From a distance of about five meters, the standing patient was hosed alternately with two streams of water, one hot, the other cold, under heavy pressure, which in addition to the thermic, must have had some mechanical effect.

In the **underwater douche massage** (or, simply, underwater douche) the patient is in a tub while a strong stream of water is directed upon and moved over the immersed area to be treated, the nozzle of the hose at a distance of a few centimeters from the skin. Little known in America, this therapy has been much used in some European countries, particularly since the development in 1939 of a pump that recycles the water of the tub (25) to produce the forceful jet of the hose. The impact of the jet is strong enough to indent the integument, stimulating the circulation in the superficial blood and lymph vessels.[3]

---

[3] The term "underwater massage" is occasionally, but improperly, used for underwater douche or for whirlpool, or even for hydromassage in general. It should be reserved for a manual massage under water: the area under treatment is either immersed or under a shower. In German-speaking countries, where underwater douche massage is extensively administered, the equivalent term has been supplanted by *Unterwasser-Druckstrahlmassage* or *Unterwasserstrahlmassage* (25, 35), terms which could indeed be properly used in their English equivalent of "underwaterjet massage."

The most frequently used hydromassage, at least in the United States, is the **whirlpool bath.** The whirlpool, in hydrotherapy, is a body of water agitated by a powered device (called agitator) which injects air. Whirlpool baths are given in tanks or tubs of various shapes and sizes, chosen according to the body parts to be treated. In the tank for total immersion of the body (Hubbard tank), there are usually two agitators. The intensity of agitation of the water and its temperature can be regulated. The therapeutic value of the whirlpool bath results no doubt from the combination of the temperature of the water, its pressure, and its movement. There are clearly massage-like effects including relaxation and improvement of circulation.

A variant of the whirlpool bath is the **bubble bath** in which a motor injects air into the water through hundreds of openings in a mat placed on the bottom of the tub. Baths in which bubbles are formed by the presence or addition of carbon dioxide gas or other chemical substances are beyond the subject of hydromassage.

The **hydrotherapy sleeve** is a portable whirlpool bath for an upper or lower limb. Very much looking like a sleeve for intermittent compression, it consists of a watertight perfusion chamber which encases the part to be treated. The sleeve is attached to a rather large cabinet which in addition to the motor contains two tanks, each of a capacity of 12 liters. "Air bubbles, which are essential to creation of air and liquid massage in whirlpool technique, are introduced by an air pump", as reported by the orthopedic surgeon-inventor who published this device in 1970 (58).

REFERENCES

1. Alexander, M. A., Wright, E. S., Wright, J. B., et al. Lymphedema treated with a linear pump: pediatric case report. *Arch. Phys. Med. Rehabil., 64:*132, 1983.
2. Amsterdam, E. A., Banas, J., Criley, J. M., et al. Clinical assessment of external pressure circulatory assistance in acute myocardial infarction. Report of a cooperative clinical trial. *Am. J. Cardiol., 45:*349, 1980.
3. Balk, R. A. More on the vibrating footpad. Letter to the Editor. *Am. Rev. Respir. Dis., 125:*782, 1982.
4. Billig, H. E. Personal communication. July 1983.
5. Billig, H. E., van Harreveld, A., and Wiersma, C. A. G. On re-innervation of paretic muscles by the use of their residual nerve supply. *J. Neuropathol. Exp. Neurol., 5:*1, 1946.
6. Bishop, B. Vibratory stimulation. *Phys. Ther., 54:*1273, 1974; 55:28, 1975; 55:139, 1975.
7. Brindley, G. S. Reflex ejaculation under vibratory stimulation in paraplegic men. *Paraplegia, 19:*299, 1981.
8. Brush, B. E., and Heldt, T. J. A device for the relief of lymphedema. *J.A.M.A., 158:*34, 1955.
9. Brush, B. E., Wylie, J. H., Beninson, J., et al. The treatment of postmastectomy lymphedema. *AMA Arch. Surg., 77:*561, 1958.
10. Brush, B. E., Wylie, J. H., Beninson, J., et al. A device for the prevention of phlebothrombosis and pulmonary embolism. *Henry Ford Hosp. Med. Bull., 7:*27, 1959.
11. Brush, B. E., Wylie, J. H., and Beninson, J. Some devices for the management of lymphedema of the extremities. *Surg. Clin. North Am., 30:*1493, 1959.
12. Collens, W. S., and Wilensky, N. D. (a) The use of intermittent venous compression in the treatment of peripheral vascular disease: A preliminary report. *Am. Heart J., 11:*705,

1936. (b) An apparatus for the production of intermittent venous compression in the treatment of peripheral vascular disease. *Am. Heart J., 11:*721, 1936.
13. Collens, W. S., and Wilensky, N. D. Intermittent venous occlusion in treatment of peripheral vascular disease. *J.A.M.A., 109:*2125, 1937.
14. Council on Physical Therapy, preliminary report of. Collens-Wilensky intermittent venous occlusion apparatus. *J.A.M.A., 109:*131, 1937.
15. Dally, N. *Cinésiologie ou Science du Mouvement dans ses Rapports avec l'Education, l'Hygiène et la Thérapie.* Paris, 1857.
16. Denton, R. Bronchial secretions in cystic fibrosis: the effects of treatment of mechanical percussion vibration. *Am. Rev. Respir. Dis., 86:*41, 1962.
17. Eck, L. Das "Lympha-mat"-Expressionsgerät zur Behandlung von Lymphödemen. *Z. Lymphol., 5:*34, 1981.
18. Flower, K. A., Eden, R. I., Lomax, L., et al. New mechanical aid to physiotherapy in cystic fibrosis. *Brit. Med. J., 2:*630, 1979.
19. Fuchs, M. Neue Methode zur Förderung der lokalen Blutzirkulation: "Synkardial Massage." Preliminary Report. *Schweiz Med. Wochenschr., 75:*542, 1945.
20. Fuchs, M. Syncardial massage. In: *Massage, Manipulation and Traction,* edited by Licht, S. New Haven, 1960.
21. Gardner, W. J., Anderson, R. M., and Lyden, M. The alternating pressure pad: An aid to the proper handling of decubitus ulcers. *Arch. Phys. Med. Rehabil., 35:*578, 1954.
22. Hagbarth, K.-E., and Eklund, G. The effects of muscle vibration in spasticity, rigidity, and cerebellar disorders. *J. Neurol. Neurosurg. Psychiat., 31:*207, 1968.
23. Hagbarth, K.-E., and Eklund, G. The muscle vibrator—a useful tool in neurological therapeutic work. *Scand. J. Rehab. Med., 1:*26, 1969.
24. Henry, J. P., Slaughter, O. L., and Greiner, T. A medical massage suit for continuous wear. *Angiology, 6:*482, 1955.
25. Hentschel, H.-D. Massage in der Hydrotherapie—von den Anfängen bis heute. *Therapiewoche, 24:*3683, 1974.
26. Herrmann, L. G. *Passive Vascular Exercises and the Conservative Management of Obliterative Arterial Diseases of the Extremities.* Lippincott, Philadelphia and London, 1936.
27. Herrmann, L. G., and Reid, M. R. The Pavaex (Passive Vascular Exercise) treatment of obliterative arterial diseases of the extremities. *J. Med., 14:*524, 1933.
28. Herrmann, L. G., and Reid, M. R. Passive vascular exercises. Treatment of peripheral obliterative arterial diseases by rhythmic alternation of environmental pressures. *Arch. Surg., 29:*697, 1934.
29. Holody, B., and Goldberg, H. S. The effect of mechanical vibration physiotherapy on arterial oxygenation in acutely ill patients with atelectasis or pneumonia. *Am. Rev. Respir. Dis., 124:*372, 1981.
30. Kamenetz, H. L. History of Massage. In: *Manipulation, Traction and Massage,* Third Ed. edited by Basmajian, J. Williams & Wilkins, Baltimore, 1985.
31. Kellogg, J. H. *The Art of Massage: Its Physiological Effects and Therapeutic Applications.* Battle Creek, 1895; 12th Ed. 1919.
32. Kirby, F., and Sampson, J. P. A new approach to movement of fluids in the extremities. Address to American Medical Association, Los Angeles, Nov. 1948.
33. Klemm, K. *Die Ärztliche Massage.* Riga, 1883.
34. de Lacroix de Lavalette, L. *La Sismothérapie ou L'Utilisation du Mouvement Vibratoire en Médecine Générale, et particulièrement en Thérapeutique Gynécologique.* Paris, 1899.
35. Ladeburg, H. Die Unterwasserstrahlmassage und ihre therapeutischen Möglichkeiten. *Therapiewoche, 2:*463, 1952.
36. Licht, S. Mechanical methods of massage. In: *Massage, Manipulation and Traction,* edited by Licht, S. New Haven, 1960.
37. McCarthy, H. H., McGuire, L. D., Johnson, A. C., et al. A new method of preventing the fatal embolus. *Surgery, 25:*891, 1949.

38. *Mercure de France.* Report of Prof. Astruc of Montpellier, pp. 677–688, April 1735.
39. Ottoson, D., Ekblom, A., and Hansson, P. Vibratory stimulation for the relief of pain of dental origin. *Pain, 10:*37, 1981.
40. Pagniez, P. De l'utilisation thérapeutique des ultra-sons. *Presse méd., 50:*741, 1942.
41. Partsch, H., Mostbeck, A., and Leitner, G. Experimentelle Untersuchungen zur Wirkung einer Druckwellenmassage (Lymphapress) beim Lymphödem. *Phlebol. Proktol., 9:*124, 1980. Reprinted in *Z. Lymphol., 5:*35, 1981.
42. Pavia, D., Thomson, M. L., and Phillipakos, D. A preliminary study of the effect of a vibrating pad on bronchial clearance. *Am. Rev. Respir. Dis., 113:*92, 1976.
43. Pflug, J. J., and Melrose, D. G. Prevention of thromboembolic disease in surgery. *Vasa, 5:*63, 1976.
44. Roberts, V. C., and Cotton, L. T. Prevention of postoperative deep vein thrombosis in patients with malignant disease. *Brit. Med. J., 1:*358, 1974.
45. Rohrbach, W. Zur Frage der Saugwellen-Therapie. *Arch. Badewesens, 11:*10, 1958. In Licht (36).
46. Russell, W. R. Percussion and vibration. In: *Massage, Manipulation and Traction,* edited by Licht, S. New Haven, 1960.
47. Russell, W. R., Espir, M. L. E., and Morganstern, F. S. Treatment of post-herpetic neuralgia. *Lancet, 1:*242, 1957.
48. Sampson, J. P., and Kirby, F. G. Evaluation of a new apparatus for the treatment of peripheral vascular disease. *Arch. Phys. Med. Rehabil., 36:*779, 1955.
49. Schreiber, J. *A Manual of Treatment by Massage and Methodical Muscle Exercise* (translated by W. Mendelson). Philadelphia, 1887.
50. Shaw, J. *The Nature and Treatment of Distortions of the Spine.* London, 1823, with Atlas (1824) and Supplement (1825).
51. Snow, M. L. H. A. (a) *Mechanical Vibration and Its Therapeutic Application.* New York, 1904. (b) *Mechanical Vibration. Its Physiological Application in Therapeutics.* New York, 1912.
52. Soroff, H. S., and Banas Jr., J. S. Pressure boot new angina aid. *Med. World News,* pp. 19–20, 1972.
53. Stillwell, G. K. The physiatric management of postoperative lymphedema. *Med. Clin. North Am., 46:*1051, 1962.
54. Strehler, E. H. *Die Druckwellentherapie.* Zurich, 1968.
55. Terrier, J. C., Wakim, K. G., and Krusen, F. H. The effects of occlusion with various pressures on the blood flow in the lower extremities. *Arch. Phys. Med., 29:*391, 1948.
56. Tinkham, R. G., and Stillwell, G. K. The role of pneumatic pumping devices in the treatment of postmastectomy lymphedema. *Arch. Phys. Med. Rehabil., 46:*193, 1965.
57. Tissot, J.-C. *Gymnastique Médicinale et Chirurgicale.* Paris, 1780.
58. Tracy, T. H. Hydrotherapy sleeve. *J. Bone Joint Surg., 52-A:*180, 1970.
59. Verleysen, J. *Histoire du Massage et de la Gymnastique Médicale.* Brussels, 1956.
60. Wakim, K. G., Martin, G. M., and Krusen, F. H. Influence of centripetal rhythmic compression on localized edema of an extremity. *Arch. Phys. Med. Rehabil., 36:*98, 1955.
61. Wilkins, R. W., Halperin, M. H., and Litter, J. The effects of various physical procedures on the circulation in human limbs. *Ann. Intern. Med., 33:*1232, 1950.
62. Wolf, H. F. Syncardial therapy in the treatment of gangrene and frostbites. Letter to the Editor. *N.Y. State J. Med., 53:*1126, 1953.
63. Zelikovski, A., Deutsch, A., and Reiss, R. The sequential pneumatic compression device in surgery for lymphedema in the limbs. *J. Cardiovasc. Surg., 24:*122, 1983.
64. Zelikovski, A., Manoach, M., Giler, S., et al. Lympha-Press. A new pneumatic device for the treatment of lymphedema of the limbs. *Lymphology, 13:*68, 1980.
65. Zelikovski, A., and Urca, I. Our experience with the Lympha-Press, a new pneumatic device for the treatment of lymphedema. *Proceedings of Seventh International Congress of Lymphology,* Florence, 1979, pp. 274–277. Prague, 1981.

Section

IV

WHAT NOW?

14

Research and Validation

JOHN V. BASMAJIAN

Among the everyday therapeutic tools that have been most widely accepted and simultaneously condemned are the topics of this book: Manipulation (including mobilization), stretching and traction, and massage in its variety of forms. They have no exclusive claim on this bizarre "love-hate" category, but lacking the drama of surgery and life-saving pharmaceuticals, and often prescribed as a last resort, these tools just get ignored by the scoffers. When confronted with good results, the skeptics fall back on a demand for double-blind controlled studies for validation of efficacy; ironically, this caution flies out the window when they are advised by their surgeons to undergo some complex operation or to take some dangerous drug.

Prejudice and human behavior aside, the need for research and validation indeed is great for any treatments that bear a cost of money, time, and human hopes. This book is based on the premise that the successful techniques described provide legitimate therapeutic services; of these, some may be based on interventions that have direct pathomechanical and pathophysiologic bases and others may have indirect (even "placebo") effects that a significant number of the patients find worthwhile.

Investigations of therapeutic efficacy of pharmaceuticals are difficult enough even though governments, drug companies, physicians, and scientists have a vested interest and where double-blinding is quite practicable. But where there are physical procedures, especially procedures where there is direct contact between patient and therapist, these add a new dimension of difficulty. This increases exponentially as the difficulty of scientifically describing the underlying disease or disorder increases. Because many of the indications for manipulation, traction, and massage are often couched in exotic language usually unknown to the medical scientist, the problem of research becomes almost—but not completely—impossible. In fact, the frequent use of glib, fallacious, or irrelevant pathomechanics to the medical problem may pose a threat that is greater to progress in research than an absence of truly scientific pathologic explanations.

311

Placebo Effects

Placebos are defined in the old sense as anything given to please the patient—for the word placebo means "I please"—with a strong suggestion that the inert substance given has a powerful therapeutic effect. The therapist or physician, in the old definition, knew that the treatment was inert but gave the patient a strong suggestion that it was an effective treatment, possibly even a powerful treatment. When the patient recovered from the symptom rapidly, or apparently as a result of the treatment, then it was said that a "placebo response" had occurred. Great emphasis was placed in this type of definition on the therapist knowing that the treatment was nonspecific and more clearly that it was by use of an inert substance or procedure. Little attention was paid to any possible psychoneurophysiologic influences that might actually have brought about an effect in the body of the patient. A more useful modern definition of the placebo response would be—

> a response in a conscious patient to the treatment of a symptom or sign (or possible a disease and/or condition) where the administrator of the treatment has no scientific basis in demonstrated fact that the treatment has a specific effect on the target, sign, symptom, disease, or condition.

From this, the definition of a placebo can be derived as the substance or procedure received by the patient for the purpose of treatment which will bring about a placebo response, whether it is planned as deliberate deception, suggestion, or in good faith without scientific proof of efficacy in advance. It can be seen from this last definition that ideas about placebos are changing. Because the purpose of this chapter is not to obtain a placebo effect, let us now examine whatever scientific basis we have for the power of the placebo in any type of treatment and, as much as possible, treatments carried out in the rehabilitation setting. Placebos and the use of placebos with strong faith on the part of the practitioner in their efficacy are as old as medicine itself. As suggested before, it is not necessary for our conception of placebos to include planned deception.

"NO MORE, GENTLEMEN!"

In 1799, as George Washington, father of his country, lay dying, some of the greatest physicians in America were gathered around his bedside. After great debate at the highest level of medical ethics and science, the physicians decided to bleed their patient. When he did not recover any strength, once more they bled him—and still once more. It was the considered opinion that he needed high colonic irrigation; so he had one or two of those as well on that same day. Finally the patient himself, mustering what strength remained, asked his concerned physicians to forbear. "No more, gentlemen", he said. And soon after, in spite of—or, perhaps, because of—the best efforts of his doctors, he died. Fresh debate ensued over whether the doctors had been remiss in their duties in not trying out further attempts to "save the President's life."

Similar stories abound in the history of medicine. And yet, ironically, the high regard for the physician in the Middle Ages and Renaissance was far beyond the regard now given doctors in modern times. Even though much of what physicians did for many centuries now is known to be absolutely contrary to physiology and scientific management, nevertheless they were credited with many cures and substantial improvements due to their activities.

How can this be? Much of what they did was inert by scientific standards, and yet it worked! Perhaps it worked better than much of what medicine does today except for the very specific target-oriented therapies such as antibiotics for specific bacteria, vaccination against specific viral and bacterial infections, replacement therapy for hormonal deficiencies, and various other specific replacement therapies. We may include some of surgery as well, while quite clearly reserving judgment on about half of the surgery done in North America; and I mean not just the "improper" surgery, as it might be called, but also the advocated and well-regarded surgery which is done for many conditions in the partial treatment of disease conditions.

Quite correctly, our defense for many of the treatment procedures used today is that it is the best state of the art. This of course is also the argument for much of what goes on in television, advertising, politics, and so on. But it is the best state of the art that we must keep on improving.

THE POWERFUL AND MYSTERIOUS PLACEBO

While rehabilitation (including the subjects of this book) does not stand alone in its use of and unknowing dependence on the art of placebo, perhaps half of what is done in therapy departments is either useless or harmful—but we don't know which half. Intensive research to determine the specific effects of everything we do is essential. While we may advocate and admire the nonspecific effects of placebo treatments, science and plain honesty demand that we learn as much about specific effects as possible while also learning to use the powerful tool of the placebo response.

PLACEBO EFFECT OF MACHINES AND MANUAL THERAPIES

Lest physical and manual therapists congratulate themselves on the fact that they do not use drugs but rather use techniques and machines, consider the placebo effect of machines. Schwitzgebel and Traugott (15) reported experiments with normal subjects who were attached by arm electrodes to electronic machines. It was implied that their performance on special tasks would be improved when the current was on and would decrease when it was off. As you will have guessed, there was no current ever turned on, and again you have guessed that the hypothesis was borne out. When the subjects thought the current was on, their performance increased markedly. And no doubt, in a manual therapy setting, the surroundings, the equipment, and the assured way in which the therapists handle the equipment have a very strong influence on the patient.

There is no question that approaches other than chemotherapy have strong placebo influences. In 1976, Henry Byerly (2) pointed out that placebos seemed to work like magic incantations in that both require an object of concentration, and virtually anything can function as an object. Further, the improvement need not be simply of a subjective nature. Byerly cites a rheumatoid arthritis study in which placebos achieved the same level of effectiveness as aspirin in objective improvement in the swelling of the joints. It is conceivable that physical agents other than ingested chemicals might have the same influence as a placebo response, as difficult as it may be for those in rehabilitation to accept.

In a research study on the treatment of back problems (1), the electronic gear of the recording devices (inserted electrodes, EMG equipment, various electronic devices, and a computer) raised the placebo response in almost 200 patients with back problems from the usual 30% (or so) for sugar pills to about 50%.

THE THERAPIST'S ROLE

The therapist—whether a physical therapist, manual therapist, or physician—is vital. It is the human being, surrounded by the mystique of a profession, who has the strongest influence. If that therapist is knowledgeable about the procedures employed, is confident, and, above all, comes in close contact with the patient, success of almost any treatment occurs in 30% to 50% of patients. If the therapist touches and manipulates the patient, this greatly enhances the effectiveness, regardless of whether the current fad is carried out correctly or incorrectly. Hence, many patients will recover from disabilities of the musculoskeletal system by having an "improper" manipulation or traction rather than the "proper" manipulation advocated by some charismatic healer. It does not seem to matter whether transcutaneous electrical nerve stimulation or acupuncture are done absolutely "correctly"—a large number of patients will achieve substantial success or cure. The important element seems to be a close contact between the patient and the therapist. This is at least as important as the specific effect of the treatment.

Normative Data On Low-Back Mobility And Activity Levels

Low-back pain represents a process which particularly requires research both for its pathomechanics and for the modes of efficacy of techniques used in manual therapies. Holt (14) found that 54% of 2000 people questioned had low-back pain. A more recent report by Fisk (7) showed that 80% of all Americans suffer from low-back pain at one time or another.

Various classifications of low-back pain including viscerogenic, vascular, neurogenic, psychogenic, and spondylogenic have been described. Yet for patients with chronic back problems, approximately 39% show radiographic evidence of disc degeneration, primarily at the fourth and fifth lumbar discs (8). Surgical management of patients with lumbar disc disease indicates that expected improvement will occur in 70% while 90% of similar patients treated conservatively will show improvement (7). Data from long-term studies reveal that only 10% of patients treated surgically demonstrate a full return to their previous lifestyles without developing a problem secondary to their original injury (11). Moreover, results of the various nonsurgical treatments, including rest, traction, physical therapy (heat and massage), trigger point stimulation, medication, occupational changes, and joint mobilization (6) indicate such procedures are at least as beneficial as surgery and, in many cases, are more effective (17).

Information about mobility and muscle activity in the back can improve our understanding of biomechanical principles underlying posture and provide valuable data that will aid in developing more appropriate treatment plans. The actions of the erector spinae, which is composed of the transversospinalis (multifidus and rotatores), and the sacrospinalis (longissimus and iliocostalis) muscle groups, have been described in some detail in Chapter 3. Careful studies have demonstrated a profound reduction of low-back EMG-activity during painful muscle spasms (1, 14, 18).

Quantification of differences in back muscle activity between normal subjects and patients with chronic back pain appears only in our study designed to obtain normative back mobility and activity from the erector spinae muscles (18). It offered clinicians at least one method for assessing dynamic low-back movements in normal or patient populations. A total of 112 adult men and women without histories of chronic low back pain, traumatic back pathology, scoliosis, or degenerative disc disease associated with pain or movement limitations served as normal subjects. They were grouped by sex within decades. Both range of motion and EMG evaluations were performed once per subject. Occasionally repeated measurements were undertaken when some doubt existed concerning the accuracy or fluidity of dynamic movements.

EMG electrode placements were determined from measurements made on dissected cadaver material. The lower electrode pair rested on the fascial cleft separating the more medial multifidus muscle from the longissimus while the upper pair were positioned on the longissimus. Therefore, recordings made from the upper electrode pair reflected activity levels of the longissimus muscle while EMG recorded from other electrode pair showed the activity from (at least) the longissimus and multifidus muscles.

RANGE-OF-MOTION MEASUREMENTS

Straight Leg Raising (SLR)

There was no significant interaction between age and sex during SLR activities; however, women showed more mobility than men across ages for both left ($p < 0.02$) and right ($p < 0.02$) legs. Mean active hip flexion measurements indicate that women had greater mobility than their male counterparts while men in the 30- to 39-year group had bilateral limitation in SLR movements (Fig. 14.1).

Spinal Forward Flexion (Vertebral Separation)

Increases in distance between the seventh cervical and first sacral spinal processes were recorded in centimeters during full forward trunk flexion with maintained knee extension. Analysis of variance by age and sex did not indicate significant interaction, but a sex effect was present with men showing a significantly greater increase in intervertebral distance during flexion ($p < 0.008$). As seen in Figure 14.2, men showed larger changes than

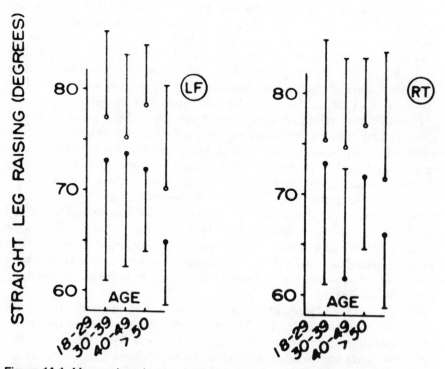

Figure 14.1. Mean values (± standard deviation) for straight leg raising in degrees (ordinate) plotted by age grouping (abscissa). *Open circles,* women; *closed circles,* men. Abbreviation: Lf = left; Rt = right (from Wolf et al. [18]).

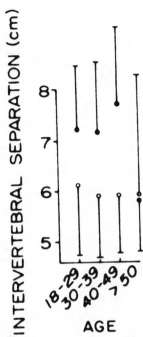

Figure 14.2. Mean values (± standard deviation) for intervertebral separation, measured in centimeters between spinous processes C7-S1 during trunk flexion (ordinate) plotted by age grouping (abscissa). *Open circles,* women; *closed circles,* men (from Wolf et al. [18]).

women and the oldest subjects showed the least amount of intervertebral separation.

Trunk Rotation

Neither a significant sex-age interaction nor a significant main effect could be detected during trunk rotation to the left or right. Figure 14.3 graphically shows that men and women of different ages performed this movement similarly.

Lateral Bending

The mean values for lateral bending to the left and right are plotted in Figure 14.4. Analysis of variance revealed a significant sex-age interaction. Significant differences between sexes occurred in the 30- to 39-year age groups upon bending to the left ($p < 0.05$) or the right ($p < 0.02$).

ELECTROMYOGRAPHIC (EMG) MEASUREMENTS

Repeated measures of EMG activity from specific electrode placements produced no significant trial effect. These findings suggest that the meth-

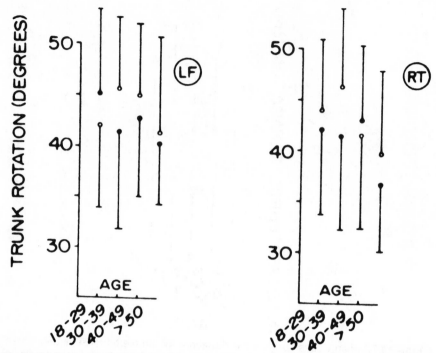

Figure 14.3. Mean values (± standard deviation) for trunk rotation in degrees (ordinate) plotted by age grouping (abscissa). *Open circles,* women; *closed circles,* men. Abbreviation: Lf = left; Rt = right (from Wolf et al. [18]).

odology of guiding subjects' movements would result in consistently reproducible integrated EMG readings during multiple trials using the same electrodes.

Trunk Flexion-Extension

Findings for the difference in EMG activity in full-trunk flexion versus extension were consistent among all subjects at each electrode placement. As expected, extension EMG activity always exceeded activity during trunk movements ($p < 0.001$). Additionally, the magnitude of these differences was not the same for each age group and a significant age-sex interaction was obtained for differences recorded at electrode placements ($p < 0.05$). Multiple comparison tests revealed that for all electrode placements the magnitude of difference between flexion and extension EMG was significantly greater ($p < 0.05$) in men than in women in the 18- to 29-year age group. EMG silence was observed when 70° of trunk flexion was exceeded and most commonly was seen between 80°–90°. This observation could be made from any electrode placement. EMG activity usually resumed after

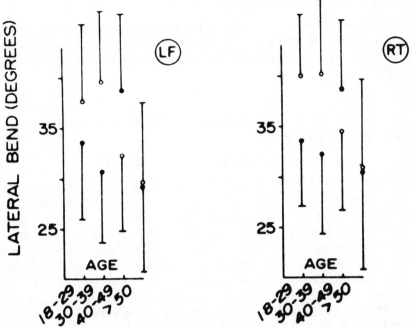

Figure 14.4. Mean values (± standard deviation) for lateral bending in degrees (ordinate) plotted by age grouping (abscissa). *Open circles,* women; *closed circles,* men. Abbreviation: Lf = left; Rt = right (from Wolf et al. [18]).

20° of extension from the fully flexed trunk position, but occurred anywhere from 90°–30° of flexion (18).

Lateral Rotation (Standing)

At one placement, the differential EMG produced a significantly negative mean score while at the second, left minus right EMG values were significantly positive and at the third and fourth, significant differences in EMG turning were not detected. Furthermore, the differences in EMG during rotation were statistically dissimilar in magnitude for men and women in the 18- to 29-year age group at the first placements ($p < 0.003$) and the second ($p < 0.0001$).

Lateral Rotation (Sitting)

The results were mixed among the sex and age groups, showing neither a significant age-sex interaction nor a significant age or sex effect within group.

Bending at the Knees (Stooping)

All electrode placements revealed consistent findings. Significant age-sex interactions were observed ($p < 0.005$) and the youngest group of women had significantly higher levels of EMG activity than their male counterparts ($p < 0.01$).

Quiet Sitting

There were no significant differences in EMG activity between men and women within any age group.

SUMMARY OF NORMATIVE STUDY (18)

This group was characterized by people whose lifestyle was primarily sedentary (even compared to older men) which might account for lower range-of-motion values (Figs. 14.1, 14.2, and 14.4). Hence, consideration of occupation and activity patterns must be incorporated into the establishment of any normative mobility profile. Generally, our mobility measurements are compatible with standards reported by other clinicians with women showing slightly greater movement than men. A significant sex effect was found during vertebral separation in trunk flexion, probably attributable to the greater excursion and larger morphology in men. Both straight leg raising and lumbar spinal flexion produced lower values than reported elsewhere (12). These limitations are probably due to tight (shortened) hamstring muscles which would restrict both movements.

Lateral bending movements produced significant sex-age interactions, and thus men and women should not be grouped within a specific age range. Because significant differences in movement to one side, but not the other, were observed in some groups and because none of our subjects showed a noticeable scoliosis or discrepancy in leg lengths our findings might be attributable to measurement error. Nonetheless, the mean ranges by sex and age group are in accord with other reports.

Movements during which EMG recordings were made can be divided into dynamic (trunk flexion-extension, lateral rotation-standing, and bending at knees) and static (quiet sitting and lateral rotation-sitting) activities. Significant sex-age interactions were observed for all dynamic activities while such occurrences were not observed during static activities. Therefore, the clinician should not group all subjects when establishing normative EMG data during these dynamic movements. On the other hand, data from men and women can be combined by age groupings during quiet sitting or rotation in a sitting position.

The significantly greater EMG activity observed in trunk extension versus flexion confirms previous EMG studies on the function of the erector spinae muscle group (Chapter 3). That the magnitude of difference between flexion and extension EMG was significantly greater in men than women at ages 18–29, might easily be attributed to the selective differences in erector spinae muscle mass for these men. Furthermore, relative quiescence in EMG activity after 70° of trunk flexion, as recorded from all electrode placements, confirms the observations reviewed in Chapter 3 that ligamentous structures and not the erector spinae support the fully flexed lumbar vertebral column.

During lateral rotation movements while standing and with the hips manually stabilized, the findings suggest that the erector spinae muscles serve to maintain the upright posture, in harmony with the gluteus maximus and stabilize the back during rotatory movements to the opposite side.

While our subjects bent over from the knees in performing this stooping motion, the posture of the back and trunk varied considerably. This variation might well account for the sex-age interactions. Several members of our youngest women group did stoop with only moderate trunk flexion, perhaps 10°–20°. This positioning will strongly activate the erector spinae muscle group and might account for the higher EMG levels for women in this age group.

The prospects for expanding the present findings appear promising. Still to be documented are patterns of EMG activity from the hip extensors or abdominal muscles. Differences in EMG levels or patterns from these muscle groups during dynamic movements in a normal population versus a back pain patient population might produce additional treatment strategies.

Research on Manipulation for Low-Back Pain

Research on the effectiveness of manipulation began in earnest during the past decade. A randomized trial of a single manipulation compared with "placebo" by Glover et al. (9) was inconclusive though it tended to favor manipulation. Doran and Newell (3) found less support, concluding that manipulation, "physiotherapy", corsets, and analgesia were all about the same in a randomized study of 456 patients. Other, more recent, randomized studies with small groups (4, 5, 13, 16) have yielded mixed conclusions.

Perhaps the latest available report is the most scientific and the most negative; in it, Godfrey et al. (10) describe a single-blind, randomized controlled clinical trial of rotational manipulation for low-back pain of recent onset in 81 adults. The control treatments which the authors believed to be a placebo (which probably it was) were minimal massage and low-level electrostimulation. Both "treated" and "control" patients improved rapidly in the 2- to 3-week observation period. At retest, there was no statistically significant difference between the improvement scores of the two groups.

No absolutely impeccable study has yet been reported on the efficacy of any treatment for low-back pain, let alone on manipulation. This important area of medical science is a morass into which the naive investigator stumbles at his own peril. Yet science must be recruited to establish the pathomechanics and pathochemistry as well as the rationale of various specific and nonspecific treatments. Meanwhile, patients rely on their own perceptions of the dollar-value of treatments received or available. As individuals, they are guided by personal results and word-of-mouth advertising of the effectiveness of this or that treatment. Dogmatism—both pro and con—is a paramount characteristic among almost all who deal with potential manipulation therapy; against that background scientific analysis remains our best hope to lead us out of the morass.

REFERENCES

1. Basmajian, J. V. Effects of cyclobenzaprine HCl on skeletal muscle spasm in the lumbar region and back: two double-blind controlled clinical studies. *Arch. Phys. Med. Rehabil.,* 59:58, 1978.
2. Byerly, H. Explaining and exploiting placebo effects. *Perspect. Biol. Med., 19:*423, 1976.
3. Doran, D. M. L., and Newell, D. J. Manipulation in treatment of low back pain: a multicentre study. *Brit. Med. J., 2:*161, 1975.
4. Evans, D. P., Burke, M. S., Lloyd, K. N., et al. Lumbar spinal manipulation on trial, part I—clinical assessment. *Rheumat. Rehabil., 17:*46, 1978.
5. Farrell, J. P., and Twomey, L. T. Acute low back pain: Comparison of two conservative approaches. *Med. J. Austral., 1:*160, 1982.
6. Finneson, B. E. *Low Back Pain.* Philadelphia, J. B. Lippincott Co., 1973.
7. Fisk, J. R. The clinical history as a diagnostic level prognostic tool in low back pain. Second Annual Conference on Physical Impairment and Disability, "Back Pain." Emory University School of Medicine, Atlanta, Georgia, November 17, 1977.
8. Friberg, S., and Hirsch, C. Anatomical and clinical studies on lumbar disc degeneration. *Acta Orthop. Scand., 19:*222, 1950.
9. Glover, J. R., Morris, J. G., and Khosla, T. Back pain; a randomized clinical trial of rotational manipulation of the trunk. *Br. J. Indust. Med., 31:*59, 1974.
10. Godfrey, C. M., Morgan, P. P., and Schatzker, J. A randomized trial of manipulation for low-back pain in a medical setting. *Spine, 9:*301, 1984.
11. Gottlieb, H., and Strite, L. Comprehensive rehabilitation of patients having chronic low back pain. *Arch. Phys. Med. Rehabil., 58:*101, 1977.
12. Guide to the Evaluation of Permanent Impairment. American Medical Association Committee on Rating Mental and Physical Impairment, pp. 43–47, Chicago, 1971.
13. Hoehler, F. K., Tobis, J. S., and Burger, A. A. Spinal manipulation. *J.A.M.A., 245:*1835, 1981.
14. Holt, L. Cervical, dorsal and lumbar spinal syndromes: A field investigation of a nonselected material of 1200 workers in different occupations with special reference to disc degeneration and so-called muscular rheumatism. *Acta Orthop. Scand.,* Suppl 17, 1954.
15. Schwitzgebel, R. K., and Traugott M. Initial note on the placebo effect of machines. *Behav. Sci., 13:*267, 1968.
16. Sims-Williams, H., Jayson, M. I. V., Young, S. M. S., et al. Controlled trial of mobilization and manipulation for patients with low back pain in general practice. *Brit. Med. J., 2:* 1338, 1978.
17. White, A. W. M. Low back pain in men receiving workmen's compensation. *Canad. Med. Assoc. J., 95:*50, 1966.
18. Wolf, S. L., Basmajian, J. V., Russe, C. T. C., et al. Normative data on low back mobility and activity levels. *Am. J. Phys. Med., 58:*217, 1979.

Index

Page numbers in italics refer to figures.

A

Abdominal bloating, in spinal manipulation, 82
Abu'Ali, 5
Acetylcholine, 259
Achilles tendon, 277
Ackerman, 284
Acupressure, 246, 263
Acupuncture, 246, 263
Adherent scars, 273
Adhesions, 135, 158, 273
Adhesive capsulitis, 135, 136
Aftertreatment, 274, 276
Albuminuria, 242
Alternating-pressure mattress and pad, 296
American Academy of Osteopathy, 17
  School of Osteopathy, 17
Amputation stumps, 282, 300
Amputees, soft tissue contracture, 161
Analgesia, local, 272
Analgesic medications, 82
Andry, 230, 231
Anesthesia, local, therapeutic, 270
Angioneurotic injury, 280
Ankle, mobilization, 150
  sprains, 260
Ankylosing spondylitis, 114
Anti-inflammatory medication, 80
Annulus fibrosus, 189
Aortic aneurysm, 191
Apotherapy, 243
Arteriosclerosis obliterans, 298
Arthritic knee, 149
Arthritis, 181, 191
  acute traumatic, 274
Arthrosis, cervical, 99
  of knee, 149
Articular cartilage, erosion, 188
Asclepiades, 265
Aseptic necrosis, Scheuermann's, 110
Asthma, 281
Atelectasis, 281
Atherosclerosis, 191
Athletes, kneading, 283
Atlas, 56
Auriculotemporal pain, 100
Axis, 56

B

Backache, psychologic, 189
  traction for, 174–179
Bain, 259
Baker University, 16
Balfour, 234
Banas, 304
Barczewski, 244
Bard, 181
Barker, 8
Barré, 105
Barré-Lieou syndrome, 105
Bauer, 188, 260
Beard, 217, 230, 263
Behrend, 264
Bell, 233
Berghmann, 237
Berne, 240, 241
Betou, 235
Beveridge, 234
Billig, 293
Billroth, 239
Bindergewebsmassage, 245
Birch twigs, 290
Bisgaard, 247, 283
Bladder paralysis, in traction, 191
Blatz, 282
Blood clot, 275
Blood flow, venous, 241
Bobath, 162
Boerhaave, 5, 231
Boigey, 247
Bon, de, 235
Boni, 263
Bone-setters, 6
Bonnet, 236
BOC-Roberts venous flow stimulator, 302
Braaf, 204
Brandt, 239
Bright, 229
Bronchiectasis, 280
Brunner, 185, 187
Brush, 300
Bubble bath, 306
Bucholz, 264
Buck's extension, 172, 191
Bugaj, 261

Bum, 241, 247
Bunnell, 159
Bursitis, trochanteric, 145

C

Caldwell, 195
Capitate navicular blockage, 143
Capsulitis, 188
Cardiac arrest, 282
Cardiac massage, 247, 248
Cardiassist, 305
Cardiovascular disease, 191
Carotid sinus massage, 260
Carpal manipulation, 142
Carrier, 259
Castel, 290
Castex, 241
Cauda equina syndrome, 124
Cazeaux, 239
Celluloperiosteomyalgic syndrome, 86, 120, 121, 135, 149
Central spinal cord syndrome, 189
Centrifugal stroking, 265
Centripetal rhythmic compression, 265
Centripetal stroking, 257, 259, 260, 264, 265
Cervical spine evaluation, 85
  traction, 173, 202
Chang, 5
Chapna, 215
Charcot, 239, 290
Chauliac, Guy de, 228
Chirac, 290
Chiropractic, 9–11, 18
Chiropractor, 123
Chomel, 231
Chorea, 236
Chrisman, 190
Christie, 175, 190, 201
Cibot, 214
Circulation, 245, 258
Circulator, 300
Clark, 259
Claw-hand, 159
Cleobury, 232
Coccygodynia, 244
Coccyx, 52, 121
Colachis, 178, 179, 181, 183, 186
Collens, 298
Colombo, 241
Connective tissue disease, 157
Connective tissue massage, 245

Contact massage, 245
Contractures, 157, 159
Copeman, 284
Corbin, 195
Cornelius, 243, 244
Corticosteroid, 82
Cosby, 172
Coste, 243
Coulter, 225, 228, 263
Counterpulsation, 305
Covalt, 188
Cracking sound, 73, 75
Cramp
  immobilization, 287
  sportsman's, 283
Crazy Sally, 8
Cream, massage with, 285
Credé, 239
Crepitus, 277
Crestal point, 113, 115
Crisp, 185, 188, 201
Crosseyed Sally, 8
Crue, 183
Cuboid, 152
Cupping, 268, 294
Cutaneous temperature, 241
Cyriax, 13–15, 174, 179, 180, 185, 188, 190, 191, 194, 201, 247

D

Dalicho, 246
Dally, 215, 216, 231
Daremberg, 217
de Bon, 235
Decroix, 105
Deep friction, 247, 271–277
  technique, 277
Deep massage, 271, 283
  technique, 277
de Lavalette, 290
Dentz, 247
Dermatomes, 39–40, 108–109
Dermatomyositis, 159
De Sèze, 180, 184, 190, 201
DeWald, 173
Dicke, 246
Direction, stroking, 265
Disc
  herniation, 119–120
  lateral blocking, *97*
  lesions, *97*

midline protrusions, 190, 191
  pathology, 187, 190
  prolapsed, 176
  protrusion, 38–39
Discograms, 187
Donders, 239
Dorsal spine, 84, 86
Drabkin, 224
Drinker, 260
Dudgeon, 215
Dupuytren, 237
Dupuytren's contracture, 159
Dural sheath, 187

E

Eck, 303
Edema, 157, 271, 274, 280, 283
  static, 247
Edgecombe, 259
Effleurage, 213, 237, 257, 264–265, 274, 280,
  283, 294
Effusions, 241, 275
Elbow
  contracture, 144
  golfer's, 277
  nursemaid's, 144
  pulled, 144
Electrical stimulation, 144
Electromassage, 241
Elkins, 260
Epicondylar pain
  lateral, 137
  medial, 144
Epicondylitis, lateral, 94, 138, 139, 140
Esmarch, 239
Estradère, 236
Eulenberg, 235
Evaluation, spinal, 32–36
Exercises, therapeutic, 82
External counterpulsation, 304
Eye, 239

F

Facets, vertebral, subluxation, 187
Falconer, 282
Femoral traction, 173
Fibrosis, 157, 158
Fibrositis, 244, 270, 284
Fielding, 179
Finger, sprain, mild, 144

Fiocco, 241
Fishbein, 11
Flowpulse, 302
Flowtron, 302
Foramina, 189
Fox, 13
Fracture, soft-tissue contracture with immo-
  bilization, 164
Fractures, 240
Françon, 263
Frankl, 240
Frazer, 185, 188, 189, 205
Friction, 232, 237, 258, 265, 273
  deep, see Deep friction
  transverse, see Transverse friction
Friction massage, 265
Fuchs, 248, 303
Fuller, 230

G

GAG, 37
Galen, 5, 228, 229, 265
Gardner, 297
Garnault, 242
Garrett, 109
Gartland, 205
Gastrocnemius, spinal pain, 93
Gelosenmassage, 244
Gelotripsy, 244
Georgii, 234, 235
Gerneck, 188
Gestation, 290
Gingivitis, 284
Gläser, 246
Glisson, 201, 230
Glycoaminoglycan, 37
Gocht, 239
Godfrey, 180, 186
Goldie, 175
Golfer's elbow, 277
Gordon, 196
Gowers, 284
Graham, 217, 222, 229, 233, 235, 238, 239,
  257–259
Granville, 241, 242, 289
Gravity, traction and, 177
Grosvenor, 232
Gurewitch, 241
Guy de Chauliac, 227
Gynecologic massage, 239, 244

H

Halo loop, 173
Halo pelvic traction, 173
Hamilton, 172
Hand splints, 167–171
Handgriffe, 241
Hartman, 282
Hartspann, 244
Hartspannmassage, 244
Hasebroek, 241
Head, 243, 246
Head halter, 192`
Headaches, 99
   auriculotemporal, 103
   cervical origin, 99–105
   migraine, 100, 105
   occipitomandibular, 103
   occipitosupraorbital, 100
   psychogenic, 99, 105
   supraorbital, 100, 103
   unilateral, 100
Heldt, 300
Helleday, 237
Hemorrhoids, 191
Henry, 300
Herrmann, 297
Hiatus hernia, 191
Hickling, 176
Hip, mobilization, 144
   pseudopain, vertebral origin, 146
Hippocrates, 1, 173, 201, 218, 265
Hirsch, 187
Histamine, 260
Hoffa, 239, 247, 264
Hoffmann, 230
Hood, 8, 13, 190
Hubbard tank, 306
Huddleston, 260
Hueter, 241
Humphrey, 186
Hutton, 8, 13
Hydrocortisone, 279
Hydromassage, 290, 305
   devices, 305
Hydrotherapy sleeve, 306
Hyperalgic reactions, 192
Hyperemia, 259
Hypertension, 191

I

Ice, use in stretching treatment, 164
Ice massage, 261

Immobilization, 82
   soft tissue contracture in, 160–161
Infection, 159
   contraindication for traction, 191
Inflammation, 157
Infraspinatus tendon, deep friction, 279
Intermittent massage, 258
   pressure systems, 297
Interspinous ligament, 83
Intervertebral derangement, minor, 82–86,
     88, 96, 106–107, 110, 113, 115, 121
   reversible, 94
   silent, 97
Intestine, large, 258
Ischemia, 157
Isometric traction, 172
Isoprenaline, 281
Isotonic traction, 172
   skeletal, 173
   skin, 172

J

Jackson, 181
Jacquet, 243
Jastrow, 213
Joint, fluid resorption, 241
Jones, 14, 179, 181
Judet, 119
Judo, 246
Judovich, 178, 180, 184, 190, 201, 202
Junghanns, 94, *95*
Jüthner, 223

K

Kamenetz, 243
Keegan, 109
Keen, 241
Keith, 233, 240
Kellgren, 266, 270
Kellogg, 241, 242, 289
Keyring, 84, *85*
Kinesitherapy, 235
Kipling, 277
Kirby, 260, 298
Kirchberg, 214, 230, 235, 236, 239, 240, 247
Kirksville, 17
Kirschner, 173
Kleen, 259
Klemm, 289
Kneading, 228, 238, 259, 264, 283

Knee, 147
  arthritic, 149
  arthrosis of, 149
  manual treatment, 147
  medial ligament, 275
  meniscal blocking, 147
  pain, 147
  proximal tibiofibular joint block, 147
  synovial entrapment, 147
Knowles, 277
Kohlrausch, 245, 246
Kottke, 179
Kouwenhoven, 247
Krogh, 259
Kroneker, 258
Krusen, 181, 195, 205, 263
Kuatsu, 246
Kung-fu, 214
Kyphosis, 110, 173

L

LaBan, 191
Lacroix de Lavalette, 243
Laisné, 236
Lamarre, 236
Laminectomy, 190
Landquist, 175
Lange, 244
Langenbeck, 239
Lasègue's sign, 119
Lassar, 241
Lavalette, 190
Lawson, 180, 186
Lazorthes, *92, 109*
Le Gentil, 212
Lee, 241
Lehman, 185, 187
Leonardon-Lapervenche, 240
Leriche, 270
Leroy, 243, 260
Leube, 245, 246
LeVay, 14
Levernieux, 180, 184, 190, 194, 201
Licht, 228
Ligament
  anterior longitudinal, pain in, 188
  chronic lesion of knee, 276
  deep friction to, 274
  knee, 275
  medial, of knee, 275
  medial collateral, 275
  minor tear, 275

posterior longitudinal, pain in, 188
  recent injury, 274
Ling, 234–238, 265, 266, 267
Lipolysis, 257
Littré, 211
Locatelli, 241
Londe, 234
Lorry, 231, 234
Louvet, 236
Lucas-Championnière, 240
Lumbago, 96, 115, 116–124, 190, 236
  acute discal, 116
  chronic discal, 117
Lumbar disc, lesions, traction, 174
Lumbar spine, tests, 86
  traction, 174, 195, 201
Luschka, joints of, 189
Lymph, 241, 260
Lympha-mat, 303
Lympha press, 303

M

Mac-Auliffe, 215, 222
Maggiora, 241, 258
Maison, 240
Maisonneuve, 237
Malgaigne, 173
Malignant tumor, contraindication for traction, 191
Manipulation
  craniosacral, 41
  criteria, 42, 44
  direct, 26, 74
  functional, 31
  history, 3
  hypotheses, 94
  indirect, 26, 74, 75
  non-thrust, 29
  OPT, 22, 24
  research, 311
  semi-indirect, 74
  spine, 25, 71
  thrust, 28
  types, 25–32
Manipulative massage, 247
March, 13
Martin, 195, 236
Massage, clinical applications, 270
  contraindications, 284–285
  creams, 285
  deep, 271, 283
  history, 211

Massage, clinical applications—*continued*
  indications, 273, 279, 280
  mechanical devices, 289
  muscle, 273
  physiological effects, 256
  roller pad, 295
  suction-roller, 291
  suction-wave, 294
Masso-electrotherapy, 242
Masturzo, 187, 190
Mathews, 176
Mattress, alternating pressure, 296
Mayor, 172
McFarland, 181
Media, 266
Meerschaert, 191
Meffert, 257
Melzack, 284
Mennell, 18, 247, 263, 265–267
Menstrual period, alteration, in spinal treatment, 82
Meralgia paresthetica, 123
Mercurialis, 229
Metastasis, spinal, 124
Metatarsophalangeal joint, 153
Meyer, 243
Mezger, 237–240, 242
Micromassage, 246, 291
Midtarsal joint, 150
Migraine, 100, 105
Millet, 237
Mitchell, 241, 242
Mitral disease, 192
Mobile segment, 94–98
Mobilization, 3, 29
  history, 3
  of limbs, 135–154
Mosengeil, 237, 241
Moss, 286
Mosso, 241
Müller, 244, 247
Mundale, 179
Murrell, 236
Muscle, deep friction to, 273
Muscles, axial, 60
  actions and functions, 66
  erector spinae, 60
  iliocostalis, 61
  longissimus, 61
  multifidus, 62, 66
  neck, 62
  rectus capitis, 64, 66
  rotatores, 61

  scalenes, 68
  semispinalis, 66
  splenius, 66
  sternomastoid, 68
  transversospinalis, 61
Myalgia, viral, 98
Myeloma, 124
Myotomes, 70

N

Nachemson, 187
Naegeli, 241, 247
Naprapathy, 11
Navicular, 152
Neck, traction of, 187
Nei Ching, 215
Nélaton, 235
Nerve
  minimal root irritation, 88
  root, pain, 188
  roots, 189
  sinuvertebral, 95, *95*
Nerve percuter, 242, 289
Nerve point massage, 244
Neumann, 235
Neuralgia, 244
  cervical brachial, 106
  cervicobrachial, 108, 124
  femoral, 121
  great occipital nerve, 103
  postherpetic, 282, 293
Neuromas, 282, 292
Neurotripsor, 293
Neurotripsy, 293
Nick, 99
Nickel, 173
Nobel, 178, 190
Norström, 240
Nuck, 201
Nursemaid's elbow, 144

O

Obesity, 282
Obstetrics, 239
Occipitomandibular pain, 100
Oger, 124
Osteoarthritis, 116, 188, 189
Osteoarticular pathology, 124
Osteopathy, 13, 15–18

Osteoporosis, 124, 191
Otitis, 100
Otolaryngology, 242

P

Paget, 13
Pagniez, 291
Pain
  acute and chronic dorsal, 110–120
  cervical, chronic, 98
  dorsal, 98, 110
  elbow, 106, 137
  gluteus medius, 145
  interscapular, 107
    cervical origin, 110
  knee, 147–149
  lateral epicondylar, 137
  low back, 98, 112–120
  metastasis, 114
  medial epicondylar, 144
  pathogenesis, 188
  posterior ramus and, 93
  pseudovisceral, 86–91
  radicular, 93
  rule of no-pain and opposite movement,
    75–78, 97–98
  shoulder, 106
  spinal, 32, 188
  subcutaneous, 93, 113
  symptomatic, 124
  tenoperiosteal, 94
Painful subcutaneous syndrome, 93
Palmer, B. J. and D. D., 9–11
Palpatory massage, 244
Palsy, 282
Panniculitis, 285
Paralysis, 259
Paraplegia, 124
Paré, 5, 229, 231
Pavaex, 298
Pemberton, 259
Peptic ulcer, 191
Percussion, 234, 258, 292
Percussors, 292
Periosteal massage, 246
Periostitis, 280
Perry, 173
Petit, 201
Pétrissage, 213, 232, 257, 259, 264, 265, 268
Phantom limb, 282

Phlebitis, 264
Physical therapy, 22
  role, 24
Pin traction, 173
Pinch and roll maneuver, 71, 91–93, 107–
    109, 113, 114, 120–122
  eyebrow, 101
  mandibular angle, 99, 103
Placebo, 270, 312
Plastic massage, 243
Plastic surgery, 286
  cramp from immunobilization, 287
  flaps, 287
  postoperative massage, 286
  preoperative massage, 286
  tubes, 287
Pneumatic appliances, Jobst, 300
Pneumatic circulator, 300
Pneumothorax, 281
Pollack, 282
Poliomyelitis, 161, 166, 260
Pope, 16
Posner, 240
Posterior ramus, 92–93, 94–95
Postural drainage, 280, 281
Pott's disease, 124
Powder, massage with, 285
Pregnancy, 191
Pressure, 234, 266
Pressure pad, alternating, 296
Prostate, 240
Pseudomeniscal syndrome, 148
Pseudopain of hip, 146
Pseudotendonitis, 145
Pseudovisceral pain, 86, 90, 91, 93
Pulled elbow, 144
Pulmonary abscess, 280
Punctural massage, 246
Push button sign, 107

Q

Quadriplegia, 124
Quellmalz, 231, 290

R

Radicular celluloperiosteomyalgic syndrome,
    86–94

Radicular celluloperiosteomyalgic syn-
drome—*continued*
  abdominal wall of vertebral origin, 122
Radicular pain, 93
Radicular myalgic syndrome, 89
Radioulnar joint and subluxation, distal,
    141, 142
Rawlins, 256
Ray, 173
Reflex massage, 243, 244, 246
Reid, 298
Reibmayr, 238, 242
Relaxation, 266, 267
Research, 311
Reveillé-Parise, 236
Rheumatoid arthritis, *170*, 191
Rhythmic stabilization, 136
Rib joints, 59
  maneuver, 111
  strains, 111
Rizet, 240
Rosacea, 284
Rosenthal, 241, 247
Rosner, 204
Rubin, 136
Ruffier, 243
Ruhmann, 244
Rule of no pain and opposite movement, *see*
    Pain, rule of
Russell, 293

S

Sabatier, 239
Sacrum, 50
Saint-Jori, 229
Saint-Pierre, 290
Sampson, 260, 298
Saugwellen-Therapie, 294
Sauna, 290
Sauter, 172
Savary, 212
Sayre, 180, 201
Scarring, 277
Scars, adherent, 272, 273
Scheuermann's aseptic necrosis, 110
Schmorl, 94
Schreiber, 289
Schultes, 5
Sciatic nerve, 282
Sciatica, 86–97, 119–121, 176, 191, 192
  discal, 119
  lumbar spine, *88*

  neurologic defect, 191
Scleroderma, 159, 257
Scoliosis, 110, 173, 233
Scott traction frame, 186
Scotch douche, 305
Sée, 236
Séguin, 236
Sepsis, 282
Shaw, 233, 289
Sheffield, 196
Shiatsu, 246, 263, 291
Shoemaker, 242
Shower massage, 305
Sinuvertebral nerves, 95, *95*
Sismothérapie, 243
Skeletal suspension, 173
Skeletal traction, 173
Skin, influence of massage, 257
Skull, 259
Smith, 172
Snow, 290
Soft-tissue contracture, 157
  amputees, 161
  Dupuytren's, 159
  fracture immobilization, 161
  heat in treatment of, 164
  ice packs used in, 164–165
  immobilization as cause of, 160
  intrinsic plus position, 159
  ischemic, 159
  neurologic disorders, 161
  poliomyelitis, 161
  spastic, 161
  stretching, 162
  traumatic, 158
  ultrasound treatment, 160, 165
  vascular involvement, 159
  Volkmann's, 159
Solon, 217
Soroff, 304
Spastic contractures, 164
Spinal manipulation, physiopathologic basis
    for, 94
  by physical therapists, 22
Spine
  anatomy, 47
    arches, 48
    bodies, 47, 52
    curves, 55
    discs, 41
    foramina, 48
    joints, 57

ligaments, 57
processes, 48–50, 55
cervical point of back, 107, 108
derangement, minor reversible intervertebral, 71
direct, manipulation, 74
disc lesions, 94
dislocation, 173
indirect manipulation, 74
intervertebral derangement, minor (see Intervertebral derangement)
manipulation
accidents in, 123
strap technique, 131
minimal root irritation, 88
motion, 52
range of, 52
movements, 52
normative data, 314
traction of, 189
treatment session, 78
manipulative thrust, 80
patient precautions, 80
placing in position, 80
reactions to, 80
sweating, 81
sympathetic reactions, 81
taking up slack, 80
unstable, 174
weight-bearing, 52
Splint, balanced suspension, 172
Splints
hand, 167–171
stretch, 167
Split traction bed, 184, 202
upright position, 184
Split traction table, 177, 196
upright position, 177
vertebral separation, 177
Spondylitis, 114
Spondylolisthesis, 190
Spondylosis, 174, 189
Sportsman's cramp, 283
Sprain, 275
anterior chondrocostal, 111
mild, 96
Star-shaped diagram, 76, 119
spinal manipulation, 76–80
Static edema, 247
Steinmann, 173
Steroid, 279
infiltration, 279

Still, A. T., 15–18
Stillwell, 299, 300
Stirling, 258
Strabo, 216, 225
Strap technique, spinal manipulation, 131
Stretch splints, 167–171
Stretching, soft-tissue contracture, 163–166
Strohm, 178, 179, 181, 183, 186
Stroking, 236, 259, 264, 265
direction of, 265
Subluxation, distal radioulnar, 141, 142
Subtalar joint, 150
Superficial massage, 271
Supraspinatus tendon, 279
Surgery, thoracic, 281
Swedish massage, 234
Swedish Massage Institute, 235
Swenson, 259
Syncardon, 248, 303
Sydenham, 230
Synovial membrane, 188

T

Tachycardia, 260
Tapotement, 213, 230, 236, 237, 268
Tappan, 263
Tapping, 268
Tarsometatarsal joint, 153
Taylor, 181
Telangiectasia, 237
Temperature, cutaneous, 241
Temporomandibular joint, 193
Tenderness, local, 33
Tendon, 276
Tendon sheath, 276
Tendonitis, 90, 94, 275, 277
trochanteric, 145
Tenomyalgic syndrome, 90
Tenoperiosteal pain, 94
Tenoperiosteal tear, 277
Tenosynovitis, 94, 276
Tension, 72
Terrier, 247, 298
Testing, motion, 33
palpation, 33
Thiele, 244
Thiersch graft, 286
Thomas, 14
Thoracolumbar junction, 93
Tibiofibular capsulitis, proximal, 149

Tibiofibular joint
  blockage, 149
  capsulitis, 149
Tibiotarsal joint, 150
Tinkham, 299
Tinnitus, 124
Tissot, 212, 229, 231, 290
Torticollis, 98
  traumatic, 76
Traction
  angle of pull, 183
  contraindications, 191–192
  home use, 194
  hydraulic device, 185, 204
  indications for, 189
  manual, 192
  motor for, 194
  principles, 177
  sitting position in, 193
  split bed, 184
  split table for, 178, 196
  supine position in, 193
  technique, 192
  treatment, 294
Transverse friction, 273
Transverse massage, 273
Trauma, 157
  fibrosis in, 158
Traxator, 294
Treatment
  duration, 43, 80, 101, 267
  frequency, 43, 80, 101, 267
Trembling armchair, 190
Trémoussoir, 242
Trigeminal nerve nucleus, 103
Trilene, 281
Trochanteric bursitis, 145
  tendonitis, 145
Trochin, 231
Tuberculosis, 191
Turner, 197, 203

U

Ulcer, 271, 283
  varicose, 247
Ultrasound, 248, 291
  treatment of soft tissue contracture, 160, 165
Unctions, 265
Underwater douche massage, 305

V

Validation, 311
Valsalva, 239
van Veen, 246
Vaquette traction table, 203
Varicose ulcer, 283
Varicose ulcers, 247
Vasodilation, 259
Vasopneumatic apparatus, 260, 298
Vastus medialis, syndrome of lumbar nerve
  root origin, 148
Veith, 214
Velpeau, 237
Verleysen, 225, 236, 239, 242
Vertebrae, see Spine
Vertebral manipulations, 71
Vertigo, 124
Vibrating helmet, 290
Vibration, 213, 237, 241, 291
Vibratory machines, 291, 295
Viral myalgia, 98
Vis a tergo, 258
Vodder, 247
Vogler, 246
Volkmann's ischemic contracture, 159
Volkmann's ischemic paralysis, 157
Voltaire, 290

W

Waghemacker, 105
Wakim, 298
Wallenberg, 105
Wallenberg syndrome, 124
Walthard, 263
Weber, 176, 237, 242
Weinberger, 176
Weinstein, 196
Wetterwald, 244
Whiplash injury, 177
Whirlpool bath, 306
Wilensky, 298
Winter, 173
Wise, 216
Wolfe grafts, 287
Wolff, 99
Wood, 263
Worden, 186
Worden's table, 196
Wrammer, 181
Wright linear pump, 303

Wylie, 214

Y

Yabuuchi, 215
Yates, 174

Z

Zabludowski, 239
Zelikovski, 303
Zygoapophyseal joints, 84